PROGRESS IN CLINICAL AND BIOLOGICAL RESEARCH

RECENT TITLES

Vol 214: **Ethnic Differences in Reactions to Drugs and Xenobiotics,** Werner Kalow, H. Werner Goedde, Dharam P. Agarwal, *Editors*

Vol 215: **Megakaryocyte Development and Function,** Richard F. Levine, Neil Williams, Jack Levin, Bruce L. Evatt, *Editors*

Vol 216: **Advances in Cancer Control: Health Care Financing and Research,** Lee E. Mortenson, Paul F. Engstrom, Paul N. Anderson, *Editors*

Vol 217: **Progress in Developmental Biology,** Harold C. Slavkin, *Editor.* Published in two volumes.

Vol 218: **Evolutionary Perspective and the New Genetics,** Henry Gershowitz, Donald L. Rucknagel, Richard E. Tashian, *Editors*

Vol 219: **Recent Advances in Arterial Diseases: Atherosclerosis, Hypertension, and Vasospasm,** Thomas N. Tulenko, Robert H. Cox, *Editors*

Vol 220: **Safety and Health Aspects of Organic Solvents,** Vesa Riihimäki, Ulf Ulfvarson, *Editors*

Vol 221: **Developments in Bladder Cancer,** Louis Denis, Tadao Niijima, George Prout, Jr., Fritz H. Schröder, *Editors*

Vol 222: **Dietary Fat and Cancer,** Clement Ip, Diane F. Birt, Adrianne E. Rogers, Curtis Mettlin, *Editors*

Vol 223: **Cancer Drug Resistance,** Thomas C. Hall, *Editor*

Vol 224: **Transplantation: Approaches to Graft Rejection,** Harold T. Meryman, *Editor*

Vol 225: **Gonadotropin Down-Regulation in Gynecological Practice,** Rune Rolland, Dev R. Chadha, Wim N.P. Willemsen, *Editors*

Vol 226: **Cellular Endocrinology: Hormonal Control of Embryonic and Cellular Differentiation,** Ginette Serrero, Jun Hayashi, *Editors*

Vol 227: **Advances in Chronobiology**, John E. Pauly, Lawrence E. Scheving, *Editors*. Published in two volumes.

Vol 228: **Environmental Toxicity and the Aging Processes,** Scott R. Baker, Marvin Rogul, *Editors*

Vol 229: **Animal Models: Assessing the Scope of Their Use in Biomedical Research,** Junichi Kawamata, Edward C. Melby, Jr., *Editors*

Vol 230: **Cardiac Electrophysiology and Pharmacology of Adenosine and ATP: Basic and Clinical Aspects,** Amir Pelleg, Eric L. Michelson, Leonard S. Dreifus, *Editors*

Vol 231: **Detection of Bacterial Endotoxins With the Limulus Amebocyte Lysate Test,** Stanley W. Watson, Jack Levin, Thomas J. Novitsky, *Editors*

Vol 232: **Enzymology and Molecular Biology of Carbonyl Metabolism: Aldehyde Dehydrogenase, Aldo-Keto Reductase, and Alcohol Dehydrogenase**, Henry Weiner, T. Geoffrey Flynn, *Editors*

Vol 233: **Developmental and Comparative Immunology,** Edwin L. Cooper, Claude Langlet, Jacques Bierne, *Editors*

Vol 234: **The Hepatitis Delta Virus and Its Infection**, Mario Rizzetto, John L. Gerin, Robert H. Purcell, *Editors*

Vol 235: **Preclinical Safety of Biotechnology Products Intended for Human Use,** Charles E. Graham, *Editor*

Vol 236: **First Vienna Shock Forum,** Günther Schlag, Heinz Redl, *Editors*. Published in two volumes: Part A: *Pathophysiological Role of Mediators and Mediator Inhibitors in Shock.* Part B: *Monitoring and Treatment of Shock.*

Vol 237: **The Use of Transrectal Ultrasound in the Diagnosis and Management of Prostate Cancer,** Fred Lee, Richard McLeary, *Editors*

Vol 238: **Avian Immunology,** W.T. Weber, D.L. Ewert, *Editors*

Vol 239: **Current Concepts and Approaches to the Study of Prostate Cancer,** Donald S. Coffey, Nicholas Bruchovsky, William A. Gardner, Jr., Martin I. Resnick, James P. Karr, *Editors*

Vol 240: **Pathophysiological Aspects of Sickle Cell Vaso-Occlusion,** Ronald L. Nagel, *Editor*

Vol 241: **Genetics and Alcoholism,** H. Werner Goedde, Dharam P. Agarwal, *Editors*

Vol 242: **Prostaglandins in Clinical Research,** Helmut Sinzinger, Karsten Schrör, *Editors*

Vol 243: **Prostate Cancer,** Gerald P. Murphy, Saad Khoury, Réne Küss, Christian Chatelain, Louis Denis, *Editors*. Published in two volumes: Part A: *Research, Endocrine Treatment, and Histopathology.* Part B: *Imaging Techniques, Radiotherapy, Chemotherapy, and Management Issues*

Vol 244: **Cellular Immunotherapy of Cancer,** Robert L. Truitt, Robert P. Gale, Mortimer M. Bortin, *Editors*

Vol 245: **Regulation and Contraction of Smooth Muscle,** Marion J. Siegman, Andrew P. Somlyo, Newman L. Stephens, *Editors*

Vol 246: **Oncology and Immunology of Down Syndrome,** Ernest E. McCoy, Charles J. Epstein, *Editors*

Vol 247: **Degenerative Retinal Disorders: Clinical and Laboratory Investigations,** Joe G. Hollyfield, Robert E. Anderson, Matthew M.LaVail, *Editors*

Vol 248: **Advances in Cancer Control: The War on Cancer—15 Years of Progress,** Paul F. Engstrom, Lee E. Mortenson, Paul N. Anderson, *Editors*

Vol 249: **Mechanisms of Signal Transduction by Hormones and Growth Factors,** Myles C. Cabot, Wallace L. McKeehan, *Editors*

Vol 250: **Kawasaki Disease,** Stanford T. Shulman, *Editor*

Vol 251: **Developmental Control of Globin Gene Expression,** George Stamatoyannopoulos, Arthur W. Nienhuis, *Editors*

Vol 252: **Cellular Calcium and Phosphate Transport in Health and Disease,** Felix Bronner, Meinrad Peterlik, *Editors*

Vol 253: **Model Systems in Neurotoxicolog Alternative Approaches to Animal Testin** Abraham Shahar, Alan M. Goldberg, *Edito*

Vol 254: **Genetics and Epithelial Cell Dysfunction in Cystic Fibrosis,** John R. Riordan, Manuel Buchwald, *Editors*

Vol 255: **Recent Aspects of Diagnosis and Treatment of Lipoprotein Disorders: Imp on Prevention of Atherosclerotic Diseases,** Kurt Widhalm, Herbert K. Naito, *Editors*

Vol 256: **Advances in Pigment Cell Resear** Joseph T. Bagnara, *Editor*

Vol 257: **Electromagnetic Fields and Neurobehavioral Function,** Mary Ellen O'Connor, Richard H. Lovely, *Editors*

Vol 258: **Membrane Biophysics III: Biolog Transport,** Mumtaz A. Dinno, William McI Armstrong, *Editors*

Vol 259: **Nutrition, Growth, and Cancer,** George P. Tryfiates, Kedar N. Prasad, *Edito*

Vol 260: **Management of Advanced Cancer Prostate and Bladder,** Philip H. Smith, Michele Pavone-Macaluso, *Editors*

Vol 261: **Nicotine Replacement: A Critical Evaluation,** Ovide F. Pomerleau, Cynthia S. Pomerleau, *Editors*

Vol 262: **Hormones, Cell Biology, and Canc Perspectives and Potentials,** W. David Hankins, David Puett, *Editors*

Vol 263: **Mechanisms in Asthma: Pharmacology, Physiology, and Manageme** Carol L. Armour, Judith L. Black, *Editors*

Vol 264: **Perspectives in Shock Research,** Robert F. Bond, *Editor*

Vol 265: **Pathogenesis and New Approaches the Study of Noninsulin-Dependent Diabete Mellitus,** Albert Y. Chang, Arthur R. Diani, *Editors*

Please contact the publisher for information about previous titles in this series.

MECHANISMS IN ASTHMA
Pharmacology, Physiology, and Management

MECHANISMS IN ASTHMA
Pharmacology, Physiology, and Management

Proceedings of a Satellite Meeting of the 10th International Congress of Pharmacology, Held at Ayers Rock, Australia, August 30–September 2, 1987

Editors

Carol L. Armour
Judith L. Black
Department of Pharmacology
The University of Sydney
New South Wales
Australia

ALAN R. LISS, INC. • NEW YORK

Address all Inquiries to the Publisher
Alan R. Liss, Inc., 41 East 11th Street, New York, NY 10003

Printed in the United States of America

Library of Congress Cataloging-in-Publication Data

Mechanisms in asthma : pharmacology, physiology, and management : proceedings of a satellite meeting of the 10th International Congress of Pharmacology, held at Ayers Rock, Australia, August 30–September 2, 1987 / editors, Carol L. Armour, Judith L. Black.
p. cm. — (Progress in clinical and biological research ; v. 263)
Includes bibliographies and index.
ISBN 0-8451-5113-4
1. Asthma—Pathophysiology—Congresses. 2. Asthma—Chemotherapy—Congresses. I. Armour, Carol L. II. Black, Judith L. III. International Congress of Pharmacology (10th : 1987 : Sydney, N.S.W.) IV. Series.
RC591.M38 1988 87-37407
616.2'38—dc19 CIP

Contents

Contributors

Sandra D. Anderson, Department of Thoracic Medicine, Royal Prince Alfred Hospital, Camperdown, N.S.W. 2050, Australia **[283]**

Jonathan P. Arm, Departments of Medicine and Respiratory Medicine, United Medical and Dental Schools, Guy's Hospital, London SE1 9RT, England **[341]**

Carol L. Armour, Department of Pharmacology, University of Sydney, N.S.W. 2006, Australia **[xv, 99, 267]**

B. Arnoux, INSERM U.200, Clamart 92140, France **[81]**

Neil Barnes, London Chest Hospital, London E2, England **[393]**

Peter J. Barnes, Department of Clinical Pharmacology, Cardiothoracic Institute, Brompton Hospital, London SW3, England **[111]**

Nicholas G. Belcher, Departments of Medicine and Respiratory Medicine, United Medical and Dental Schools, Guy's Hospital, London SE1 9RT, England **[341]**

J. Benveniste, INSERM U.200, Clamart 92140, France **[81]**

Jerry M. Bergen, Department of Physiology, Faculty of Medicine, University of Manitoba, Winnipeg R3E 0W3, Canada **[219]**

Judith L. Black, Department of Pharmacology, University of Sydney, N.S.W. 2006, Australia **[xv, 99, 267]**

D. Benjamin Borson, Cardiovascular Research Institute and Departments of Medicine and Physiology, University of California-San Francisco, San Francisco, CA 94143 **[123]**

John P. Boyle, Department of Physiological Sciences, University of Manchester Medical School, Manchester M13 9PT, England **[205]**

S.D. Brain, Section of Vascular Biology, MRC Clinical Research Centre, Harrow, Middlesex HA1 3UJ, England **[55]**

David H. Bryant, Department of Thoracic Medicine, St. Vincent's Hospital, Sydney, N.S.W. 2010, Australia **[379]**

John F. Burka, Department of Anatomy and Physiology, Atlantic Veterinary College, University of Prince Edward Island, Charlottetown, P.E.I., Canada C1A 4P3 **[35]**

The numbers in brackets are the opening page numbers of the contributors' articles.

Alan R. Burns, Pulmonary Research Laboratory, St. Paul's Hospital, Department of Pathology, U.B.C. Vancouver, British Columbia, Canada V6Z 1Y6 **[25]**

Martin K. Church, Immunopharmacology Research Group, Clinical Pharmacology, Centre Block, Southampton General Hospital, Southampton SO9 4XY, England **[15,159]**

Dolores M. Conroy, Department of Pharmacology, Hunterian Institute, Royal College of Surgeons, London WC2A 3PN, England **[47]**

John Costello, Department of Thoracic Medicine, King's College School of Medicine and Dentistry, London SE5, England **[393]**

E.E. Daniel, Department of Neurosciences, McMaster University, Faculty of Health Sciences, Hamilton, Ontario L8N 3Z5, Canada **[3,167,179]**

Jane M. Davies, Department of Physiological Sciences, University of Manchester Medical School, Manchester M13 9PT, England **[205]**

Johan C. de Jongste, Department of Pediatric Pulmonology, University Hospital Rotterdam/Sophia Children's Hospital, Rotterdam, The Netherlands **[255]**

A. Denjean, Laboratoire d'Explorations Fonctionnelles, Clamart 92140, France **[81]**

William L. Eschenbacher, Department of Internal Medicine/Pulmonary, University of Michigan Medical Center, Ann Arbor, MI 48109 **[355]**

Jane Evans, Department of Thoracic Medicine, King's College School of Medicine and Dentistry, London SE5, England **[393]**

Lynette B. Fernandes, Department of Pharmacology, University of Western Australia, Perth, Nedlands 6009, Australia **[317]**

Robert W. Foster, Department of Physiological Sciences, University of Manchester Medical School, Manchester Ml3 9PT, England **[205]**

Roy G. Goldie, Department of Pharmacology, University of Western Australia, Perth, Nedlands 6009, Australia **[317]**

Thomas R. Gravelyn, Department of Internal Medicine/Pulmonary, University of Michigan Medical Center, Ann Arbor, MI 48109 **[355]**

P.G. Hellewell, Section of Vascular Biology, MRC Clinical Research Centre, Harrow, Middlesex HA1 3UJ, England **[55]**

Stephen T. Holgate, Immunopharmacology Research Group, Centre Block, Southampton General Hospital, Southampton SO9 4XY, England **[159]**

Alan L. James, Department of Pulmonary Physiology, Sir Charles Gairdner Hospital, Perth, Australia **[301]**

Peter R.A. Johnson, Department of Pharmacology, University of Sydney, N.S.W. 2006, Australia **[99,267]**

G.L. Jones, Departments of Medicine and Neurosciences, McMaster University, Hamilton, Ontario, Canada **[3]**

P.J. Jose, Section of Vascular Biology, MRC Clinical Research Centre, Harrow, Middlesex HA1 3UJ, England **[55]**

J. Jury, Department of Neurosciences, McMaster University, Faculty of Health Sciences, Hamilton, Ontario L8N 3Z5, Canada **[167]**

Karel F. Kerrebijn, Department of Pediatric Pulmonology, University Hospital Rotterdam/Sophia Children's Hospital, Rotterdam, The Netherlands **[255]**

S.K. Kong, Department of Physiology, Faculty of Medicine, University of Manitoba, Winnipeg, Manitoba R3E 0W3, Canada **[231]**

Edwin A. Kroeger, Department of Physiology, Faculty of Medicine, University of Manitoba, Winnipeg R3E 0W3, Canada **[219]**

C.G. Lane, Departments of Medicine and Neurosciences, McMaster University, Hamilton, Ontario, Canada **[3]**

Tak H. Lee, Departments of Medicine and Respiratory Medicine, United Medical and Dental Schools, Guy's Hospital, London SE1 9RT, England **[341]**

Gordon L. Letts, Department of Pharmacology, Merck Frosst Canada Inc., Pointe Claire-Dorval, Quebec H9R 4P8, Canada **[91]**

David A. Lindsay, Department of Medicine, Gold Coast Hospital, Southport, Queensland, Australia **[421]**

Jennifer Maclagan, Pharmacology Department, Royal Free Hospital Medical School, London NW3, England **[149]**

Roger Marthan, Department of Pharmacology, University of Sydney, N.S.W. 2006, Australia **[267]**

Cyril S. McFarlane, Department of Pharmacology, Merck Frosst Canada Inc., Pointe Claire-Dorval, Quebec H9R 4P8, Canada **[91]**

Richard W. Mitchell, Department of Physiology, Faculty of Medicine, University of Manitoba, Winnipeg R3E 0W3, Canada **[219]**

Jay A. Nadel, Cardiovascular Research Institute and Departments of Medicine and Physiology, University of California-San Francisco, San Francisco, CA 94143 **[123,331]**

S. Nourshargh, Section of Vascular Biology, MRC Clinical Research Centre, Harrow, Middlesex HA1 3UJ, England **[55]**

P.M. O'Byrne, Departments of Neurosciences and Medicine, McMaster University, Faculty of Health Sciences, Hamilton, Ontario L8N 3Z5, Canada **[3,167]**

Stephen P. O'Hickey, Departments of Medicine and Respiratory Medicine, United Medical and Dental Schools, Guy's Hospital, London SE1 9RT, England **[341]**

Clive P. Page, Department of Pharmacology, King's College, London University, London SW3, England **[71]**

Peter D. Paré, St. Paul's Hospital Pulmonary Research Laboratory, University of British Columbia, Vancouver, Canada **[301]**

M. Pashley, Department of Neurosciences, McMaster University, Faculty of Health Sciences, Hamilton, Ontario L8N 3Z5, Canada **[3,167]**

James W. Paterson, Department of Pharmacology, University of Western Australia, Perth, Nedlands 6009, Australia **[317]**

Priscilla J. Piper, Department of Pharmacology, Hunterian Institute, Royal College of Surgeons, London WC2A 3PN, England **[47,393]**

Louise Plowman, Department of Thoracic Medicine, David Read Laboratory, University of Sydney, N.S.W. 2006, Australia **[131]**

M. Rampart, Section of Vascular Biology, MRC Clinical Research Centre, Harrow, Middlesex HA1 3UJ, England **[55]**

Paul J. Rigby, Department of Pharmacology, University of Western Australia, Perth, Nedlands 6009, Australia **[317]**

Deirdre N. Robertson, Department of Pharmacology, King's College, London University, London SW3, England **[71]**

Richard E. Ruffin, Department of Respiratory Medicine, Flinders Medical Centre, Bedford Park, South Australia 5042, Australia **[427]**

Cheryl M. Salome, Department of Medicine, University of Sydney, N.S.W. 2006, Australia **[405]**

Marwa N. Samhoun, Department of Pharmacology, Hunterian Institute, Royal College of Surgeons, London WC2A 3PN, England **[47]**

Tethys Scheibner, Department of Thoracic Medicine, David Read Laboratory, University of Sydney, N.S.W. 2006, Australia **[131]**

J. Paul Seale, Department of Pharmacology, University of Sydney and Department of Thoracic Medicine, Royal Prince Alfred Hospital, Camperdown 2050, Australia **[367]**

Cheryl J. Sedgwick, Department of Medicine, University of Sydney, N.S.W. 2006, Australia **[405]**

C.Y. Seow, Department of Physiology, Faculty of Medicine, University of Manitoba, Winnipeg, Manitoba R3E 0W3, Canada **[231]**

R. Serio, Department of Neurosciences, McMaster University, Faculty of Health Sciences, Hamilton, Ontario L8N 3Z5, Canada **[167]**

Roger C. Small, Department of Physiological Sciences, University of Manchester Medical School, Manchester M13 9PT, England **[205]**

Christine M. Smith, Department of Thoracic Medicine, Royal Prince Alfred Hospital, Camperdown, N.S.W. 2050, Australia **[283]**

Newman L. Stephens, Department of Physiology, Faculty of Medicine, University of Manitoba, Winnipeg, Manitoba R3E 0W3, Canada **[231]**

Colin E. Sullivan, Department of Thoracic Medicine, David Read Laboratory, University of Sydney, N.S.W. 2006, Australia **[131]**

David C. Walker, Pulmonary Research Laboratory, St. Paul's Hospital, Department of Pathology, U.B.C. Vancouver, British Columbia V6Z 1Y6, Canada **[25]**

T.J. Williams, Section of Vascular Biology, MRC Clinical Research Centre, Harrow, Middlesex HA1 3UJ, England **[55]**

Ann J. Woolcock, Department of Medicine, University of Sydney, N.S.W. 2006, Australia **[405]**

Wendy Wright, Department of Medicine, University of Sydney, N.S.W. 2006, Australia **[405]**

Jerzy Zakrzewski, Department of Thoracic Medicine, King's College School of Medicine and Dentistry, London SE5, England **[393]**

Preface

In August 1987 a group of pharmacologists, physiologists, and thoracic physicians from twelve countries met at Ayers Rock in the centre of Australia to attend "AIRWAYS 87," an official satellite of the 10th International Congress of Pharmacology. Their common interest was asthma—a disease entity with a high prevalence, morbidity, and mortality in Australia. The aim of the meeting was to integrate knowledge and research from these different disciplines with a view to a further understanding of asthma and a more rational approach to its management.

The meeting was made possible by a generous grant-in-aid from Boehringer-Ingelheim, which enabled us to bring delegates to such a remote area. We thank Associate Professor Diana M. Temple and Dr. Sandra D. Anderson for their assistance in the organisation of the meeting and in the preparation of this volume.

Carol L. Armour
Judith L. Black

Inflammation—Cells and Mediators

Mechanisms in Asthma: Pharmacology, Physiology, and Management, pages 3–13

NEURAL TRANSMISSION DURING OZONE-INDUCED AIRWAY HYPERRESPONSIVENESS.

P.M. O'Byrne, G.L. Jones, C.G. Lane, M. Pashley and E.E. Daniel.
Departments of Medicine and Neurosciences, McMaster University, Hamilton, Ontario, Canada.

INTRODUCTION

Airway hyperresponsiveness is an important feature in patients with clinical asthma (Hargreave et al, 1981), which appears to relate to the severity of the disease (Juniper et al, 1981). Airway hyperresponsiveness can be induced in a number of animal preparations after inhalation of stimuli, such as allergen or ozone, which also cause airway hyperresponsiveness in human subjects. These observations have allowed investigation of the pathogenesis of airway hyperresponsiveness in ways which are not possible in asthmatic subjects.

Airway hyperresponsiveness develops in dogs (Holtzman et al, 1983) and rats (Lee et al, 1985) as well as in human subjects (Golden et al, 1978) after inhalation of ozone. In human subjects and dogs, the development of airway hyperresponsiveness is temporally related to an influx of inflammatory cells as part of the development of an acute inflammatory response in the airways (Holtzman et al, 1983; Seltzer et al, 1986). Also, in dogs the depletion of inflammatory cells, such as neutrophils, prevents the development of airway hyperresponsiveness after inhaled ozone (O'Byrne et al, 1984). Therefore, airway inflammation and subsequent release of inflammatory mediators, appear to play an important role in the pathogenesis of airway hyperresponsiveness after ozone.

The chemical mediators responsible for the development of airway hyperresponsiveness have also been studied in dogs, after airway hyperresponsiveness has been induced using a number of different stimuli, including ozone, allergen, leukotriene B_4 (LTB_4) and platelet activating factor (PAF). Initial studies indicated that the cyclooxygenase inhibitor, indomethacin, prevented the development of airway hyperresponsiveness after inhalation of ozone (O'Byrne et al, 1984b). This suggested that a cyclooxygenase product released during the inflammatory response after ozone, was causing airway hyperresponsiveness. Subsequently, increased levels of thromboxane B_2, the metabolite of thromboxane A_2, was measured in bronchoalveolar lavage fluid from dogs with airway hyperresponsiveness after LTB_4 (O'Byrne et al, 1985). Lastly, the thromboxane-synthetase inhibitor, OKY 046, has been demonstrated to effectively inhibit the development of airway hyperresponsiveness after inhaled allergen (Chung et al, 1986), ozone (Aizawa et al, 1985), LTB_4 (O'Byrne et al, 1985), and PAF (Chung et al, 1986) in dogs. One potential problem with the interpretation of results using thromboxane-synthetase inhibitors is that shunting within the cyclooxygenase pathway is known to occur resulting in the production of prostacyclin (PGI_2) and/or prostaglandin E_2 (Chung et al, 1986). To circumvent this problem, we have recently examined the ability of a thromboxane receptor antagonist, L655,240 (Hall et al, 1987) to protect against ozone-induced airway hyperresponsiveness. The doses of L655,240 used were initially demonstrated to antagonise the bronchoconstrictor responses to inhaled U46619. L655,240 significantly inhibited the development of airway hyperresponsiveness after ozone, although this inhibition was not complete. The study,however, supported the hypothesis that airway hyperresponsiveness after ozone was, in part at least, caused by thromboxane release in the airways. This hypothesis for the pathogenesis of airway hyperresponsiveness in dogs after inhalation of allergen or ozone is represented in Fig. 1.

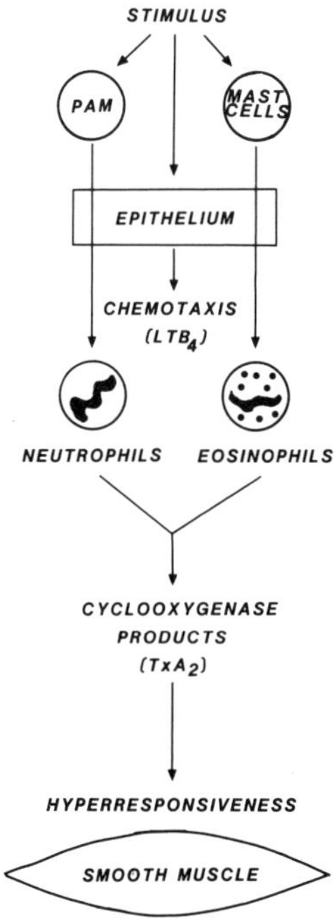

Figure 1. Hypothesis to explain the development of airway hyperresponsiveness following the inhalation of ozone or allergen in dogs.

The mechanism by which inflammatory mediators, such as thromboxane, cause airway hyperresponsiveness is not yet known, but possible mechanisms include heightened reflex bronchoconstriction, presynaptic modulation of acetylcholine release, effects on local axonal reflexes, or an effect on airway smooth muscle. Recent studies using dogs with airway hyperresponsiveness after inhaled ozone have addressed some of these possible mechanisms.

REFLEX BRONCHOCONSTRICTION

It has been suggested that airway hyperresponsiveness after stimuli such as ozone and upper respiratory viral infections is mediated via parasympathetic reflex mechanisms.

Golden et al (1978) demonstrated that the muscurinic receptor antagonist, atropine, prevents ozone-induced hyperresponsiveness in healthy subjects. Also, Holtzman et al (1979) studied the effects of ozone in atopic and non-atopic subjects. In both groups of individuals airway hyperresponsiveness induced by ozone was prevented by treatment with atropine. These investigators concluded that ozone increases bronchial reactivity via cholinergic postganglionic pathways and was unrelated to the immunological status of the subject. In addition, Empey et al (1976) demonstrated that atropine prevents airway hyperresponsiveness after viral infections.

Other studies, however, have suggested that airway hyperresponsiveness in human subjects is not mediated via cholinergic reflex mechanisms. Inhaled hexamethonium, a nicotinic receptor antagonist which inhibits transmission through autonomic ganglia, abolished airway hyperresponsiveness to inhaled histamine but not to methacholine in allergic subjects (Holtzman, 1980). These results suggested that histamine was causing bronchoconstriction entirely through reflex mechanisms but the abnormality causing airway hyperresponsiveness to methacholine in human subjects was in the efferent parasympathetic pathway distal to the ganglion. Also, inhaled atropine provides only a minor degree of protection against the response to inhaled allergen (Boulet et al, 1984), or cold air (O'Byrne et al, 1985b) in asthmatic subjects. In addition, inhaled atropine does not prevent the development of airway hyperresponsiveness induced by allergen (Boulet et al, 1984).

One potential problem with the studies demonstrating a lack of effect of inhibition of reflex pathways to prevent airway hyperresponsiveness after stimuli such as ozone, is either that the doses of the antagonist administered are inadequate or the drug is not reaching the necessary site of action in the airways. To further address the question of the importance of reflex bronchoconstriction in ozone-induced airway hyperresponsiveness, Jones et al (1987) have pretreated dogs with doses of hexamethonium which they have demonstrated adequately blocks autonomic ganglionic transmission in dogs. This study demonstrated that autonomic ganglionic blockade did not inhibit the development of airway hyperresponsiveness to either acetylcholine or histamine after inhalation of ozone. Therefore, as in human subjects after inhaled allergen, a parasympathetic reflex mechanism does not play a major role in the development of airway hyperresponsiveness induced by inhalation of ozone in dogs.

PRESYNAPTIC MODULATION OF ACETYLCHOLINE RELEASE.

The first indication that presynaptic modulation of acetylcholine release may be altered in dogs with airway hyperresponsiveness after inhaled ozone came from studies by Walters et al (1986). When trachealis muscle from dogs with airway hyperresponsiveness in vivo was studied in the organ bath, the responses to electrical field stimulation were increased when compared to control dogs. By contrast, the responses to exogenous acetylcholine were not different between the two groups of dogs. These results suggested that trachealis muscle itself was not different in dogs with airway hyperresponsiveness after ozone, but that the amounts of acetylcholine being released in response to nerve stimulation was increased.

These results are consistent with the known effects of thromboxane on the responses of canine trachealis in vitro. Munoz et al (1986) have demonstrated that pretreatment with a thromboxane mimetic, U46619, causes a time-dependent increase in the responses to vagal nerve stimulation, but not to exogenous acetylcholine and that this effect was, therefore, prejunctional. In addition, aggregated platelets in an organ bath release thromboxane which can increase the responses to electrical field stimulation, as does U46619 (Tamoki et al, 1987). The differential effect of U46619 on smooth muscle responses to field stimulation and acetylcholine may not, however, necessarily be caused by increased amounts of acetylcholine released from the nerve terminal. For example, Serio and Daniel (submitted) have demonstrated that while U46619 increases the responses to electrical field stimulation in canine trachealis, this is not associated with increases in the amplitude or duration of associated excitatory junctional potentials (EJPs), but rather with an increase in the number of secondary oscillations which follow the EJP. These results suggest that thromboxane does not enhance the amount of acetylcholine release per se, but rather the duration of release or improves the propagation of activity through the muscle. Therefore, thromboxane released as part of the airway inflammatory response after inhaled ozone may be responsible for the alterations in the responses to nerve stimulation in the ozone treated tissues.

To further examine this possibility that presynaptic modulation is altered in dogs with airway hyperresponsiveness after inhaled ozone, we have repeated the studies of Walters et al (1986). In addition, we have measured EJPs, using both single and double sucrose gap, in these muscle strips, to evaluate the release of acetylcholine. These studies have confirmed the results of Walters et al (1986) that the responses to electrical field stimulation are increased in ozone treated dogs when compared to control dogs. However EJPs, whether measured by the single or double sucrose gap, were not different between the two groups of dogs. These results were qualitatively similar to the results of Serio and Daniel of the effects of U46619 on the responses to field stimulation. These results suggest that something other than an increase in the initial amounts of acetylcholine released is responsible for the increased response to field stimulation in muscle strips from dogs with airway hyperresponsiveness in vivo.

EFFECTS ON AIRWAYS SMOOTH MUSCLE

To examine the possibility that airway smooth muscle responses to constrictor mediators is increased in dogs with airway hyperresponsiveness after inhaling ozone, we have measured the responses to exogenous acetylcholine and potassium chloride (KCl) in canine trachealis from dogs with airway hyperresponsiveness after ozone. The responses to exogenous acetylcholine, as measured by changes in active tension, were increased in trachealis muscle from hyperresponsive dogs compared to control dogs. This increased responsiveness in vitro was not present, however, to exogenous KCl. These results suggest that a post-junctional abnormality exists in muscle strips from dogs with airway hyperresponsiveness in vivo. In addition, as KCl causes smooth muscle contraction by Ca^{2+} movement through voltage dependent Ca^{2+} channels, it is unlikely that an increased influx of extracellular Ca^{2+} through voltage dependent channels is responsible for airway hyperresponsiveness associated with ozone inhalation.

CONCLUSION

Airway hyperresponsiveness after inhaled ozone in dogs occurs as a result of an acute inflammatory response in the airways. Thromboxane is an important mediator in causing airway hyperresponsiveness, which may act through presynaptic modulation of acetylcholine release. However, an abnormality may also exist in airway smooth muscle as well as in presynaptic modulation of acetylcholine release, which together accounts for the presence of airway hyperresponsiveness after inhaled ozone.

REFERENCES

Aizawa H, Chung KF, Leikauf GD, Ueki I, Bethel RA, O'Byrne PM, Hirose T, Nadel JA (1985). Significance of thromboxane generation in ozone-induced airway hyperresponsiveness in dogs. J Appl Physiol 59:1918-1923.

Boulet LP, Latimer KM, Roberts RS, Juniper EF, Cockcroft DW, Thomson NC, Daniel EE, Hargreave FE (1984). The effect of atropine on allergen-induced increases in bronchial responsiveness to histamine. Am Rev Respir Dis 130:368-372.

Chung KF, Aizawa H, Becker AB, Frick O, Gold WM, Nadel JA (1986). Inhibition of antigen-induced airway hyperresponsiveness by a thromboxane synthetase inhibitor (OKY 046) in allergic dogs. Am Rev Respir Dis 134:258-261.

Chung KF, Aizawa H, Leikauf GD, Ueki IF, Evans TW, Nadel JA (1986). Airway hyperresponsiveness induced by platelet-activating factor: role of thromboxane generation. J Pharmacol Exp Ther 236:580-584.

Empey DW, Laitinen LA, Jacobs L, Gold WM, Nadel JA (1976). Mechanisms of bronchial hyperreactivity in normal subjects after upper respiratory tract infections. Am Rev Respir Dis 113:131-139.

Golden JA, Nadel JA, Boushey HA (1978). Bronchial hyperirritability in healthy subjects after exposure to ozone. Am Rev Respir Dis 118:287-294.

Hall RA, Gillard J, Guindon Y, Letts G, Campion E, Ethier D, Evans J, Ford-Hutchinson AW, Fortin R, Jones TR, Lord A, Morton HE, Rokach J, Yoakim C (1987). Pharmacology of L-655,240 (3-[1-(4-chlorobenzyl)-5-flouro-3-methyl-indol-2-yl]2,2 -dimethylpropanoic acid); a potent selective thromboxane/prostaglandin endoperoxide antagonist. Eur J Pharm (in press).

Hargreave FE, Ryan G, Thomson NC, O'Byrne PM, Latimer K, Juniper EF, Dolovich J (1981). Bronchial responsiveness to histamine or methacholine in asthma: measurement and clinical significance. J Allergy Clin Immunol 68:347-355.

Holtzman MJ, Cunningham JH, Sheller JR, Irsigler GB, Nadel JA, Boushey HA (1979). Effect of ozone on bronchial reactivity in atopic and non-atopic subjects. Am Rev Respir Dis 120:1059-1067.

Holtzman MJ, Fabbri LM, O'Byrne PM, Gold BD, Aizawa H, Walters EH, Alpert SE, Nadel JA (1983). Importance of airway inflammation for hyperresponsiveness induced by ozone. Am Rev Respir Dis 127:686-690.

Holtzman MJ, Sheller JR, Dimeo M, Nadel JA, Boushey HA (1980). Effect of ganglionic blockade on bronchial reactivity in atopic subjects. Am Rev Respir Dis 122:17-25.

Jones GL, Lane CG, Manning PJ, O'Byrne PM (1987). Role of the parasympathetic nervous system in airway hyperresponsiveness after ozone. J Appl Physiol (Inpress).

Juniper EF, Frith PA, Hargreave FE (1981). Airway responsiveness to histamine and methacholine: relationship to minimum treatment to control symptoms of asthma. Thorax 36:575-579.

Lee HK, Murlas C (1985). Ozone-induced bronchial hyperreactivity in guinea pigs is abolished by BW 755C or FPL 55712 but not by indomethacin. Am Rev Respir Dis 132:1005-1009.

Munoz NM, Shioya T, Murphy TM, Primack S, Dame C, Sands MF, Leff AR (1986). Potentiation of vagal contractile response by thromboxane mimetic U-46619. J Appl Physiol 61:1173-1179.

O'Byrne PM, Leikauf GD, Aizawa H, Bethel RA, Ueki IF, Holtzman MJ, Nadel JA (1985). Leukotriene B_4 induced airway hyperresponsiveness in dogs. J Appl Physiol 59:1941-1946.

O'Byrne PM, Thomson NC, Latimer KM, Roberts RS, Morris MM, Daniel EE, Hargreave FE (1985). The effect of inhaled hexamethonium bromide and atropine sulphate on airway responsiveness to histamine. J Allergy Clin Immunol 76:97-103.

O'Byrne PM, Walters EH, Aizawa H, Fabbri LM, Holtzman MJ, Nadel JA (1984). Indomethacin inhibits the airway hyperresponsiveness but not the neutrophil influx induced by ozone in dogs. Am Rev Respir Dis 130:220-224.

O'Byrne PM, Walters EH, Gold BD, Aizawa HA, Fabbri LM, Alpert SE, Nadel JA, Holtzman MJ (1984). Neutrophil depletion inhibits airway hyperresponsiveness induced by ozone exposure. Am Rev Respir Dis 130:214-219.

Seltzer J, Bigby BG, Stulbarg M, Holtzman MJ, Ueki IF, Leikauf GD, Goetzl EJ, Boushey HA (1986). Ozone induced change in bronchial reactivity to methacholine and airway inflammation in humans. J Appl Physiol 60:1321-1326.
Serio R, Daniel EE. Thromboxanes and other inflammatory modulators of canine trachealis neuromuscular function (Submitted).
Tamaoki J, Sekizawa K, Osborne ML, Ueki IF, Graf PD, Nadel JA (1987). Platelet aggregation increases cholinergic neurotransmission in canine airways. J Appl Physiol 62:2246-2251.
Walters EH, O'Byrne PM, Graf PD, Fabbri LM, Nadel JA (1986). The responsiveness of airway smooth muscle in vitro from dogs with airway hyper-responsiveness in vivo. Clin Science 71:605-611.

DISCUSSION

Benveniste: Most of these mediators act in sequences. The fact that you find an effect with inhibitors doesn't mean that the whole job is done by this mediator. You might have a series of mediators in cascade. Secondly, it is clear that thromboxane blockers do not change reactivity in man - so why do these experiments?

O'Byrne: Firstly, I don't think that it's very clear at all that thromboxane blockers don't alter airway responsiveness in man. I'm not aware that this study has been done. We have recently shown that indomethacin will inhibit the development of airway hyperresponsiveness after inhaled allergen in allergic subjects. To answer your first point, I agree with you in that this is almost certainly a cascade - but one of the mediators in this model is thromboxane A_2.

Walters: What was the washout and delay time in your experiments? This may be important when you consider that picomolar amounts of prostanoid seem to have substantial effects on smooth muscle in vitro.

O'Byrne: We studied the tissues as quickly as possible - generally it was an hour or less between when the animals were euthanized and the studies in the bath. Another important point is that only if we express the results as tension/g wet weight do we get the sorts of differences I've discussed.

Stephens: Do you know what was happening to the activity of the postsynaptic acetylcholinesterase, because that might give you an increased response to acetylcholine? In a different model we have evidence that it is in fact reduced.

O'Byrne: No, I don't know.

Barnes: Can you comment on the role of airway epithelium in this model, because ozone is well known to damage epithelium and could be releasing mediators or inducing loss of a relaxant factor.

O'Byrne: Ed Daniel will be presenting data showing that actually there is much less damage to the epithelium than you would think after ozone. He's looked at the ultrastructure very carefully. We've also tried in a functional way to look at the effect of epithelium. The responses to a number of exogenous mediators were not different in the trachea of the ozone-treated dogs.

Mechanisms in Asthma: Pharmacology,
Physiology, and Management, pages 15–23

MAST CELL HETEROGENEITY

Martin K. Church

Immunopharmacology Research Group, Clinical Pharmacology, Centre Block, Southampton General Hospital, Southampton SO9 4XY, U.K.

Mast cells were initially identified and named by Paul Ehrlich in 1876 after their characteristic ability to stain metachromatically with aniline dyes. For 50 years they were believed to be a homogeneous population of cells whose function was largely unknown until the pioneering studies of Dale and colleagues (Best *et al.*, 1927) linked mast cells with anaphylaxis and allergy. In the early 1900's Maximow (1906) suggested that mast cells were not indeed homogeneous but cells obtained from different sites showed different morphological characteristics. These studies were, however, largely forgotten until the great upsurge in the interest of the association of the mast cell with allergic reactions such as asthma, hay fever, gastro-intestinal allergy and urticaria in the 1960's. Then in 1966 Enerback produced a series of classic papers in which he conclusively demonstrated that there were two sub-populations of rodent mast cell which could be differentiated not only by their fixation and staining characteristics but also by their monoamine content and their ability to respond to secretagogues (Enerback, 1960a,b,c,d). The mast cell from the peritoneum or connective tissue mast cell (CTMC) he found to be resistant to formalin fixation and stained with safranin O rather than alcian blue. The cell associated with the mucosal surface of the gastro-intestinal tract or mucosal mast cell (MMC), however, could not be stained when fixed with formalin and when fixed with alternative fixatives such as Carnoy's fixative it stained with alcian blue rather than safranin. Subsequent studies have shown as much about the mechanisms of development and the properties of these two types of rodent mast cell (Enerback, 1986). However, we do not know for certain whether or not these findings can be extrapolated to human mast cells.

SOURCE AND DEVELOPMENT OF RODENT MAST CELLS

Mast cell precursors are found in the bone marrow from where they enter the circulation and are distributed to the tissues where they mature and can be identified. Although it was initially considered that the CTMC and MMC were derived from different precursor cells i.e. genetically determined, it has recently been demonstrated by the studies of Kitamura and colleagues that the environmental factors prevailing in the tissue of deposition determine the development of the phenotype (Nakano *et al.*, 1985). In elegant experiments in mice, they demonstrated that mast cell precursors from mouse bone marrow transplanted into mast cell deficient W/W^v mice developed into CTMC if implanted into the skin or MMC if implanted into the intestine. Furthermore, they showed that mature CTMC removed from the skin and implanted into the mucosal layer of the intestine changed their characteristics to CTMC (Kitamura *et al.*, 1986).

Studies in parasitized rats and in tissue culture have shown that the development of the mucosal mast cell is dependent on T-lymphocyte products (Haig *et al.*, 1982) particularly interleukin-3 (Ihle *et al.*, 1983) and that there is a dramatic rise in MMC numbers during parasite infections. In contrast, the numbers of CTMC are unaffected by T-cell products. The development of these cells is dependent on other factors, possibly fibroblast products. This then raises the possibility that MMC are likely to be of more importance than CTMC in allergic diseases because of their specific accumulation at the focus of an allergic reaction.

HETEROGENEITY OF RAT MAST CELLS

The properties of rat CTMC and MMC are summarized in Table 1. These differences may be divided for convenience into five areas, staining characteristics, granule

TABLE 1. Heterogeneity of rodent mast cells

	Connective Tissue Mast Cells	Mucosal Mast Cells
Fixation	Formaldehyde	Carnoys
Staining	Safranin O	Alcian Blue
Granule Content		
Proteoglycan	Heparin	Heparin E
Protease	RMCPI	RMCP II
Histamine	10 pg	1 pg
5-HT	+	-
Newly Generated Mediators		
PGD_2	+ + +	+
LTC_4	+	+ +
Secretagogues		
Antigen	+ +	+ +
A23187	+ + +	+ +
Co 48/80	+ + +	-
Substance P	+ +	±
Morphine	+ +	-
Inhibitors		
Cromoglycate	+ +	-
Theophylline	+ +	-
β-agonist	-	?

content, profile of eicosanoid generation, response to secretagogues and modulation by drugs. In rats the differences between mast cells within each of these areas correlate neatly to enable a clear sub-division to be made between CTMC and MMC. As mentioned earlier the mast cell sub-populations may be readily distinguished under the microscope by their size, number of granules, fixation sensitivity to formalin and by their staining. The fixation and staining characteristics are determined by the proteoglycan backbone present in the cell. The high molecular weight heparin (750,000 d) of the connective tissue mast cell does not readily interact with the copper phthalocyanin dyes such as alcian blue dye. Conversely the undersulphated heparin E of the MMC does stain with alcian blue (Enerback, 1986). The cells may also be distinguished immunocytochemically by their different proteases (Woodbury and Miller, 1982) and biochemically by their histamine and 5-HT content. When stimulated the connective tissue mast cell produces large amounts of PGD_2 but little LTC_4 (Stevens *et al.*, 1986). The converse is true for the MMC. Functionally, CTMC may be stimulated to secrete mediators by compound 48/80, peptides and morphine and secretion is inhibited by sodium cromoglycate (Pearce, 1986). The MMC is unaffected by any of these agents.

EVIDENCE FOR HETEROGENEITY IN HUMAN MAST CELLS

Although it is clear from a number of lines of evidence that there is heterogeneity amongst human mast cells it does not appear to be a simple sub-division into two sub-populations as seen in the rat.

In our experience, mast cells isolated from human lung, skin, intestinal muscle and intestinal mucosa all have a similar monophasic size distribution with no obvious evidence of two sub-populations. Also the histamine content of mast cells from these sources is similar, 3-5 pg/cell. When viewed under the electron microscope all human mast cells have a similar crystalline structure which is quite distinct from the amorphous appearance of the rat mast cell granule. With respect to morphology and histamine content then, human mast cels would appear to be homogeneous.

The most clear cut evidence of heterogeneity within human mast cells derives from the immunocytochemical studies of their protease content performed by Schwartz, Schechter and colleagues (Irani *et al.*, 1986; Schwartz *et al.*, 1987). Mast cells of the intestinal mucosa and from all areas of the lung contain tryptase as their neutral protease. In contrast, the mast cells of the skin and the sub-mucosal layers of the intestine contain chymase in addition to tryptase. Like rat MMC, human tryptase containing mast cells are dependent on T-cell factors for their development as evidenced by their absence in T-lymphocyte deficiency diseases (Irani *et al.*, 1987).

There have been numerous publications on the sensitivity of human mast cells to formalin fixation and alcian blue staining. These, however, are confused and do not appear to correlate with the protease content of the cells. For example, both human lung and skin have been reported to contain sizable quantities of cells with both fixation and staining characteristics. I would be surprised, however, if techniques developed to discriminate between the different species of heparin in rat mast cells was readily extrapolatable to heparin of human cells which are quite different (Stevens *et al.*, 1986). In our experience mast cell activation greatly influences the sensitivity of human mast cells to formalin fixation and alcian blue dyes. Despite these comments, there is one study which demonstrates a great proliferation of formalin-sensitive alcian blue staining mast cells in the nasal mucosa during the hay fever season (Otsuka *et al.*, 1985). Furthermore, the development of these cells is prevented by corticosteroids (Otsuka *et al.*, 1986), a finding similar to that made with rat MMC following parasitic infection (King *et al.*, 1985). This is highly suggestive of the proliferation of a T-cell dependent mast cell in allergic reactions.

Rat CTMC produce predominantly PGD_2 whilst MMC produce mainly LTC_4. However, in response to stimulation with calcium ionophore A23187, mast cells of human skin and lung produce similar amounts of PGD_2 (Holgate *et al.*, 1984; Benyon *et al.*, 1987). Also the findings by Murray *et al.* (1986) that large quantities of PGD_2 are found in bronchoalveolar lavage fluid following antigen challenge would argue against the mast cells of the bronchial lumen being different from those dispersed from lung parenchyma.

Functional studies have also demonstrated heterogeneity amongst human mast cells, but these do not correlate with either protease content or staining (Lowman *et al.*, 1987). Skin mast cells, which contain both tryptase and chymase secrete histamine in response to peptides whereas mast cells from lung, adenoids, tonsils, intestinal mucosa and intestinal sub-mucosa (the latter also containing both tryptase and chymase) do not.

Extrapolation of studies from rat mast cells would suggest that the human skin, but not the lung mast cell, would be susceptible to inhibition by sodium cromoglycate

(Pearce, 1986). In fact the converse is true, the human skin mast cell being totally unresponsive (Clegg *et al.*, 1985) whereas the lung mast cell shows some susceptibility (Church and Hiroi, 1987). Furthermore, sodium cromoglycate is a more effective inhibitor of mediator release from mast cells recovered by bronchoalveolar lavage (BAL) than those dispersed by enzymatic digeston of lung tissue. Furthermore, no tachyphylaxis to the drug is obvious in BAL mast cells whereas it is readily demonstrable in dispersed mast cells and lung fragments (Flint *et al.*, 1985). Whether this represents true mast cell heterogeneity or the state of cell activation is not known.

CONCLUSIONS

There are two clear sub-populations of mast cells in rodents whereas in man the picture is much less clear. In view of the complex effects of the local environment and immunological factors on mast cell development, it is likely that the site of mast cell deposition which determines its development into its mature phenotype. Major differences are observed between organs e.g. lung and skin where the constituent mast cells may be modified to perform a particular function relevant to that organ e.g. defence against parasites at a mucosal surface or control of blood flow deep within the skin. However, the migration of a mast cell through a tissue e.g. from the lung parenchyma to the mucosal surface may also induce subtle changes in its characteristics and function as exemplified by the disparate actions of sodium cromoglycate on mast cells dispersed from lung tissue and recovered by BAL. A knowledge of the complex mixture of cytokines which determine mast cell differentiation and maturation will enable the culture of human mast cells and allow studies of the effects of tissue factors and even disease states on the function of mast cells.

ACKNOWLEDGEMENTS

This work was supported in part by a grant from the Medical Research Council. I would like to thank all my colleagues whose studies and labours have contributed towards this manuscript.

REFERENCES

Benyon RC, Robinson C, Holgate ST, Church MK (1987). Prostaglandin D_2 release from human skin mast cells in response to ionophore A23187. Br J Pharmacol In Press.

Best CH, Dale HH, Dudley HW (1927). The nature of vasodilator constituents of certain tissue extracts. J Physiol (Lond) 62: 397-417.

Church MK, Hiroi J (1987). Inhibition of IgE-dependent histamine release from human dispersed lung mast cells by anti-allergic drugs and salbutamol. Br J Pharmacol 90: 421-429.

Ehrlich P (1876). Beitrage zur kenntnis der anilinfarbungen und ihrer verwengung in der mikroskopischen technik. Arch Mikr Anat 13: 263-277.

Enerback L (1966a). Mast cells in the gastrointestinal mucosa. I. Effects of fixation. Acta Path Microbiol Scand 66: 289-302.

Enerback L (1966b). Mast cells in the gastrointestinal mucosa. II. Dye binding and metachromatic properties. Acta Path Microbiol Scand 66: 303-312.

Enerback L (1966c). Mast cells in the gastrointestinal mucosa. III. Reactivity towards compound 48/80. Acta Path Microbiol Scand 66: 313-322.

Enerback L (1966d). Mast cells in the gastrointestinal mucosa. IV. Monoamine storing capacity. Acta Path Microbiol Scand 67: 365-379.

Enerback L (1986). Mast cell heterogeneity: The evolution of the concept of a specific mucosal mast cell. In Befus AD, Bienenstock J, Denburg JA (eds): "Mast Cell Differentiation and Heterogeneity," New York: Raven Press, p 1-26.

Flint KC, Leung KBP, Pearce FL, Hudspith BN, Brostoff J, Johnson NMcI (1985). Human mast cells recovered from bronchoalveolar lavage: their morphology, histamine release and effects of sodium cromoglycate. Clin Sci 68: 427-432.

Haig DM, McKee TA, Jarrett EEE, Woodbury R, Miller HRP (1982). Generation of mucosal mast cells is stimulated in in vitro by factors derived from T cells of helminth infected rats. Nature 300: 188-190.

Holgate ST, Burns GB, Robinson C, Church MK (1984). Anaphylactic and calcium dependent generation of prostaglandin D_2 (PGD_2), thromboxane B_2 and other cyclooxygenase products of arachidonic acid by dispersed

human lung cells and relationship to histamine release. J Immunol, 133, 2138-2144.
Ihle JN, Keller J, Oroszlan S, Henderson LE, Copeland TD, Fitch F, Prytsowsky MB, Goldwasser E, Schrader JW, Palaszynski E, Dy M, Lebel B (1983). Biological properties of homogenous interleukin 3: Demonstration of WEHI-3 growth factor activity, mast cell growth factor activity, P-cell stimulating factor activity, colony-stimulating activity and histamine producing cell stimulating factor activity. J Immunol 131: 282-287.
Irani AA, Schechter NM, Craig S, DeBlois G, Schwartz LB (1986). Two types of human mast cells that have distinct neutral protease compositions. Proc Natl Acad Sci USA 83: 4464-4468.
Irani AA, Buckley R, Haynes B, Schechter NM, Schwartz LB (1987). Selective depletion of T mast cells in intestinal mucosa of patients with defective lymphocyte function [Abstract]. J Allergy Clin Immunol 79: 178.
King SJ, Miller HR, Newlands GF, Woodbury RG (1985). Depletion of mucosal mast cell protease by glucocorticosteroids: effect on intestinal anaphylaxis in the rat. Proc Natl Acad Sci USA 82: 1214-1218.
Kitamura Y, Nakano T, Kanakura Y, Matsuda H (1986). Factors influencing mast cell differention. In Reed CE (ed) "Proceedings of the XII International Congress of Allergy and Clinical Immunology", St. Louis: CV Mosby, J Allergy Clin Immunol 154-8.
Lowman MA, Rees PH, Benyon RC, Church MK (1987). Human mast cell heterogeneity: Histamine release from mast cells dispersed from skin, lung, adenoids, tonsils and intestinal mucosa in response to IgE-dependent and non-immunological stimuli. J Allergy Clin Immunol In Press.
Murray JJ, Tonel AB, Brash AR, Roberts LJ, Gosset P, Workman R, Capron A, Oates JA (1986). Release of prostaglandin D2 into human airways during acute antigen challenge. N Engl J Med 315: 800-804.
Nakano T, Sonoda T, Hayashi C, Yamatodani A, Kanayama Y, Yamamura T, Asai H, Yonezawa T, Kitamura Y, Galli SJ (1985). Fate of bone marrow-derived cultured mast cells after intracutaneous, intraperitoneal and intravenous transfer into genetically mast cell deficient W/Wv mice: evidence that cultured mast cells can give rise to both connective tissue type and mucosal mast cells. J Exp Med 162: 1025-1043.
Otsuka H, Denburg JA, Befus AD, Hitch D, Lapp P, Rajan RS, Bienenstock JA, Dolovich J (1986). Effect of

beclomethasone dipropionate on nasal metachromatic subpopulations. Clin Allergy 16: 589-595.
Otsuka H, Denburg J, Dolovich J, Hitch D, Lapp P, Rajan RS, Bienenstock J, Befus D (1985). Heterogeneity of metachromatic cells in human nose: significance of mucosal mast cells. J Allergy Clin Immunol 76: 695-702.
Schwartz LB, Irani AM, Roller K, Castells M, Schechter NM (1987). Quantitation of histamine, tryptase, and chymase in dispersed human T and CT mast cells. J Immunol 138: 2611-2615.
Woodbury RG, Miller HRP (1982). Quantitative analysis of mucosal mast cell protease in the intestine of Nippostrongylus-injected rats. Immunology 46: 487-495.

DISCUSSION

Nadel: I would suggest that as this evolves, you're going to find that differentiation of one kind of cell like the mast cell is going to be potently affected by the cells surrounding it. I don't think you should limit yourself to the fibroblast, proximity to sensory nerves, ganglia or glands may all influence the type of mast cell developed rather than the source like skin or penis.

Church: I agree with your comments entirely.

Benveniste: We have recently shown that PAF-acether can control the proliferation of thymocytes. This is an example of what J. Nadel suggested, i.e. a peripheral mediator controlling cell proliferation.

Mechanisms in Asthma: Pharmacology, Physiology, and Management, pages 25–34

THE MECHANISM OF CIGARETTE SMOKE INDUCED INCREASED EPITHELIAL PERMEABILITY IN GUINEA PIG AIRWAYS

David C. Walker, Alan R. Burns

Pulmonary Research Laboratory
St. Paul's Hospital, Dept. of Pathology, U.B.C.
Vancouver, British Columbia, Canada V6Z 1Y6

INTRODUCTION

Increased epithelial permeability is a demonstrable early response to cigarette smoke in humans (Jones et al., 1980; Minty et al., 1981; Mason et al., 1983; Kennedy et al., 1984) and guinea pigs (Simani et al., 1974; Boucher et al., 1980; Hulbert et al, 1981; Burns et al., 1987). Localization of HRP between epithelial cells of guinea pig tracheas and bronchioles suggested that epithelial tight junction opening might contribute to the increased permeability (Simani et al., 1974). While qualitative observations suggested that disruption of tight junctions did occur with cigarette smoke exposure, (Boucher et al., 1980), this was not supported by quantitative studies (Walker et al., 1984). In normal guinea pig tracheal epithelium, mucous cell tight junctions were described as being more loosely organized than those between non-secretory cells (Inoue and Hogg, 1977). Counting studies suggested that the number of mucous cells in the tracheal epithelium of guinea pigs declines immediately following cigarette smoke exposure. This was attributed to emptying of mucous cells by traumatic secretory activity (Hulbert et al., 1981). Treatment of tracheal epithelia with DMSO produced traumatic lumenal mucous cell activity (Walker and Hosford, 1986). The avenue of permeability to HRP involved secretory cell breakdown without tight junction penetration. This study also showed that HRP could enter intercellular spaces by crossing at disrupted secretory cells and diffuse laterally.

These observations led to the present cigarette smoke exposure study which focused on epithelial mucus and permeability to HRP. Morphometric analysis showed no decline in epithelial mucus (Walker et al., 1987). Quantitative measurement of HRP penetration patterns reported here do not support tight junction permeability changes and a new explanation and mechanism are suggested.

METHODS

Thirty Hartley guinea pigs (Male n=19 and Female n=11) of similar size (control 459g+66SD, treated 466g+91SD) were used for this study. Treated animals were exposed to 15-20 (n=5), 45-50 (n=5) and 90-100 (n=5) puffs of whole cigarette smoke as in previous studies (Simani et al., 1974). Control animals were sham exposed in the same apparatus (n=5/group) for equivalent periods of time. All animals were sacrificed by an intraperitoneal overdose of pentabarbital sodium so that tracheas could be excised within 7 minutes of the end of exposure. Excised tracheal segments were immersed in HRP (10mg/ml Tyrodes buffer, pH 7.4) for 2 minutes then fixed (2.5% glutaraldehyde in 0.1M cacodylate buffer at pH 7.4) for 2h at RT. This was followed by DAB and H_2O_2 to localize HRP and then processed for transmission electron microscopy and light microscopy.

Three blocks of tissue from each of the 30 tracheas were thin sectioned and viewed unstained. Tight junctions were assessed for the presence of HRP within and below the tight junctions with the aid of a goniometer stage on a Philips 400 TEM. Epithelial lesions were photographed when present.

RESULTS

Of the 4,145 tight junctions observed in the 45 sections from the 15 control animals, 17 tight junctions contained HRP (Table 1). All of these penetrated junctions were between cells in a single epithelial lesion in one section. Similarly, 26 of the 4,282 tight junctions from the smoke exposed animals contained HRP (Table 1). As in the controls these 26 penetrated

Table 1
HRP Within Tight Junctions

		Exposure (cigarettes) 1	3	6
Smokers	W	0	0	26
	NW	1,184	1,576	1,499
Controls	W	0	17	0
	NW	1,248	1,402	1,478

W = Within, NW = Not Within

junctions were between the cells of 2 epithelial lesions in a single section. All 3 of these lesions were characterised by the absence of ciliate and mucous cells suggesting that regeneration was under way (Fig.1) and that

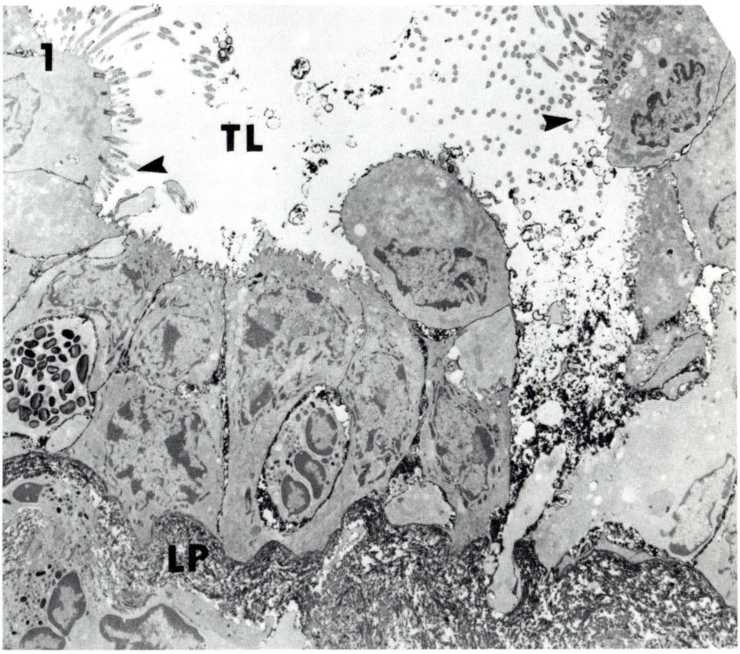

Figure 1. Older epithelial lesion with essentially cuboidal cells neither cilitate nor secretroy. Unstained section showing DAB stained HRP in traceal lumen (TL), between cells and in lamina propria (LP). Lesion margins are at ciliate cells (arrowhead). 2,650X.

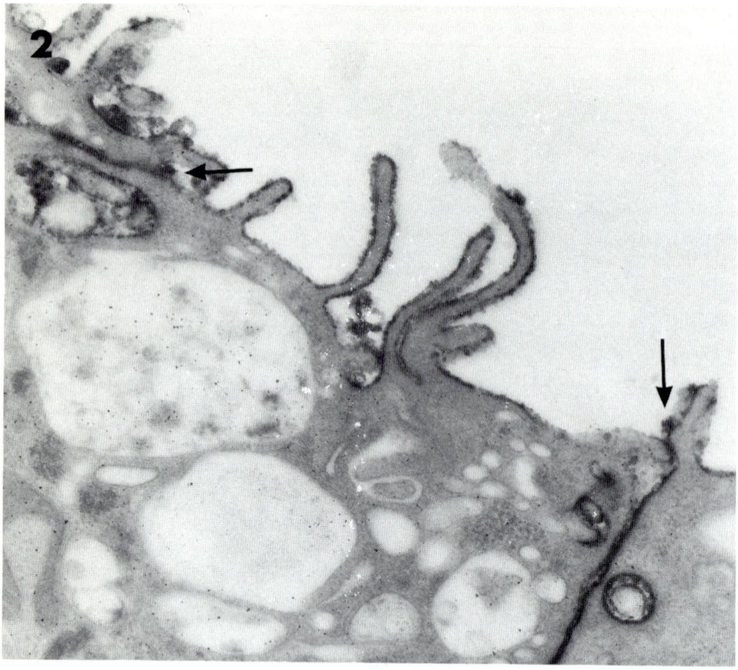

Figure 2. Free surface and penetrated epithelial tight junctions (arrow) from older lesion. Unstained section with DAB localization of HRP. 32,250X.

the junctions penetrated were between undifferentiated cells (Fig.2). HRP also filled intercellular spaces below tight junctions in and around these lesions (Fig.1). This interstitial filling extended laterally between epithelial cells well away from the lesions to the extent that all basal-lateral spaces of the section containing a lesion contained HRP. HRP was not observed in tight junctions away from the lesions. Two other lesions were found in one section where only a few epithelial cells were missing. Adjacent cells appeared fine and there was no evidence of repair (Fig.3). This type of lesion also provided HRP direct access to intercellular spaces through lateral diffusion and no adjacent junctions were penetrated (Fig.3, arrowheads). This is presumed to be a recent lesion. Some migratory cells appear to have reached the epithelial surface through this hole (Fig.3). As in previous studies HRP

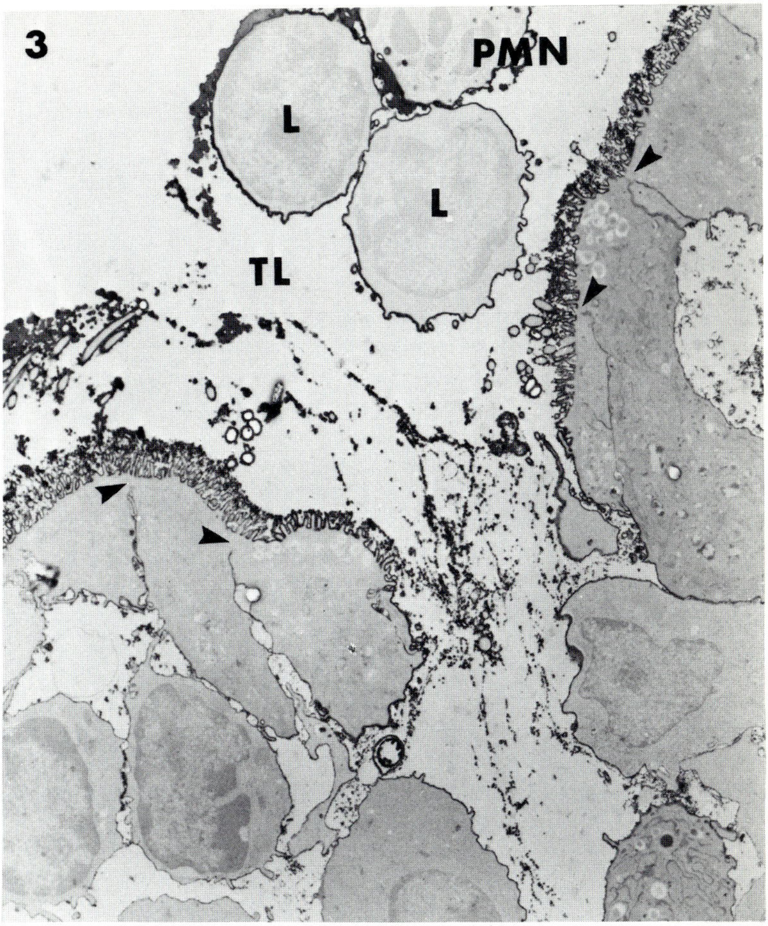

Figure 3. More recent epithelial lesion with differentiated epithelial cells to either side. Free lymphocytes (L) and PMN above epithelium. Section is unstained and HRP free tight junctions (arrowheads) are clear over backfilled intercellular spaces. 4,400X.

was also found below tight junctions and not associated with a lesion. HRP was present in 808 of the 4,215 intercellular spaces observed between cells of smoke exposed animals (Table 2). A similar but slightly smaller number of intercellular spaces, 638 out of 4,146, contained HRP in the controls (Table 2). A

Table 2
HRP Below Tight Junctions

		Exposure (cigarettes)		
		1	3	6
Smokers	B	157	281	370
	NB	1,018	1,292	1,097
Controls	B	109	307	162
	NB	1,138	1,049	1,321

B = Below, NB = Not Below

t-test suggests that the number of HRP containing intercellular spaces is not significantly larger for the smoke exposed animals.

DISCUSSION

The most important observation made here is the obvious lack of HRP within the tight junctions of epithelial cells in either the cigarette smoke exposed or control animal tracheas (Table 1). Increased amounts of HRP below tight junctions of the tracheal epithelial cells (Simani et al., 1974; Boucher et al., 1980; Hulbert et al., 1981) have been correlated with cigarette smoke exposure in the guinea pig. Only one of these studies claims to demonstrate HRP within a tight junction (Simani et al., 1974). This observation was from an obliquely sectioned tight junction (Simani et al., 1974, Fig. 7) which may have only appeared to be penetrated by HRP since sectioned membranes viewed en face or obliquely are more electron dense (Hayat, 1975). The 43 apparently penetrated tight junctions observed here were between undifferentiated epithelial cells presumably forming a repair epithelium (Figs. 1&2). Tight junctions of undifferentiated epithelia have been demonstrated to be incomplete (Marin et al., 1979; Luciano et al., 1979; Feltkamp and Waerden, 1983) and penetrable (Gonzalez-Marisca et al., 1985). However, since these cells are only separated from each other by nanometer distances and the lesions are on the order of micrometers across it would seem that the latter would be more significant as an avenue for HRP penetration. Therefore, it seems improbable that the penetrated junctions observed within relatively large epithelial lesions could contribute significantly to the amounts of HRP between epithelial cells. The absence of penetrated tight junctions away from lesions also argues against their playing a significant role in cigarette smoke induced permeability changes. The occurrence of HRP between epithelial cells of smoke exposed and control tracheas seems best explained by the presence of lesions nearby but not included in the particular plane of section. This is supported by the fact that areas where HRP occurs between epithelial cells are focal like the lesions rather than generally distributed. This interpretation is further supported by our ability to create similar patterns of HRP penetration by focally damaging mucous cells with DMSO (Walker and Hosford 1986). Even apparently dead mucous cells retained tight junctions impermeable to HRP while permitting penetration into intercellular spaces to back-fill them to the bottoms of the junctional complexes (Walker and Hosford 1986).

The data presented here strongly suggest that intercellular HRP in the guinea pig tracheal epithelium is present because of epithelial lesions in smokers and controls. Furthermore, the repair areas suggest that these lesions may not be directly related to cigarette smoke insult. This led to our re-examination of bronchiolar and alveolar epithelia with the tracer FITC-dextran (Burns et al., 1987a). These studies have shown that smoking focuses deposition of nebulized FITC-dextran at bronchioloalveolar junctions and that the mechanism of increased permeability appears to be type I pneumocyte damage (Burns et al., 1987b).

ACKNOWLEDGEMENTS

This work was supported by the B.C. Lung Association and the B.C. Health Care Foundation.

REFERENCES

Boucher RC, Johnson J, Inoue S, Hulbert WC, Hogg JC (1980). The effect of cigarette smoke on the permeability of guinea pig airways. Lab Invest 43:94-100.

Burns AR, Van Oostdam J, Walker DC, Hogg JC (1987a). Effect of urethane anesthesia on cigarette smoke-induced airway injury in guinea pig. J Appl Physiol. 63:84-91.

Burns AR, Walker DC, Hosford S, Hogg JC (1987b). A study of respiratory epithelial permeability to fluresce-inisothiocyanate dextran (FITC-D) following cigarette smoke exposure in the guinea pig. Fed Proc 46:815 abs.

Feltkamp CA, van de Waerden AWM (1983). Junction formation between cultured normal rat hepatocytes. J Cell Sci 63:271-286.

Gonzalez-Mariscal L, Chavez de Remirez B, Cereijido M (1985). Tight junction formation in cultured epithelial cells (MDCK). J Membrane Biol 86:113-125.

Hayat MA (1975). Positive staining for electron microscopy. van Norstrand Reinhold Co. N.Y., Pp. 361.

Hulbert WC, Walker DC, Jackson A, Hogg JC (1981). Airway permeability to horseradish peroxidase in guinea pig: the repair phase after injury by cigarette smoke. Am Rev Respir Dis 123:320-326.

Inoue S, Hogg JC (1977). Freeze-etch study of the tracheal epithelium of normal guinea pigs with particular reference to intercellular junctions. J Ultrastruct Res 61:89-99.

Jones JG, Lawler P, Crawley JCW, Minty BD, Hulands G, Veall N (1980). Increased alveolar epithelial permeability in cigarette smokers. Lancet i:66-68.

Kennedy SM, Elwood RK, Wiggs BJR, Pare PD, Hogg JC (1984).
Increased airway mucosal permeability of smokers. Am Rev Respir Dis 129:143-148.

Luciano LJ, Thiele J, Reale E (1979). Development of follicles and of occluding junctions between the folicular cells of the thyroid gland. J Ultrastruct Res 66:164-181.

Marin ML, Gordon RE, Lane BP (1979). Development of tight junctions in rat tracheal epithelium during the early hours after mechanical injury. Am Rev Respir Dis 119:101-106.

Mason GR, Uszler JM, Effros RM, Reid E (1983). Rapidly reversable alternations of pulmonary epithelial permeability induced by smoking. Chest 83:6-11.
Minty BD, Jordan C, Jones JG (1981). Rapid improvement in abnormal pulmonary epithelial permeability after stopping cigarettes. British Med J 282:1183-1186.
Simani AS, Inoue S, Hogg JC (1974). Penetration of the respiratory epithelium of guinea pigs following exposure to cigarette smoke. Laboratory Invest 31:75-81.
Walker DC, Hosford S (1986). Mucous cells secretion and epithelial permeability. Fed Proc 45:786 abs.
Walker DC, Hosford S, Burns AR (1987). Tracheal lumen mucous cell activity during cigarette smoke exposure in guinea pigs. Fed Proc 46:815 abs.
Walker DC, Mackenzie A, Wiggs BRJ, Hulbert WC, Hogg JC (1984). The structure of tight junctions in the tracheal epithelium may not correlate with permeability. Cell Tissue Res 235:607-613.

DISCUSSION

Fuller: Your evidence suggesting that the main lesions were out in the alveolus implies that this was due to the gas rather than particulate phase of cigarette smoke. Do you have any direct evidence to support this?

Walker: We haven't done any work looking at the gas phase with particulates removed. The dextran was nebulized at the end of cigarette smoke exposure so we may be looking at a change in focal deposition, but I don't know the mechanism.

Kerrebijn: In humans there are two distinct clinical pictures after smoking. One is hypersecretion only and the other is hypersecretion with wheezing. Have any studies like yours been done in humans and related to their clinical syndrome?

Walker: I know that increased permeability following cigarette smoke has been documented in humans, however it's impossible to study this tissue morphologically.

Holma: Do you know if cigarette smoke changes the pH of the mucous?

Walker: I suspect there may be a change in the source of mucous following cigarette smoke. Submucosal glands may become the main source - but whether this alters the pH I don't know.

Holma: A decreased pH of the mucous will alter the permeability of the epithelial layer and some asthmatics have acidic mucous.

Walker: There is definitely a heterogeneity in mucous cell populations in the airways and how the source alters with different pathology may be very relevant.

Mechanisms in Asthma: Pharmacology,
Physiology, and Management, pages 35–46

ROLE OF EICOSANOIDS IN AIRWAY SMOOTH MUSCLE TONE

John F. Burka

Department of Anatomy and Physiology,
Atlantic Veterinary College,
University of Prince Edward Island,
Charlottetown, P.E.I., Canada C1A 4P3.

INTRODUCTION

Although the effects of lipid substances from seminal fluid on uterine smooth muscle were first described in the 1930's (Kurzrok and Lieb, 1930; von Euler, 1934), the structure of these compounds, coined "prostaglandins", and their origin from arachidonic acid was not described until 1957 (Bergstrom and Sjovall, 1957). The discovery of prostaglandin (PG) $F_{2\alpha}$ in sheep and pig lungs (Bergstrom et al., 1962) has stimulated intense investigation of eicosanoids on respiratory and pulmonary vascular smooth muscle over the last 25 years. Reviews on this topic have been published (Mathe, 1977; Hyman et al., 1978). The more recent characterization of the bronchoconstrictor compound, slow reacting substance of anaphylaxis (SRS-A), as a series of eicosanoids called leukotrienes (LTs)(Murphy et al., 1979; Morris et al., 1980) has again sparked interest in the physiological and pathological roles of eicosanoids in the airways.

This paper will concern itself primarily with the role of prostaglandins and thromboxanes, products of the cyclooxygenase pathway of arachidonic acid metabolism, on airway tone. The accompanying paper by Dr. Piper will deal with the leukotrienes, products of the lipoxygenase pathway. However, is not possible to separate the two groups of compounds entirely and some overlap is inevitable.

RELEASE AND EFFECTS OF EICOSANOIDS ON THE AIRWAYS

Various eicosanoids are released from diverse cells in lung tissue, the proportion depending on the stimulus, the cell type, and the species. Challenge of passively-sensitized human lung parenchymal tissue with specific antigen in vitro results in the release of the following PGs, in order of quantity released: $PGD_2 \simeq PGI_2 >> PGF_{2}\alpha > PGE_2 \simeq TXA2$, whereas the following order of release is observed from bronchi: $PGI_2 > PGE_2 \simeq PGF2\alpha > PGD_2 > TXA_2$ (Schulman et al., 1982). In contrast, sensitized guinea pig lung parenchyma releases considerable quantities of TXA_2 and PGI_2 when challenged with specific antigen (Boot et al., 1978), whereas the major prostanoid released from trachea is PGE_2 (Burka et al., 1981). The source and activities of cyclooxygenase products released in the lungs is indicated in Table 1. A number of the cells, such as platelets and leukocytes, are not part of the integral structure of the lung, but migrate through the lung. Especially under pathological conditions such as inflammation, leukocytes will be induced to synthesize vast quantities of eicosanoids, particularly leukotrienes.

The physiological role of eicosanoids in the airways is still not clear. The hypothesis that eicosanoids are 'local hormones' that maintain intrinsic tone as well as balance metabolic function is particularly appealing, since both bronchoconstrictor and dilator eicosanoids are produced in the airways and inhibition of their synthesis is not generally life threatening. The 'gross' control of airway tone is likely due to neural influences, particularly the balance between the constrictor vagal cholinergic and the dilator nonadrenergic noncholinergic stimulation and circulating catecholamines. The 'fine tuning' would be provided by the eicosanoids.

In vitro, human and guinea pig airways display intrinsic tone, which can be reduced with cyclooxygenase inhibition. PGE_2 is likely the major contributor to the intrinsic tone observed in guinea pig trachea. This is the major prostanoid synthesized in trachea, even spontaneously, and low concentrations of PGE_2 are contractile (Burka and Paterson, 1980; Gardiner and Collier, 1980; Burka et al., 1981). However, substances in

TABLE 1. Source, activities, and metabolism of prostanoids produced in the lung.

Eicosa-noid	Source	Activity: Pulmonary Vasculature	Activity: Airway Smooth Muscle	Activity: Mucous Secretion	Activity: Platelet Aggregation	Metabolism
PGI_2	vascular endothelium	--	(-)	+	--	hydrolysis to 6-keto $PGF_{1\alpha}$
PGD_2	lung mast cell, platelets	+	++	+	-	enzymatically to PGF derivatives
PGE_2	various cell types	-	$\pm$	-	-	PGDH to 15-keto PGE_2
$PGF_{2\alpha}$	various cell types	+	+	+		PGDH to 15-keto $PGF_{2\alpha}$
TXA_2	platelets, monocytes, neutrophils	++	++		++	hydrolysis to TXB_2

PGDH prostaglandin dehydrogenase
+ constrictor or inductive
- dilator or inhibitory

addition to cyclooxygenase products probably also contribute to intrinsic airway tone. Lipoxygenase inhibitors are known to decrease tone in guinea pig trachea (Saad and Burka, 1983; Mansour and Daniel, 1986) and airways smooth muscle that has already been treated with indomethacin can be further relaxed with the LTD_4 receptor antagonists, L-649,923 and LY163443 (Fig. 1). Thus, LTs may also contribute to intrinsic tone.

The role of eicosanoids on tone is further exemplified by the observations of hyperreactivity to other agonists in the presence of cyclooxygenase inhibition. Orehek et al. (1973; 1975) first noted that indomethacin enhanced the responses of guinea pig trachea to histamine, acetylcholine, serotonin, barium, and potassium, while simultaneously decreasing PGE_2 synthesis. In the absence of indomethacin, the bronchoconstrictor agonists were inducing the synthesis of PGE_2, which in this situation was at a concentration high enough to be bronchodilatory. Inhibition of PGE_2 synthesis resulted in enhanced contractions due to removal of the negative feedback effects of PGE_2. This enhancement is not observed with LTD_4 (Fig. 2). Several explanations can be provided. First, the maximal contraction of LTD_4 may not have been achieved at 10^{-7}M due to limited availability of LTD_4. Secondly, LTD_4 induces the synthesis of TXA_2 , a bronchoconstrictor (Piper and Samhoun, 1981). Inhibition of TXA_2 synthesis, in this case, would result in a reduction in contractility, which was observed at low concentration of the agonist.

The enhancement of contractions to histamine and carbachol and inhibition of the contraction to LTD_4 with the lipoxygenase inhibitor, nordihydroguaiaretic acid (NDGA) (Fig. 2), was unexpected. It is possible that NDGA was exerting some cyclooxygenase inhibitory activity at the concentration used. However, the possible inhibition of a bronchodilator or modulatory lipoxygenase product cannot be ruled out. It also remains to be determined whether selective LT receptor blockers also modulate contractility to other agonists.

During inflammatory conditions, including asthma, the proportion of eicosanoids released changes and the carefully maintained balance in tone no longer exists. The tendency is towards increased production of bronchoconstrictor eicosanoids and thus, in vivo, increased airway resistance and decreased pulmonary compliance results. Changes in the responsiveness of airway smooth muscle, both dependent and independent of eicosanoids also occur, resulting in hyperreactivity. TXA_2, LTB_4, and LTE_4 have all been implicated in inducing airway hyperreactivity in several species (O´Byrne et al., 1985; Aizawa et al., 1985; Lee et al., 1984).

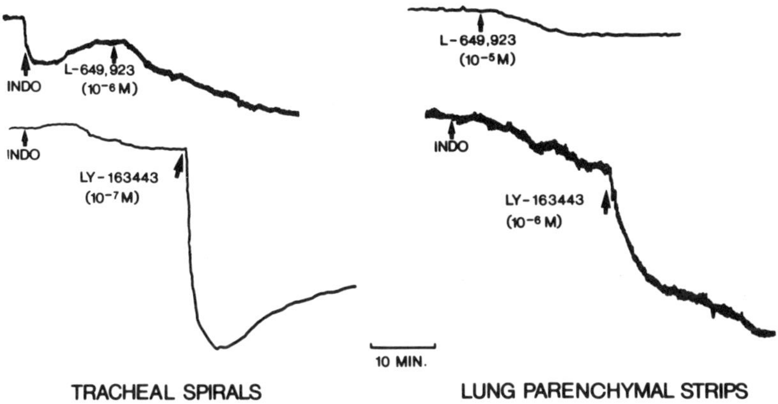

Fig. 1. Relaxation of airways with spontaneous tone with indomethacin (8.5 μM) and L-649,923 and LY-163443.

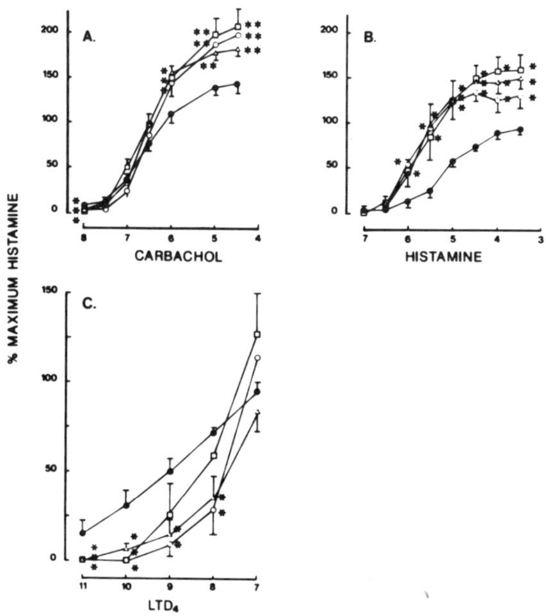

Fig. 2. Concentration-response curves to agonists on guinea pig tracheal spirals after pretreatment with indomethacin (8.5 μM) (□), NDGA (30 μM) (△), and phenidone (185 μM) (○). Concentrations are expressed as -log Molar. Values are mean ± SEM (n=5). Significant differences from paired controls: $*p<0.05$ and $**p<0.01$.

The contribution of cyclooxygenase products to asthma is not clear, since inhibitors of their synthesis are ineffective antiasthmatic agents and, in fact, exacerbate the bronchoconstriction in "aspirin-sensitive" asthmatic patients. Despite this observation, it is well documented that prostanoids are released in inflammatory responses and contribute to smooth muscle contraction, mucous secretion, neutrophil infiltration, increased permeability, etc. (Table 1). PGD_2 is the major prostanoid released from human lung mast cells on antigenic challenge (Lewis et al., 1982). It is 3.5 times more potent that $PGF_{2\alpha}$ in inducing bronchoconstriction in man and produces a greater decrease in specific airway conductance in asthmatic, than in normal, subjects (Hardy et al., 1984). Thus, PGD_2 and, to a lesser extent, $PGF_{2\alpha}$ have been implicated as major contributors to allergic bronchoconstriction in man.

TXA_2 is also a potent bronchoconstrictor, but is released in fairly low proportions in man (Schulman et al., 1982). It may contribute to allergic bronchoconstriction, but may also contract pulmonary vessels and induce intravascular platelet aggregation which can lead to the release of other spasmogens, such as serotonin. As noted above, TXA_2 may contribute to airway hyperreactivity. Recent studies in Nadel's laboratory have shown that the TXA_2-mimic, U-46619, at subthreshold doses causes a fourfold increase in airway responsiveness to acetylcholine in dogs (Aizawa et al., 1985).

The role of PGI_2 is somewhat more equivocal. As noted above, quantities of PGI_2 are released from both human bronchi and lung parenchyma and guinea pig lung parenchyma on immunological stimulation. It is a weak bronchodilator of guinea pig airways in vitro (Burka, 1983) and has no consistent effect on airway caliber in man (Hardy et al., 1985). The activity of PGI_2 may be predominant in pulmonary vascular bed, and indeed it has been demonstrated that there is a high probability that the PGI_2 receptors linked to adenylate cyclase in the lung are located on vascular tissue and not on airways (MacDermot et al., 1981). PGI_2 is a potent pulmonary vasodilator and its role may be to maintain adequate blood flow for gaseous exchange in situations where the supply of oxygen through the airways is compromised. Its presence would also be necessary to counteract the pulmonary vasoconstrictor effects of TXA_2, PGD_2, and the LTs, and the platelet aggregation induced by TXA_2.

The concentrations of PGE_2 released immunologically from lung and airways is sufficient to induce bronchodilation (Burka et al., 1981; Schulman et al., 1982). Thus, this prostaglandin may be the major eicosanoid opposing the bronchoconstrictor effects of its relatives. Schulman et al. (1982) suggested that the PGI_2 levels in human airways may also reach levels high enough to be bronchodilator. PGE_2 is also unique among prostanoids released in lung in that it is the only one which inhibits mucous secretion (Marom et al., 1981).

MECHANISMS OF ACTION

a) Receptors

Studies on the actions of prostaglandins have been hampered by the lack of a clear definition of receptors and availability of receptor blockers. Most compounds with clearly defined receptors and specific receptor antagonists contain an amide group. This includes the LTs, for which selective antagonists are now available. In contrast, the prostanoids are fatty acid derivatives with only a carboxylic end group. Only the location of hydroxy and keto groups on the molecule create distinctions between the molecules. Yet these are sufficient to allow each molecule to have distinct activities, which suggests that some sort of receptors must exist. Gardiner and Collier (1980) categorized three types of receptors for prostanoids in the airways: a contractant, a relaxant, and an irritant receptor. To date this definition has held up quite well. However, blockers have been synthesized for only the contractile receptor. One such agent is SK&F 88046, which blocks the bronchconstrictor effects of TXA_2, $PGF_{2}\alpha$, and PGD_2 (Weichman et al., 1984). Compounds such as this may be useful in asthma, blocking only the bronchoconstrictor effects of the prostanoids, but leaving the bronchodilator effects untouched. Prostanoids may have different affinities for these receptors, although this has not yet been shown with binding studies. For example, low concentrations of PGE_2 are contractile in guinea pig airways, whereas higher concentrations relax (Burka and Paterson, 1980; Gardiner and Collier, 1980). The dual effect of PGE_2 is also seen following inhalation of PGE_2 by human subjects (Walters and Davies, 1982). The weak effect of PGI_2 on airways may reflect low affinity for the relaxant receptor, such that much higher concentrations of PGI_2 are required to relax this tissue.

b) Intracellular mechanisms

The relaxant effects of both PGE_2 and PGI_2 appear to be linked to intracellular increases in cyclic AMP (MacDermot et al., 1981; Burka and Saad, 1984). However, the hypothesis that cyclic AMP is the second messenger leading to bronchodilation is still unproven due to several discrepancies. For example, indomethacin reduces the relaxant effects of PGE_2 on guinea pig lung parenchymal strips (Burka and Saad, 1984), canine trachealis (Yamaguchi et al., 1976), and human airways (Walters et al., 1982), but does not decrease adenylate cyclase activity (Burka and Saad, 1984). This lack of correlation between PG activity and cyclic AMP is not limited to airways tissues (Samuelsson et al., 1978). Thus further mechanisms will have to be sought for the effects of these compounds.

An attractive hypothesis for the intracellular mechanism for the contractile effects of the prostanoids is hydrolysis of inositol lipids. This has already been shown to be a mechanism of signal transduction for LTD_4 receptors in guinea pig lung (Mong et al., 1987) and for acetylcholine receptors in canine trachea (Baron et al., 1984). Phosphatidylinositol turnover may be part of a receptor transduction process controlling membrane calcium channels and intracellular release of calcium.

ACKNOWLEDGEMENTS: This work was supported by a grant from the Medical Research Council of Canada. Some of the work reported was carried out by Dr. M.H. Saad for his Ph.D. thesis.

REFERENCES

Aizawa H, Chung KF, Leikauf GD, Ueki I, Bethel RA, O'Byrne PM, Hirose T, Nadel JA (1985). Significance of thromboxane generation in ozone-induced airway hyper-responsiveness in dogs. J Appl Physiol 59: 1918-1923.

Baron CB, Cunningham M, Strauss JF, Coburn RF (1984). Pharmacomechanical coupling in smooth muscle may involve phosphatidylinositol metabolism. Proc Natl Acad Sci USA 81: 6899-6903.

Bergstrom S, Sjovall J (1957). The isolation of prostaglandin. Acta Chem Scand 17: S282-S287.

Bergstrom S, Dressler F, Krabisch L, Ryhage R, Sjovall J (1962). The isolation and structure of a smooth muscle stimulating factor in normal sheep and pig lungs. Arkiv Kem 20: 63-66.

Boot JR, Cockerill AF, Dawson W, Mallen DNB, Osborne DJ (1978). Modification of prostaglandin and thromboxane release by immunological sensitisation and successive immunological challenges from guinea-pig lung. Int Archs Allergy Appl Immun 57: 159-164.

Burka JF (1983). Effects of selected bronchodilators on antigen- and A23187-induced contraction of guinea pig trachea. J Pharmacol Exp Ther 225: 427-435.

Burka JF, Ali M, McDonald JWD, Paterson NAM (1981). Immunological and non-immunological synthesis and release of prostaglandins and thromboxanes from isolated guinea-pig trachea. Prostaglandins 22: 683-691.

Burka JF, Paterson NAM (1980. Evidence for lipoxygenase pathway involvement in allergic tracheal contraction. Prostaglandins 19: 499-515.

Burka JF, Saad MH (1984). Bronchodilator-mediated relaxation of normal and ovalbumin-sensitized guinea-pig airways: lack of correlation with lung adenylate cyclase activation. Br J Pharmac 83: 645-655.

Gardiner PJ, Collier HOJ (1980). Specific receptors for prostaglandins in airways. Prostaglandins 19: 819-841.

Hardy CC, Robinson C, Tattersfield AE, Holgate ST (1984). The bronchoconstrictor effect of inhaled prostaglandin D_2 in normal and asthmatic men. New Engl J Med 311: 209-213.

Hardy C, Robinson C, Lewis RA, Tattersfield AE, Holgate ST (1985). Airway and cardiovascular responses to inhaled prostacyclin in normal and asthmatic subjects. Am Rev Respir Dis 131: 18-21.

Hyman AL, Mathe AA, Lippton HL, Kadowitz PJ (1981). Prostaglandins and the lung. Med Clin N Amer 65: 789-808.
Kurzrok R, Lieb CC (1930). Biochemical studies of human semen. II. The action of semen on the human uterus. Proc Soc Exp Biol Med 28: 268-272.
Lee TH, Austen KF, Corey EJ, Drazen JM (1984). Leukotriene E_4-induced airway hyperresponsiveness of guinea-pig trachea smooth muscle to histamine and evidence for three separate sufidopeptide leukotriene receptors. Proc Natl Acad Sci USA 81: 4922-4925.
Lewis RA, Soter NA, Diamond PT, Austen KF, Oates JA, Roberts LJ (1982). Prostaglandin D_2 release after activation of rat and human mast cells with anti-IgE. J Immunol 129: 1627-1631.
MacDermot J, Barnes PJ, Waddell KA, Dollery CT, Blair IA (1981). Prostacyclin binding to guinea pig pulmonary receptors. Eur J Pharmacol 75: 127-130.
Mansour S, Daniel EE (1986). Maintenance of tone, role of arachidonate metabolites, and effects of sensitization in guinea pig trachea. Can J Physiol Pharmacol 64: 1096-1103.
Marom Z, Shelhamer JH, Kaliner M (1981). The effects of arachidonic acid, monohydroxyeicosatetraenoic acid, and prostaglandins on the release of mucous glycoproteins from human airways in vitro. J Clin Invest 67: 1695-1703.
Mathe AA (1977). Prostaglandins and the lung. In Ramwell PW (ed): "The Prostaglandins, Vol. 3", New York: Plenum, pp 169-224.
Moncada S, Vane JR (1978). Unstable metabolites of arachidonic acid and their role in haemostasis and thrombosis. Br Med Bull 34: 129-135.
Mong S, Hoffman K, Wu H-L, Crooke ST (1987). Leukotriene-induced hydrolysis of inositol lipids in guinea pig lung: mechanism of signal transduction for leukotriene D_4 receptors. Mol Pharmacol 31: 35-41.
Morris HR, Taylor GW, Piper, PJ, Tippins JR (1980). Structure of slow-reacting substance of anaphylaxis from guinea-pig lung. Nature 285: 104-106.
Murphy RC, Hammarstrom S, Samuelsson B (1979). Leukotriene C. A slow-reacting substance from murine mastocytoma cells. Proc Natl Acad Sci USA 76: 4275-4279.

O'Byrne PM, Leikauf GD, Aizawa H, Bethel, RA, Ueki IF, Holtzman MJ, Nadel JA (1985). Leukotriene B_4 induces airway hyperresponsiveness in dogs. J Appl Physiol 59: 1941-1946.
Orehek J, Douglas JS, Bouhuys A (1975). Contractile responses of the guinea-pig trachea in vitro: Modification by prostaglandin synthesis-inhibiting drugs. J Pharmacol Exp Ther 194: 554-564.
Orehek J, Douglas JS, Lewis AJ, Bouhuys A (1973). Prostaglandin regulation of airway smooth muscle tone. Nature New Biol 245: 84-85.
Piper PJ, Samhoun MN (1981). The mechanism of action of leukotriene C_4 and D_4 in guinea pig isolated perfused lung and parenchymal strips of guinea pig, rabbit and rat. Prostaglandins 21: 793-803.
Saad MH, Burka JF (1983). Effects of immunological sensitization on the responses and sensitivity of guinea pig airways to bronchoconstrictors. Modulation by selective inhibition of arachidonic acid metabolism. Can J Physiol Pharmacol 61: 876-887.
Samuelsson B, Goldyne M, Granstrom E, Hamberg M, Hammarstrom S, Malmsten C (1978). Prostaglandins and thromboxanes. Ann Rev Biochem 47: 997-1029.
Schulman ES, Adkinson NF, Newball HH (1982). Cyclooxygenase metabolites in human lung anaphylaxis: airway vs. parenchyma. J Appl Physiol 53: 589-595.
Von Euler US (1934). Zur Kenntnis der pharmakologischen Wirkungen von Nativsekreten und Extrackten mannlicher accessorischer Geschlechtsdrusen. Arch Exp Pathol Pharmakol 175: 78-84.
Walters EH, Davies BH (1982). Dual effect of prostaglandin E_2 on normal airways smooth muscle in vivo. Thorax 37: 918-922.
Walters EH, Bevan M, Davies BH (1982). The effects of oral propranolol and indomethacin on the response to inhaled PGE_2 in normal human subjects. Prostaglandins Leukotrienes Med 8: 141-150.
Weichman BM, Wasserman MA, Gleason JG (1984). SK&F 88046: A unique pharmacologic antagonist of bronchoconstriction induced by leukotriene D_4, thromboxane and prostaglandins $F_2\alpha$ and D_2 in vitro. J Pharmacol Exp Ther 228: 128-132.
Yamaguchi T, Hitzjb B, Coburn RF (1976). Endogenous prostaglandins and mechanical tension in canine trachealis muscle. Am J Physiol 230: 1737-1743.

DISCUSSION

Nadel: LTC_4, LTD_4, bradykinin and eosinophil major basic protein have been shown in several species to release PGE_2 from airway epithelium when introduced onto the epithelial but not the submucosal surface.

Thompson: In 1984 we investigated the relaxing activity of aspirin or indomethacin, compared it to BW755C, and found that they were similar. Gardiner and Collier have shown that indomethacin will produce a relaxation of guinea-pig trachea equivalent to a maximal isoprenaline response. This suggests that there is no muscle tone after indomethacin.

Burka: We've never been able to get a full relaxation with indomethacin, however we've always measured changes isotonically. Maybe our differences are due to methodology.

Mechanisms in Asthma: Pharmacology,
Physiology, and Management, pages 47–54

LEUKOTRIENES AND AIRWAY SMOOTH MUSCLE TONE

Priscilla J Piper, Marwa N Samhoun and

Dolores M Conroy Dept of Pharmacology, Hunterian

Institute, Royal College of Surgeons, London WC2A 3PN

INTRODUCTION

Inflammation of the airways may be an important mechanism in the pathophysiology of various respiratory diseases such as asthma. There is increasing evidence that phospholipid-derived mediators play significant roles in inflammatory conditions. Such naturally-occurring phospholipid metabolites include the leukotrienes (LTs), prostaglandins (PGs), thromboxanes (Txs) and platelet-activating factor (PAF). In some species, there are significant interactions between mediators, for instance between LTs and cyclo-oxygenase products.

The leukotrienes can be divided, on the basis of their chemical structures and pharmacological actions, into LTB_4, which is devoid of an amino acid (aa) residue and the cysteinyl-containing LTs, LTC_4, LTD_4, LTE_4 and LTF_4. These products are generated by the enzymatic conversion of the highly unstable allylic epoxide, LTA_4, yielding either LTB_4 or the C-6 aa-substituted metabolite LTC_4, following the action of a hydrolase or glutathione-s-transferase respectively. LTC_4 can undergo conversion to the highly active compound LTD_4 upon enzymatic hydrolysis of its peptide side chain by a γ-glutamyltranspeptidase (γ-GT) which, as yet, has not been identified. Further metabolism of these cysteinyl-containing LTs by a dipeptidase results in loss of a glycine molecule from LTD_4 and leads to generation of LTE_4 which possesses a single aa residue, cysteine, at C-6.

LTF_4 was shown to be synthesized from LTE_4 in the

presence of glutathione and γ-GT (Anderson et al., 1982). LTF_4 has not yet been detected in biological fluids but it might be formed in vivo since this would be analogous to the formation of γ-glutamylcysteine from cysteine (Griffith et al., 1981). N-acetylation of LTs occurs in rodents and the N-acetylated product of these LTs has been isolated in subcellular fractions of liver and, in smaller quantities, in microsomal preparations of spleen, kidney, skin and lung in the rat (Bernstrom & Hammarstrom, 1986). N-acetyl LTE_4 has been shown to be the major endogenous LT metabolite in rat bile (Hagmann et al., 1986). The enzymatic conversions of LTC_4 do not necessarily represent a series of detoxification steps, since N-acetyl LTE_4 possesses considerable biological activity. Metabolism of LTB_4, on the other hand, results in loss of biological activity. LTB_4 rapidly undergoes ω-oxidation to 20-OH LTB_4 and 20-COOH LTB_4 during incubation with human blood polymorphonuclear leukocytes (PMNs). Whereas 20-COOH LTB_4 has little biological activity, 20-OH LTB_4 is active in some systems (Borgeat, 1986). In the cynomolgous monkey, the major pathway of LTB_4 metabolism is complete ω-oxidative degradation where the main products are water and 20-OH LTB_4 (Serafin et al., 1984).

LEUKOTRIENES IN RESPIRATORY TISSUES

Leukotrienes C_4, D_4 and E_4 collectively account for the biological activity of SRS-A, which has long been proposed as an important mediator of allergic bronchoconstriction in man. In addition to LTD_4, which accounts for the main biological activity of guinea-pig SRS-A, LTB_4 is also found in appreciable amounts in perfusates from guinea-pig lung collected during anaphylaxis.

Generation of leukotrienes from different regions

It is well known that LTs are released during antigen challenge of sensitized guinea-pig or human lung, but the exact cellular origin of LTs is unclear. Since LTs are putative mediators of asthma, it is of interest that antigen challenge of chopped lung tissue from asthmatic patients in vitro, in the presence of arachidonic acid, results in the generation of LTs. LTs C_4, D_4 and E_4 are formed in addition to relatively higher concentrations of cyclo-oxygenase (Dahlen et al., 1983). Stimulation of lung tissue with A23187 releases LTB_4 in addition to cysteinyl-containing LTs and cyclo-oxygenase products, suggesting that the enzymes activated vary with the stimulus applied. In addition, the enzymes which form the individual LTs may be located in different parts of the lung. In another study, division of human chopped unsensitized lung tissue into bronchi and parenchyma, followed by challenge with A23187, results in generation of LTs from both pulmonary structures with higher levels of LTB_4 released from the parenchyma. Differences in generation of LTs also occur during antigen or A23187 challenge of guinea-pig chopped trachea or parenchyma: both LTB_4 and cysteinyl-containing LTs are released from the parenchyma, whereas mainly LTB_4 is produced by the trachea (Barnett & Piper, 1985). Since parenchyma contains a large amount of microvessels in addition to small airways, vascular tissue may be an important source of the LTs released.

Actions in airways from various species

Considerable species variation exists in the responses of airways to LTs.

Guinea-pig isolated tissues

LTs C_4 and D_4 contract guinea-pig trachea (GPT) and lung parenchyma (GPP), preparations of large and small airways respectively, in vitro, at picomolar doses and are approximately 1000 times more active than histamine (see Piper, 1983).

Tracheal strips: LTs E_4 and F_4 are equiactive and about 10 times less active than LTD_4 on GPT. Responses elicited by all cysteinyl-containing LTs are, however, indistinguishable, being identical in onset and duration and longer-lasting than those due to other agonists, including histamine and the TxA_2 mimetic agent, U-44069. In contrast, LTB_4 has no effect on the trachea (Samhoun & Piper, 1986). Recent observations with N-acetyl LTE_4 show that this compound retains considerable biological activity and induces protracted responses on GPT in comparison with histamine. It is about 2 orders of magnitude less active than LTD_4 but still approximately 100 times more active than histamine (Conroy et al., 1987).

Lung parenchymal strips: Actions of LTC_4, LTD_4 and LTE_4 have been extensively investigated on this airway preparation (see Piper, 1983). Recent comparative studies of the cysteinyl-containing LTs demonstrate a marked similarity with respect to potency and contractions induced between LTC_4 and LTD_4 on the one hand and LTE_4 and LTF_4 on the other. LTC_4 and LTD_4 are approximately 10 times more active than LTE_4 and LTF_4 but contractions elicited by LTE_4 and LTF_4 are longer in duration, in some cases up to 4 times (Samhoun & Piper, 1984a). Although LTB_4 has very little smooth muscle stimulating activity, it contracts the GPP, being approximately similar in potency and duration of action to LTC_4 and LTD_4 (Samhoun & Piper, 1984b). N-acetyl LTE_4 displays a pharmacological profile almost identical with that of LTE_4 or, indeed, LTF_4 (Conroy et al.,1987). Comparative investigations with other naturally-occurring inflammatory mediators show that LTD_4 is about 2, 3 and 4-5 orders of magnitude more active on the lung strip than histamine, acetylcholine and the undecapeptide, Substance P, respectively (Samhoun & Piper, 1986; Samhoun et al., 1987). It is interesting to note that, with respect to their putative role in allergic bronchoconstriction, none of the cysteinyl-containing LTs induces tachyphylaxis in either GPT or GPP. However, tachyphylaxis rapidly occurs when LTB_4 is administered in successive doses to the GPP (Samhoun & Piper, 1984b; 1986).

Human isolated tissues

Leukotrienes C_4 and D_4 are approximately 3 orders of magnitude more active than histamine or $PGF_{2\alpha}$ in contracting strips of human bronchus and lung parenchyma (Dahlen et al., 1980; Hedqvist et al., 1980). They are more active on strips of bronchus and bronchioles, which contract following administration of bolus doses as low as 3 pmol, than on parenchyma (Samhoun & Piper, 1984c). As in the guinea pig, LTC_4 and LTD_4 induce contractions which are indistinguishable in macroscopically normal human tissues (Samhoun & Piper, 1984c) or in isolated airways from asthmatic patients (Dahlen et al., 1983). A recent study suggests that both LTs occupy the same receptors in human intralobar airways, partly because contractions elicited by LTC_4 were very similar to those due to LTD_4 and were unchanged in the presence of L-serine borate complex, which inhibits the action of γ-GT and hence the metabolic transformation of LTC_4 into LTD_4 (Buckner et al., 1986).

In some studies, LTE_4 has been found to be equiactive with LTC_4 or LTD_4 (Dahlen et al.,1983; Buckner et al.,1984) however, when tested in comparison with either LTC_4 or LTD_4 on the same preparations of isolated bronchus or lung parenchyma in a superfusion cascade, LTE_4 is about 1-2 orders of magnitude less active than either of its parent metabolites. Further, as in GPP, LTE_4 induces sustained contractions which last at least twice as long as those due to LTC_4 or LTD_4. In addition, N-acetyl LTE_4 causes long-lasting contractions of human bronchus which are very similar to those of LTE_4 (Samhoun & Piper, 1984c). It is of interest that our above studies of the pharmacological profile of LTC_4, $LTD_4$and LTE_4 in human isolated airways are in close agreement with those obtained in man in vivo (see Barnes & Costello, 1987).

Since LTE_4 is more stable than LTC_4 or LTD_4, if LTs have a role in inflammation of the airways, LTE_4 may be present in the airways as a degradation product of cysteinyl-containing LTs and might prolong bronchoconstriction initiated by LTC_4 or LTD_4.

Inflammation and hyperreactivity

LTs B_4, C_4 and D_4 have been detected and quantitated in sputum from patients with various respiratory diseases, including asthma (Zakrzewski et al., 1985). The presence of LTE_4 was not investigated but this LT is also likely to occur in sputum. Prostanoids are also present in sputum ((Zakrzewski et al., 1987) and may synergize with LTB_4 and cysteinyl-containing LTs to induce plasma exudation and oedema of bronchial mucosa while LTB_4 is chemotactic for inflammatory cells such as PMNs.

Phospholipid-derived mediators may contribute to the hyperreactivity of the airways, which is a characteristic of asthma. Inhalation of PAF by normal subjects leads to hypperreactivity to methacholine lasting up to two weeks (Cuss et al., 1986). Inhaled LTE_4 sensitizes airways of asthmatics but not normal subjects to the effects of inhaled histamine (Arm et al., 1987).

CONCLUSIONS

Cysteinyl-containing LTs have potent spasmogenic actions on human and guinea-pig airway smooth muscle and are active in both large and small airways. Even the more stable metabolites of LTC_4 such as LTE_4 and N-acetyl LTE_4

are 10-100 times more active than histamine. The possibility therefore arises that LTs released in close proximity to respiratory smooth muscle or into the airways may contribute to bronchoconstriction in allergic and other respiratory diseases.

ACKNOWLEDGEMENTS

We thank the Frances and Augustus Newman Foundation for financial support and Dr J Rokach, Merck Frosst, Canada for leukotrienes.

REFERENCES

Anderson ME, Allison RD, Meister A. (1982) Interconversion of leukotrienes catalysed by purified γ-glutamyltranspeptidase; concomitant formation of leukotriene D_4 and γ-glutamyl amino acids. Proc.Natl.Acad.Sci. USA 79:1088-91

Arm JP, Spur BW, Lee TH (1987). Leukotriene E_4 (LTE_4) enhances airway histamine responsiveness in asthmatic subjects. Thorax 42:220.

Barnes NC, Costello JF (1987). Airway hyperresponsiveness and inflammation. Br Med Bull 43:445-449.

Barnett K, Piper PJ (1985). The release of leukotrienes from large and small airways of guinea pig and man. Br J Pharmac 86:642P.

Bernstrom K, Hammarstrom S (1986). Metabolism of LTE_4 by rat tissues: formation of N-acetyl leukotriene E_4. Arch Biochem Biophys 244:486-491.

Borgeat P (1986). Biochemistry of leukotrienes. In: Piper PJ, ed. The Leukotrienes: their biological significance. New York: Raven Press, pp 1-14.

Buckner CK, Krell RD, Laravuso RB, Coursin DB, Bernstein PR, Will JA (1986). Pharmacological evidence that human intralobar airways do not contain different receptors that mediate contractions to leukotriene C_4 and leukotriene D_4. J Pharm exp Ther 237:558-562.

Conroy DM, Piper PJ, Samhoun MN (1987). The effect of N-acetyl leukotriene E_4 on guinea pig airway smooth muscle in vitro. Br J Pharmac 91:365P.

Cuss FM, Dixon CMS, Barnes PJ (1986) Effects of inhaled platelet activating factor on pulmonary function and bronchial responsiveness in man. Lancet ii: 189-192

Dahlen S-E, Hansson G, Hedqvist P, Bjorck T, Granstrom E, Dahlen B (1983). Allergen challenge of lung tissue from asthmatics elicits bronchial contraction that correlates with release of leukotrienes C_4, D_4 and E_4. Proc Natl Acad Sci 80:1712-1716.

Dahlen S-E, Hedqvist P, Hammarstrom S, Samuelsson B (1980). Leukotrienes are potent constrictors of human bronchi. Nature (London) 288:484-486.

Griffith OW, Bridges RJ, Meister A (1981). Formation of γ-glutamylcyst(e)ine in vivo is catalysed by γ-glutamyltranspeptidase. Proc Natl Acad Sci 78:2777-2781.

Hagmann W, Denzlinger C, Rapp S, Weckbecker G, Keppler D (1986). Identification of the major endogenous leukotriene metabolite in the bile of rats as N-acetyl leukotriene E_4. Prostaglandins 31:239-251.

Hedqvist P, Dahlen S-E, Gustafsson L, Hammarstrom S, Samuelsson B (1980). Biological profile of leukotrienes C_4 and D_4. Acta Physiol Scand 110:331-333.

Piper PJ (1983). Pharmacology of leukotrienes. Br Med Bull 39:255-259

Samhoun MN, Conroy DM, Piper PJ, Yiangou Y, Bloom SR (1987) The differential effect of vasoactive intestinal peptide on contractions induced by leukotriene D_4, histamine and acetylcholine in guinea-pig lung parenchyma in vitro. Prostaglandin, Thromboxane and Leukotriene Research, Vol.17. New York: Raven Press pp 1023-1027.

Samhoun MN, Piper PJ (1984a). Leukotriene F_4 : comparison of its pharmacological profile with that of the other cysteinyl-containing leukotrienes in guinea-pig ileum and lung parenchyma in vitro. Prostaglandins 28:623-628.

Samhoun MN, Piper PJ (1984b). The combined use of isolated strips of guinea-pig lung parenchyma and ileum as a sensitive and selective bioassay for leukotriene B_4. Prostaglandins 27:711-24.

Samhoun MN, Piper PJ (1984c). Actions and interactions of lipoxygenase and cyclo-oxygenase products in respiratory and vascular tissues. Prostaglandins, Leukotrienes and Medicine 13:79-87

Samhoun MN, Piper PJ (1986). Actions of leukotrienes in non-human respiratory tissues. In: Piper PJ ed. The leukotrienes: their biological significance. New York: Raven Press, pp 151-160.

Serafin WE, Oates JA, Hubbard WC (1984). Metabolism of leukotriene B_4 in the monkey. Identification of the principal non-volatile metabolite in the urine. Prostaglandins 27:899-911.

Zakrzewski JT, Barnes NC, Piper PJ, Costello JF (1985). Quantitation of leukotrienes and prostanoids in asthmatic sputum. Br J Clin Pharmacol 19:549.

Zakrzewski JT,Barnes NC,Piper PJ,Costello JF (1987). Detection of sputum eicosanoids in cystic fibrosis and in normal saliva by bioassay and radioimmunoassay. Br J Clin Pharmac 23:19-27

DISCUSSION

de Jongste: A recent study by P. Sterk has shown that inhalation of LTD_4 will potentiate subsequent responses to methacholine in humans (Am. Review Respir. Dis. 1987, 135, A89).

Piper: Thank you, that agrees with our results.

Coburn: I would like to know about the timing in your studies. You sensitize to the leukotrienes and then you challenge; are the leukotrienes still present?

Piper: N. Barnes will be able to give you the exact timing.

N. Barnes: It's just a few minutes between leukotriene inhalation and subsequent challenge with methacholine. T. Lee has demonstrated there are also clear differences between the way normals and asthmatics respond to LTD_4.

Lee: Since LTC_4, LTD_4 are converted to LTE_4, we did our human studies with LTE_4 to avoid confusion by bioconversion. We administered LTE_4 to asthmatics and normals by inhalation in a dose-related manner to produce either a 35% decrease in SGaw or less than 10% decrease in SGaw. We found that if asthmatics inhaled LTE_4 and then SGaw was allowed to return to baseline, 60 min later the subsequent bronchoconstrictior response to histamine was enhanced. This occurred in a dose and time-dependent manner. The maximal effect occurred 7 hours after inhalation of LTE_4 and persisted for 1 week. The mechanism is unknown; LTE_4 is not chemotactic so we were surprised at this result. There was no enhancement of reactivity by LTE_4 in normals even when it was given in a dose that gave the same degree of bronchoconstriction as in the asthmatics.

Nadel: What is the half-life of the sulfidopeptide leukotrienes in the airways of normals, asthmatics and cystic fibrosis patients.

Piper: I don't know the answer to that.

Mechanisms in Asthma: Pharmacology,
Physiology, and Management, pages 55–69

ALTERATION IN MICROVASCULAR PERMEABILITY INDUCED BY PRODUCTS RELEASED DURING INFLAMMATION

T.J. Williams, S.D. Brain, P.G. Hellewell,
P.J. Jose, S. Nourshargh and M. Rampart

Section of Vascular Biology, MRC Clinical
Research Centre, Harrow, Middlesex HA1 3UJ, U.K.

INTRODUCTION

Under physiological conditions a dynamic fluid equilibrium exists in tissues. The net hydrostatic pressure tending to move water and small solutes from blood microvessels to interstitium is approximately balanced by an osmotic pressure exerted in the opposite direction by virtue of a high intravascular protein concentration. Any excess outflow is compensated for by lymphatic clearance. This equilibrium is dependent on a low permeability of the vascular endothelium to macromolecules. The level of permeability varies from tissue to tissue, and this is related to the differing morphology of endothelial cells and inter-endothelial cell junctions.

The hydrostatic pressure at a given point within the blood microvessel lumen is dependent on the systemic arterial/venous blood pressure difference and local vessel tone. Both of these determine tissue blood flow. In most tissues local blood flow is controlled largely by arteriolar tone. Arteriolar tone can be regulated by several factors e.g. (a) a myogenic effect that lowers tone to maintain flow when systemic arterial pressure falls (autoregulation); (b) local factors such as gas tensions and metabolite levels; (c) neurotransmitters released to subserve the specialised functions of a particular organ (e.g. as in 'functional hyperaemia'), or to regulate total peripheral vascular resistance to maintain systemic arterial blood pressure and (d) circulating hormones.

In response to a local inflammatory stimulus, e.g. the presence of potentially harmful microbes, these physiological control systems are overridden for the essential function of local host defence. The inflammatory response of microvessels has three characteristic components. Firstly, arterial and arteriolar vasodilatation occurs resulting in hyperaemia, sometimes after a short initial period of vasospasm. Secondly, the permeability of the microvascular endothelium rises dramatically. This eliminates the preexisting fluid equilibrium, resulting in protein-rich fluid leakage from microvessels which causes tissue swelling. Thirdly, leukocytes, typically neutrophils in the acute phases, adhere to the endothelium and migrate into the tissue.

These three features of the inflammatory response are brought about by the release of chemical mediators in the tissue. Investigations of the mechanisms of action of mediators have revealed a relationship between leukocyte accumulation and protein leakage from microvessels, and how these events can be affected by mediators acting on vascular tone. In this chapter the activities of a range of inflammatory mediators will be briefly discussed to present some of the current ideas concerning inflammatory mechanisms. These mechanisms have been derived from studies of various models often in animal skin for technical convenience. Detailed analysis of inflammatory mechanisms in the lung is difficult, but where possible the relevance of the observations to the lung microvasculature will be included.

HISTAMINE AND BRADYKININ - DIRECT ACTION MEDIATORS

Histamine, as the oldest known mediator, has a special place in studies of mediator mechanisms. It was originally shown by Thomas Lewis (1927) and his associates that histamine was able to cause a wheal and flare reaction in human skin that mimicked the response to mild trauma. Later studies with intravenous albumin-bound dye showed that histamine was able to cause protein leakage from microvessels and the expression 'increased capillary permeability' came into common use. In the early 60's the classical studies of Majno and colleagues (Majno et al, 1961) using carbon and mercuric sulphide labelling in the rat cremaster muscle showed that histamine, in fact, causes leakage from postcapillary venules. This was later shown for the nonapeptide, bradykinin (Majno et al, 1969) and in this study endothelial cell bulging was observed suggesting that endothelial cell contraction was involved in opening inter-endothelial cell junctions.

Because of its historical position, histamine has been assigned more importance in inflammation than it probably deserves. Release of histamine from mast cells and basophils often contributes to the very acute phases of inflammatory reactions, but the amine is unlikely to be involved in protracted phases of oedema formation. Release and action of histamine are of short duration; released histamine is quickly degraded by histaminases in tissues, and tachyphylaxis to prolonged exposure rapidly occurs.

In animal test systems increased venular permeability induced by histamine involves H_1 receptors so that the contribution of endogenous histamine to a particular inflammatory reaction can be readily determined using H_1 receptor antagonists.

In the dog, rat, guinea pig and sheep, intravenously-injected histamine induces increased permeability of bronchial venules as indicated by carbon labelling (Pietra et al, 1971; Gabbiani et al, 1970). Both the submucosal and peribronchial plexuses are affected, but no effect is seen in the pulmonary microcirculation.

In most test systems bradykinin is more potent than histamine in increasing permeability. There is evidence for bradykinin generation in some inflammatory models (e.g. paw oedema induced by carrageenan in the rat). Although kallikrein inhibitors that suppress kinin generation have been known for some time, prototype receptor antagonists have only recently become available. Two types of bradykinin receptor have been recognised, and increased venular permeability is mediated via the B_2 receptor (Regoli & Baraba, 1980). In the lung the bronchial microcirculation is affected by bradykinin, but not the pulmonary vessels (Gabbiani et al, 1970).

To distinguish mediators such as bradykinin and histamine that act directly on endothelial cells from those that have an indirect effect (see below) the former have been termed 'direct-action mediators' (Wedmore & Williams, 1981a).

C5a AND NEUTROPHIL-DEPENDENT MEDIATORS

The protein fragments C3a and C5a are split from C3 and C5 respectively during activation of the complement system in extracellular tissue fluid. Both peptides release histamine from mast cells and, in addition, C5a is a very potent chemoattractant for neutrophils. The link between the complement system and inflammatory changes in microvessels was thought to be because of mast cell histamine release, but studies in the rabbit showed that intradermally-injected complement-activated plasma in the presence of vasodilator prostaglandins (see next section) induces oedema that is resistant to antihistamines (Jose et al, 1978). Further, it was shown that purified rabbit C5a has the same activity (Williams & Jose, 1981) and that human C5a without its carboxyl terminal arginine (i.e. C5a des Arg), which is essential for histamine-releasing activity, is also potent in inducing oedema (Jose et al, 1981).

C5a des Arg, although less potent than the intact molecule, is active as a neutrophil chemoattractant, suggesting a link between this activity and increased microvascular permeability. Accordingly, it was discovered that depletion of circulating neutrophils in rabbits abolishes oedema induced by C5a (and C5a des Arg), but not that induced by histamine and bradykinin (Wedmore & Williams, 1981a). This 'neutrophil-dependent oedema' is rapid in onset (within 5-6 minutes) and has a long duration of action ($t_{\frac{1}{2}}$ = 100 minutes) in rabbit skin. The onset time of responses to histamine and bradykinin are very short (1-2 minutes) as is their duration of action ($t_{\frac{1}{2}}$ = 4-6 minutes).

The mechanisms whereby neutrophils increase permeability as they interact with microvascular endothelium are the subject of considerable speculation. Recently, it was reported that intra-articular injection of interleukin-1 in rabbits causes neutrophil accumulation without joint swelling (Pettipher et al, 1986) and intradermal injection causes neutrophil accumulation with little increased microvascular permeability (Pettipher et al, 1986; Rampart & Williams, unpublished). This suggests that it is not merely the passage of neutrophils through inter-endothelial cell junctions that causes leakage. It is postulated that C5a causes neutrophil accumulation and then triggers the cells to release a secondary factor that increases the permeability of the endothelium.

Other neutrophil chemoattractants have been shown to increase microvascular permeability e.g. formyl-peptides and leukotriene B_4 (Wedmore & Williams, 1981a; see later section). Synergistic effects of chemoattractants and endotoxin on neutrophils have been observed in vitro (Dahinden et al, 1983) and recent studies have demonstrated that this synergistic effect also occurs in vivo to increase neutrophil sequestration and neutrophil-dependent oedema in rabbit lung (Haslett et al, 1987; Worthen et al, 1987).

PROSTAGLANDINS AND SYNERGISM DEPENDENT ON VASODILATATION

In early studies of prostaglandins in guinea pig skin, it was observed that these substances are poor in inducing oedema, but that PGE_1 and PGE_2 are able to potentiate oedema induced by histamine and bradykinin (Williams & Morley, 1973). This activity of different prostaglandins as potentiators correlates with their vasodilator activity. Further studies demonstrated that endogenous prostaglandins act synergistically with endogenous permeability-increasing mediators in acute inflammatory reactions (Williams & Peck, 1977). Subsequently, it was shown that prostacyclin also has potent oedema-potentiating activity related to its vasodilator action (Peck & Williams, 1978; Williams, 1979). The oedema potentiating effect has now been shown to be a general property of vasodilators that can be demonstrated together with both direct-acting permeability-increasing mediators and neutrophil-dependent mediators such as C5a. The phenomenon is most apparent when the basal blood flow of a tissue is low (as in skin) and the permeability-increasing mediator itself has no, or weak (as with histamine and bradykinin), vasodilator activity. Thus, the tone of arterioles can have a profound effect on the rate of plasma protein leakage from venules downstream. Further, arteriolar dilators can also increase neutrophil emigration (Issekutz, 1981). It is not known how important this type of synergism is in the lung, although such an effect has been reported for prostaglandins and C5a (Henson et al, 1982).

PAF AND ITS POSSIBLE IMPORTANCE IN LUNG INFLAMMATION

The phospholipid platelet-activating factor (PAF) was shown to induce oedema in the rat paw (Vargaftig & Ferreira, 1981). In rabbit skin, PAF increases permeability and acts synergistically with prostaglandins to induce oedema (Wedmore & Williams, 1981b; Hellewell & Williams, 1986).

Oedema responses to PAF are unaffected by systemic neutrophil-depletion or platelet depletion (Wedmore & Williams, 1981b; Pirotzky et al, 1984). It was suggested that PAF could be the endogenous secondary factor released from neutrophils by C5a to induce increased microvascular permeability (Wedmore & Williams, 1981b). However, studies with receptor antagonists for PAF showed no inhibition of responses to C5a in vivo (Hellewell & Williams, 1986). PAF antagonists are ineffective in reducing oedema in IgE-mediated passive cutaneous anaphylactic reactions in rabbits (Hellewell et al, 1987), but partially suppress oedema in Arthus reactions initiated by immune complex deposition around vessel walls (Hellewell & Williams, 1986). Similar suppression of Arthus reactions in the rat has also been observed (Camussi et al, 1987). Interestingly, injection of preformed immune complexes induces oedema that is unaffected by PAF antagonists (Hellewell & Williams, 1986). A sequence of events has been proposed to explain these results. Complexes close to the vessel wall will activate complement and generate C5a. C5a generation has been detected in an Arthus reaction using radioimmunoassay (Jose et al, 1983). C5a will cause neutrophil accumulation and these cells will then phagocytose complexes which stimulates PAF release. The PAF then acts on the endothelium to increase permeability. PAF is unstable in tissue fluid so that it may be important that it is released very close to its target cell.

A similar sequence may occur in the lung, although it is not clear which part of the microcirculation is responsive to PAF. Intravenous PAF appears to increase microvascular permeability in the lung of the sheep in vivo as indicated by increased lymph protein concentrations (Burhop et al, 1986). Intravenous PAF has been shown to increase permeability in the tracheal and bronchial circulation of the guinea pig, as indicated by carbon labelling (O'Donnell & Barnett, 1987). Little labelling of pulmonary microvessels was observed in these experiments, although leakage has been detected in isolated rabbit lung perfused with PAF via the pulmonary artery using an isotopic system (Seale et al, unpublished). As in the skin, plasma protein leakage induced by PAF in the airways can be blocked by PAF antagonists (Barnes et al, 1986).

LEUKOTRIENES

Certain cyclo-oxygenase metabolites of arachidonic acid

can enhance oedema induced by other mediators because of their arteriolar dilator activity (PGE_2, PGI_2), but in most tissues these substances alone are weak in increasing microvascular permeability. Thus, aspirin-like compounds, which inhibit cyclo-oxygenase, can suppress oedema by removing the potentiating effect of prostaglandins (Williams & Peck, 1977). On the other hand, arachidonic metabolites produced by the aspirin-insensitive 5-lipoxygenase pathway can have potent effects on permeability. Leukotrienes C_4 and D_4 are components of SRS-A released from isolated sensitised guinea pig lung perfused with antigen. Leukotriene D_4 increases permeability by direct-action (Peck et al, 1981; Dahlen et al, 1981). Leukotriene C_4 also increases permeability in some tissues (Dahlen et al, 1981), but is noted for its potent vasoconstrictor action, which can attenuate oedema (Peck et al, 1981). Intravenous LTC_4 and LTD_4 have been shown to cause plasma protein leakage in the bronchial circulation of the guinea pig (O'Donnell & Wholohan, 1984; Hua et al, 1985).

Leukotriene B_4 is a potent chemoattractant for neutrophils (Ford-Hutchinson et al, 1980) and increases microvascular permeability by a neutrophil-dependent process (Wedmore & Williams, 1981a). Inhibitors of 5-lipoxygenase have been developed so that the possible involvement of metabolites in experimental lung inflammation can be investigated. There are few studies on the effects of LTB_4 in the lung. Intravenous LTB_4 in sheep has been reported to induce neutropenia associated with a small increase in microvascular permeability in the lung (Noonan et al, 1985).

NEUROPEPTIDES AND NEUROGENIC INFLAMMATION

Antidromal electrical stimulation of sensory afferent nerves was shown in early studies to induce local inflammation in the rat (Jancso et al, 1968). Much attention has been focussed on the 11 amino acid substance P which is present in C fibres. Substance P has three major activities. Firstly, it has vasodilator activity which is often dependent on endothelial-derived relaxant factor (EDRF) (Furchgott & Zawadzki, 1980; Tanaka & Grunstein, 1985). Secondly, substance P releases mast cell histamine. Thirdly, substance P has a direct effect in increasing permeability. Intradermal injection of substance P in man induces a wheal and flare reaction due to a combination of these activities. More recently other tachykinins related to substance P have been detected in sensory nerves, neurokinins A and B. NKA and NKB induce increased permeability and are vasodilators, but both are weak histamine releasers.

The 28 amino acid vasoactive intestinal polypeptide (VIP) is contained in certain autonomic efferent nerves. VIP releases mast cell histamine in some species. VIP is a potent dilator of arterioles and potentiates oedema induced by permeability-increasing mediators in skin models (Williams, 1982). Like substance P, VIP induces a wheal and flare reaction in human skin.

Calcitonin gene-related peptide (CGRP) is a 37 amino acid polypeptide that has been detected, sometimes co-stored with substance P, in sensory nerve fibres. The pattern of activity of CGRP is rather different from that of substance P and VIP. CGRP is a very weak releaser of mast cell histamine. It has no intrinsic permeability-increasing activity, and does not induce a wheal and flare reaction in human skin, except at very high doses. CGRP is a very potent arteriolar vasodilator and it produces intense and protracted local erythema when injected into human skin (Brain et al, 1985; Brain et al, 1986). CGRP is a potent potentiator of oedema in rabbit skin experiments (Brain & Williams, 1985) and in rat skin synergism between CGRP and substance P has been demonstrated (Brain & Williams, 1985; Gamse & Saria, 1985).

In the lung a possible role for neuropeptides in the induction of local oedema has been investigated in experimental animals by electrical stimulation of the vagus nerve, by use of capsaicin which releases peptides from C fibres, and by studying the effects of exogenous peptides (Lundberg & Saria, 1987; Persson et al, 1986). Many of these studies have been carried out in the trachea. Tachykinins, especially substance P, are potent in causing plasma protein leakage whereas CGRP, as in skin, increases flow without itself increasing permeability. Stimulation of the vagus or application of capsaicin causes plasma protein leakage in the rat and guinea pig, but not in the cat and dog (Lundberg & Saria, 1987). Cigarette smoke causes leakage that appears to be dependent on the release of tachykinins (Lundberg et al, 1983). Further, part of the permeability effect of histamine and bradykinin in the lung also seems to be dependent on the release of tachykinins (Widdicombe, 1981; Lundberg & Saria, 1987).

DISCUSSION

It is self-evident that inflammatory mechanisms are complex. Each mediator can have a single action or a combination of actions. Mediator activities may be animal species specific, and within a species a particular mediator may have differing effects in different organs. Moreover, molecules quite chemically distinct can have identical activities. This complexity is a consequence of the fundamental importance of inflammation to host survival. This necessitates the development of replicate mediator mechanisms in animals to compensate for the evolution of chemical evasion systems by microbes.

Studies of inflammatory mechanisms have revealed some of the basic principles of mediator action. Firstly, in most tissues the extravasation of plasma proteins and leukocytes takes place from small venules (an exception may be the pulmonary microcirculation where capillaries are possibly involved). Secondly, protein leakage and leukocyte accumulation are dependent on arteriolar tone. Thus arteriolar dilators can have a profound enhancing effect on leukocyte accumulation and oedema formation induced by other mediators. This effect is most dramatic in tissues with a low basal blood flow. Thirdly, some mediators act directly on venular endothelial cells to increase permeability, whereas others (neutrophil chemoattractants such as C5a) increase permeability as a consequence of a rapid neutrophil/endothelial cell interaction. This does not appear to be merely a consequence of opening of inter-endothelial cell junctions by neutrophils, as interleukin-1 can cause neutrophil emigration with little protein leakage.

Inflammatory swelling of a tissue is often regarded as a consequence of microvascular injury. That complex mechanisms have evolved to initiate and regulate protein leakage implies an important function. Increased endothelial permeability has a vital role in that it facilitates the supply of plasma proteins containing, for example, complement and antibodies to an infected tissue to facilitate local host defence reactions. This process is probably continually occurring undetected in focal areas of tissue. When protein leakage occurs on a large scale this can compromise the functioning of the affected tissue. This is clearly of special importance in the lung. A large increase in lung interstitial fluid will interfere with gas exchange. Further, blood proteins in high concentrations in contact with airway smooth muscle may contribute to the airway hyper-reactivity which is a feature of asthma (Persson, 1987).

REFERENCES

Barnes PJ, Chung KF, Evans TW, Rogers DF (1986). Increased airway vascular permeability induced by platelet activating factor: effect of specific antagonism and platelet depletion. Brit J Pharmac 89:764P.

Brain SD, Tippins JR, Morris HR, MacIntyre I, Williams TJ (1986). The potent vasodilator activity of calcitonin gene-related peptide in human skin. J Invest Derm 87: 533-536.

Brain SD, Williams TJ (1985). Inflammatory oedema induced by synergism between calcitonin gene-related peptide (CGRP) and mediators of increased vascular permeability. Br J Pharmac 86:855-860.

Brain SD, Williams TJ, Tippins JR, Morris HR, MacIntyre I (1985). Calcitonin gene-related peptide (CGRP) is a potent vasodilator. Nature 313:54-56.

Burhop KE, Garcia JGN, Selig WM, LO SK, van der Zee H, Kaplan JE, Malik AB (1986). Platelet-activating factor increases lung vascular permeability to protein. J Appl Physiol 61:2210-2217.

Camussi G, Pawlowski I, Saunders R, Brentjens J, Andres G (1987). Receptor antagonist of platelet activating factor inhibits inflammatory injury induced by in situ formation of immune complexes in renal glomeruli and in the skin. J Lab Clin Med 110:196-206.

Dahlen SE, Bjork J, Hedqvist P, Arfors KE, Hammerstrom S, Lindgren J-A, Samuelsson B (1981). Leukotrienes promote plasma leakage and leukocyte adhesion in postcapillary venules: In vivo effects with relevance to the acute inflammatory response. Proc Natl Acad Sci 78:1887-1891.

Dahinden C, Galands C, Fehr J (1983). Granulocyte activation by endotoxin. I. Correlation between adherence and other granulocyte functions, and the role of endotoxin structure on biologic activity. J Immunol 130:857-862.

Ford-Hutchinson AW, Bray MA, Doig MV, Shipley ME, Smith MJH (1980). Leukotriene B, a potent chemokinetic and aggregating substance released from polymorphonuclear leukocytes. Nature 286:264-265.

Furchgott RF, Zawadzki JV (1980). The obligatory role of endothelial cells in the relaxation of arterial smooth muscle by acetylcholine. Nature 288:373-376.

Gabbiani G, Badonnel MC, Majno G (1970). Intra-arterial injection of histamine, serotonin, or bradykinin. A topographic study of vascular leakage. Proc Soc Exp Biol Med 135:447.

Gamse R, Saria A (1985). Potentiation of tachykinin-induced plasma protein extravasation by calcitonin gene-related peptide. Eur J Pharmacol 114:61-66.

Haslett C, Worthen GS, Giclas PC, Morrison DC, Henson JE, Henson PM (1987). The pulmonary vascular sequestration of neutrophils in endotoxemia is initiated by an effect of endotoxin on the neutrophil in the rabbit. Am Rev Respir Dis 136:9-18.

Hellewell PG, Jose PJ, Williams TJ (1987). Mediators of IgE-dependent local anaphylactic reactions in rabbit skin. Brit J Pharmac 91:317P.

Hellewell PG, Williams TJ (1986). A specific antagonist of platelet-activating factor suppresses oedema formation in an Arthus reaction but not oedema induced by leukocyte chemoattractants in rabbit skin. J Immunol 137:302-307.

Henson PM, Larsen GL, Webster RO, Mitchell RC, Goins AJ, Henson JE (1982). Pulmonary microvascular alterations and injury induced by complement fragments: Synergistic effect of complement activation, neutrophils sequestration, and prostaglandins. Ann N Y Acad Sci 384:287-300.

Hua X-Y, Dahlen S-E, Lundberg JM, Hammarstrom S, Hedqvist P (1985). Leukotrienes C_4, D_4 and E_4 cause widespread and extensive plasma extravasation in the guinea-pig. Naunyn-Schmiedeb Arch Pharmacol 330:136.

Issekutz AC (1981). Effect of vasoactive agents on polymorphonuclear leukocyte emigration in vivo. Lab Invest 45:235.

Jancso N, Jancso-Gabor A, Szolcsanyi I (1968). The role of sensory nerve endings in neurogenic inflammation induced in human skin and in the eye and paw of the rat. Br J Pharmacol Chemother 32:32-41.

Jose PJ, Forrest MJ, Williams TJ (1981). Human C5a des Arg increases vascular permeability. J Immunol 127:1276-1280.

Jose PJ, Forrest MJ, Williams TJ (1983). Detection of the complement fragment C5a in inflammatory exudates from the rabbit peritoneal cavity using radioimmunoassay. J Exp Med 158:2177-2182.

Jose PJ, Peck MJ, Robinson C, Williams TJ (1978). Characterization of a histamine-independent vascular permeability-increasing factor generated on exposure of rabbit plasma to zymosan. J Physiol (Lond) 281:13-14P.

Lewis T (1927). The blood vessels of the human skin and their responses. Shaw & Sons London.

Lundberg JM, Saria A (1983). Capsaicin-induced desensitization of airway mucosa to cigarette smoke, mechanical and chemical irritants. Nature 302:251-253.

Lundberg JM, Saria A (1987). Polypeptide-containing neurons in airway smooth muscle. Ann Rev Physiol 49:557-572.

Majno G, Schoefl GI, Palade G (1961). Studies on inflammation. II. The site of action of histamine and serotonin on the vascular tree; a topographic study. J Biophys Biochem Cytol 11:607-626.

Majno G, Shea SM, Leventhal M (1969). Endothelial contraction induced by histamine-type mediators. An Electron microscopic study. J Cell Biol 42:647.

Noonan TC, Kern DF, Malik AB (1985). Pulmonary microcirculation responses to leukotrienes B_4, C_4 and D_4 in sheep. Prostaglandins 30:419-434.

O'Donnell SR, Barnett CJK (1987). Microvascular leakage to platelet activating factor in guïnea pig trachea and bronchi. Eur J Pharmacol 138:385-396.

O'Donnell SR, Wholohan T (1984). Microvascular leakage induced by histamine and leukotriene D_4 in guinea-pig trachea and bronchi: A pharmacological study. In Courtice FC, Garlick DG, Perry MA (eds): "Progress in Microcirculation Research II", Comm Postgrad Med Educ. Univ of NSW, p.465.

Peck MJ, Piper PJ Williams TJ (1981). The effect of leukotrienes C_4 and D_4 on the microvasculature of guinea pig skin. Prostaglandins 21:315-321.

Peck MJ, Williams TJ (1978). Prostacyclin (PGI_2) potentiates bradykinin-induced plasma exudation in rabbit skin. Br J Pharmac 62:464-465P.

Persson CGA (1987). Leakage of macromolecules from the tracheobronchial microcirculation. Am Rev Resp Dis 135:371-375.

Persson CGA, Erjefalt I, Andersson P (1986). Leakage of macromolecules from guinea-pig tracheobronchial microcirculation. Effects of allergen, leukotrienes, tachykinins and antiasthma drugs. Acta Physiol Scand 127:95-105.

Pettipher ER, Higgs GA, Henderson B (1986). Interleukin 1 induces leukocyte infiltration and cartilage proteoglycan degradation in the synovial joint. Proc Natl Acad Sci USA 83:8749-8753.

Pietra GG, Szidon JP, Leventhal MM, Fishman AP (1971). Histamine and interstitial edema in the dog. Circ Res 29:337.

Pirotzky E, Page CP, Roubin R, Pfister A, Paul W, Bonnet J Benveniste J (1984). PAF-acether-induced plasma exudation in rat skin is independent of platelets and neutrophils. Microcirc Endothel Lymph 1:107.

Regoli D, Barabe J (1980). Pharmacology of bradykinin and related kinins. Pharmacol Rev 32:1-46.

Tanaka DT, Grunstein MM (1985). Vasoactive effects of substance P on isolated rabbit pulmonary artery. J Appl Physiol 58:1291-1297.

Vargaftig BB, Ferreira SH (1981). Blockade on the inflammatory effects of platelet-activating factor by cyclooxygenase inhibitors. Bra J Med Res 14:187-189.

Wedmore CV, Williams TJ (1981a). Control of vascular permeability by polymorphonuclear leukocytes in inflammation. Nature 289:646-650.

Wedmore CV, Williams TJ (1981b). Platelet-activating factor (PAF), a secretory product of polymorphonuclear leukocytes, increases vascular permeability in rabbit skin. Br J Pharm 74:916-917.

Widdicombe J (1981). Nervous receptors in the respiratory tract and lungs. In Hornbeim T (ed): "Lung Biology in Health and Disease", 17:429-472.

Williams TJ (1979). Prostaglandin E_2, prostaglandin I_2 and the vascular changes in inflammation. Br J Pharmac 65:517-524.

Williams TJ (1982). Vasoactive intestinal polypeptide is more potent than prostaglandin E_2 as a vasodilator and oedema potentiator in rabbit skin. Br J Pharmac 77:505-509.

Williams TJ, Jose PJ (1981). Mediation of increased vascular permeability after complement activation: Histamine-independent action of rabbit C5a. J Exp Med 153:136-153.

Williams TJ, Morley J (1973). Prostaglandins as potentiators of increased vascular permeability in inflammation. Nature 246:215-217.

Williams TJ, Peck MJ (1977). Role of prostaglandin-mediated vasodilatation in inflammation. Nature 270:530-532.

Worthen GS, Haslett C, Rees AJ, Gumbay RS, Henson JE, Henson PM (1987). Neutrophil-mediated Pulmonary Vascular Injury. Synergistic effect of trace amounts of lipopolysaccharide and neutrophil stimuli on vascular permeability and neutrophil sequestration in the lung. Am Rev Respir Dis 136:19-28.

DISCUSSION

P. Barnes: There are marked differences between circulations in respect to leakage and the relevant circulation to asthma would be the bronchial circulation. Many people believe that increased leakage from the bronchial microcirculation may be important in asthma, leading to oedema and plasma exudation into the airway. We have been looking at airway microvasculature leakage and our results are different from those you describe for the skin, e.g. allergen challenge in sensitized guinea-pigs, which causes marked leakage, is almost completely blocked by a leukotriene antagonist. Also, whereas PAF is a potent endogenous source of leakage, we don't see any effects with a PAF antagonist on allergen-induced leakage. We don't observe the synergistic effects you describe e.g. with CGRP we don't get enhancement of substance P-induced leakage. These different results may be explained by the fact that bloodlfow is much higher in airways than in the skin and we should be careful in interpreting the data.

Williams: I agree. When you have high basal blood flow, dilators are unlikely to make any difference to the amount of flow and also to the amount of leakage of plasma protein. But there may be other instances where one of your mediators actually reduces the basal blood flow and there the addition of a dilator will have an effect. P. Henson has shown that in the lung C_{5a} does actually cause a vascular constriction and when you add a prostaglandin you reverse this effect. So P. Henson has seen this interaction between prostaglandins and C_{5a} in the lung - although admittedly it is less dramatic. To answer your point about allergen-induced effects: I suspect this has something to do with the sensitization procedure. There are instances where differences in results have been obtained in passively and actively sensitized animals, and also between IgE and IgG_1 mediated effects. With respect to PAF antagonists - we get the same results as you. If we look at the anaphylactic reactions both IgE-mediated in the rabbit or IgG in the guinea-pig, the PAF antagonists have no effect on leakage, the only situation in which we see an effect is in the Arthus-type reaction.

Benveniste: I was surprised to find that you needed PGE_2 to see any effect with PAF-acether. We have shown that it has an effect alone.

Williams: If you're studying something like blue-dye leakage then certainly in guinea-pigs you can see an effect of PAF. There are species differences, the effect is less prominent in the guinea-pig or rat, but marked in the rabbit and I think that the modulation by PGE_2 may depend on the basal blood flow which may differ between species.

Nadel: Have you looked at a 2-stage reaction with neutrophils? You seem to think it's got to be an intimate relationship, but what about activating the neutrophil, taking the supernatant and perfusing the microvasculature bed?

Williams: We have tried that. We have also taken neutrophil depleted animals which don't respond to intradermal C_{5a}, taken neutrophils in vitro and incubated them with C_{5a} and taken that supernatant and tested it in those animals - but we get no activity. But we may need an intimate relationship between the endothelial cell and the neutrophil - they may need to be very close together and there may be something very transiently active. So we haven't been able to generate this factor in vitro.

Mechanisms in Asthma: Pharmacology,
Physiology, and Management, pages 71–80

THE ROLE OF PAF IN ALTERED AIRWAY RESPONSIVENESS

Clive P. Page and Deirdre N. Robertson

Department of Pharmacology, King's College,
London University, Manresa Road, London SW3.

INTRODUCTION

Increased airway responsiveness to a wide range of stimuli is considered to be a characteristic feature of asthma (Hargreave et al., 1986). However, the mechanisms involved in the pathogenesis of bronchial hyperresponsiveness are insufficiently understood. Certainly asthma is now considered to be a disease associated with inflammatory events occuring within the airways (Fabbri, 1985) and cellular infiltration into the lungs accompanies late-onset airways obstruction (de Monchy et al, 1985) and increased airways responsiveness following allergen inhalation in allergic asthmatics (Cartier et al., 1982). Examination of bronchoalveolar lavage fluid and sputum has demonstrated that the predominant cell present is the eosinophil (de Monchy et al., 1985; Frigas & Gleich, 1986). Pathological observations of individuals dying of status asthmaticus and of material biopsied from living asthmatics has also revealed accompanying sub-mucosal oedema, shedding of the ciliated epithelial cell layer, mucus plugs and bronchial smooth muscle hyperplasia (Hogg, 1985; Laitinen et al, 1985).

Platelet activating factor (PAF) is an extremely potent endogenously produced phospholipid that has recently been implicated in the pathogenesis of asthma and allergic disease particularly because this substance induces eosinophil recruitment and bronchial hyperresponsiveness (Morley et al., 1984; Barnes et al., in press). This review will summarise the evidence for the involvement of PAF in airway hyperresponsiveness.

AIRWAY HYPERRESPONSIVENESS AND INFLAMMATION

Airway hyperresponsiveness is associated with airways inflammation in man and several animal species, particularly after exposure to sensitising chemicals such as toluene diisocyanate (TDI), the oxidant gases ozone or nitrogen dioxide, and after exposure to allergens (Fabbri, 1985).

Eosinophils are the major inflammatory cell type found in the lungs of asthmatics at autopsy (Dunhill, 1978) and there seems to be a correlation between the presence of eosinophilia and bronchial hyperresponsiveness (Durham & Kay, 1985). The mechanisms of this selective cell influx, and the precise role of these eosinophils in bronchial hyperresponsiveness and asthma are unclear. Eosinophils are more commonly associated with the expulsion of parasites from the body, although this defence reaction is IgE dependent and has many similarities to an allergic reaction (Frigas & Gleich, 1986). Activated eosinophils release a number of toxic agents which are cytotoxic for the invading parasite and other mammalian cells. Eosinophil cationic protein (ECP) is is one such agent, and is also able to destroy respiratory mucosal cells and activate basophils, mast cells and lymphocytes. Major basic protein (MBP) has been shown to be cytotoxic for respiratory epithelial cells (Frigas & Gleich, 1986) and loss of respiratory epithelium has been associated with increased responsiveness of airway smooth muscle <u>in vitro</u> (Barnes, 1986). Eosinophils have thus been implicated in the epithelial damage observed in the asthmatic lung (Frigas & Gleich, 1986) which may in part contribute to the airway hyperresponsiveness by the loss of the proposed epithelial relaxant factor or by activation of local axon reflexes caused by exposure of sensory nerve endings (Barnes, 1986).

PLATELET ACTIVATING FACTOR (PAF)

PAF is produced by a wide variety of inflammatory cells including platelets, macrophages, neutrophils and eosinophils (Morley et al, 1984). PAF is an extemely potent bronchoconstrictor in both experimental animals (Vargaftig et al, 1980) and man (Cuss et al, 1986) but unlike other putative mediators of asthma, PAF can also mimic all the other pathological features of this disease. PAF has been shown to cause increased microvascular permeability (O'Donnell & Barnett, 1987; Evans et al, 1987), mucus production (Steiger et al, 1987), inflammatory cell infiltration (Cammussi et al, 1983; Archer et al, 1985; Henocq & Vargaftig, 1986) and in particular, PAF has been demonstrated to produce a long-lasting and non-specific bronchial hyperresponsiveness in experimental animals (Mazzoni et al, 1985; Chung et al, 1986; Barnes et al, 1987; Christman et al, 1987) and man (Cuss et al, 1986). The magnitude and time course of PAF-induced bronchial hyperresponsiveness is similar to that seen in allergic asthmatics following allergen challenge. Direct evidence for a role for PAF in allergen-induced bronchial hyperresponsiveness is suggested by the observations that pretreatment of sensitised guinea pigs (Page et al, 1987) or rabbits (Coyle et al, 1987) with the selective PAF antagonist BN 52021, reduces the non-specific bronchial hyperresponsiveness induced following exposure to antigen.

Exposure of animals to PAF has been shown to produce recruitment of eosinophils and platelets into the airways reminiscent of the histopathological changes observed following treatment of allergic animals with allergen (Lellouch-Tubiana et al, 1986; 1987; Metzger et al, 1985; 1987; Robertson & Page, 1987). Such histological studies have shown extravasation of both these cell types, and in particular platelets have been observed lying in close apposition to bronchial smooth muscle cells. Bronchoalveolar lavage studies of guinea pigs exposed to an aerosol of PAF or antigen have demonstrated a selective increase in the number of eosinophils at 24 hours. This eosinophil accumulation and coincident bronchial hyperresponsiveness are prevented by pretreatment with BN 52021 (Page et al, 1987). Furthermore, antigen-induced cell recruitment in sensitised rabbits is inhibited by prior treatment with the PAF antagonist BN 52021 (Coyle et al, 1987).

Bronchial hyperresponsiveness induced by an intravenous infusion of PAF is accompanied by a pulmonary accumulation of platelets (Robertson & Page, 1987) and has been shown to be dependent upon the presence of circulating platelets since, guinea-pigs made thrombocytopenic by administration of an anti-platelet anti-serum, do not exhibit bronchial hyperresponsiveness after infusion of PAF (Mazzoni et al, 1985). In contrast, selective immune depletion of neutrophils is without effect on PAF-induced bronchial hyperresponsiveness (Morley et al, 1985). The mechanisms responsible for this platelet-dependent bronchial hyperresponsiveness are unknown, but infusion of other platelet agonists such as ADP, collagen or U46619 (a thromboxane mimetic) do not result in hyperresponsiveness of the airways despite similar pulmonary platelet accumulation (Robertson & Page, 1987). These results demonstrate that bronchial hyperresponsiveness is not secondary to pulmonary platelet recruitment per se or to the release of ADP or thromboxane. However, it is of interest that ADP does not cause an extravascular platelet recruitment or eosinophil infiltration as has been observed following PAF administration (Lellouch-Tubiana et al., 1985) which may provide a clue as to why one platelet agonist (PAF) induces bronchial hyperresponsiveness whereas another (ADP) does not.

It is of considerable interest that platelets have also been demonstrated to possess IgE receptors on their surface, and that IgE activated platelets release cytotoxic free radicals in sufficient amounts to kill parasites, a novel form of platelet activation independent of platelet aggregation (Capron et al., 1986). Platelets are also capable of undergoing phagocytosis and chemotaxis similar to other inflammatory cells, although consideration of platelets as inflammatory cells is not widespread. Whether this type of platelet activation is linked to the induction of bronchial hyperresponsiveness is as yet unknown but recently, platelet depletion has been observed to significantly reduce the eosinophil accumulation following administration of either PAF or antigen (Lellouch-Tubiana et al, 1987b). This observation suggests that the platelet is a necassary intermediary for eosinophil activation and provides a partial explanation for how platelet depletion may modify PAF-induced bronchial hyperresponsiveness in this species (Mazzoni et al, 1985). Certainly platelet activation is now recognised as a feature not just of allergic inflammation (e.g. parasitemia) but also of allergic asthma (Reviewed by Gresele et al., 1987) and just as there are similarities between the role of the eosinophil in the removal of parasites and the tissue damage observed in asthma, so it is equally plausible that the role of the platelet in the defence of the body against parasitic invasion, when inappropriatley activated may contribute to pathological events such as the bronchial hyperresponsiveness observed in asthma.

PAF AND ASTHMA

PAF was originally described as a participant of acute IgE anaphylaxis in the rabbit as it could be detected in plasma by bioassay during an allergic response and mimicked the anaphylactic response in this species (Henson & Pinckard, 1977). Comparable studies have now been performed in allergic asthmatics where a PAF-like material has been detected in plasma following allergen challenge (Thompson et al, 1985; Beer, 1985; Nakamura et al, 1987). Unfortunatley, at the moment there is no convenient assay for the determination of PAF in biological fluids and all the studies to date have relied upon modifications of the bioassay procedure originally utilised by Henson and Pinckard in 1977. PAF anti-bodies have recently been described (Smal et al., 1987), and it is anticipated that the emergance of an RIA like assay for PAF in the near future will greatly aid our understanding of this molecule in health and disease.

CONCLUSION

PAF mimicks the features of asthma more closely than any other endogenous substance and as such should be considered an important mediator of this disease. The ultimate verification of this hypothesis will be dependent on the clinical success of the various selective PAF antagonists now available. BN 52063, a mixture of ginkolides containing BN 52021 as the major active component has recently been observed to act as a selective PAF antagonist in man (Chung et al., 1987) and perhaps more importantly to inhibit the late-onset allergic response in the skin of atopic volunteers (Roberts et al., 1987). Since the pharmacological sensitivity of cutaneous responses to allergen are similar to that observed in the lung of allergic asthmatics, these preliminary clinical findings suggest that PAF should be considered as a possible mediator contributing to the late-onset airways obstruction associated with exacerbations of bronchial hyperresponsiveness in asthmatics.

REFERENCES

Archer CB, Page CP, Morley J, MacDonald DM (1985). Accumulation of inflammatory cells in response to intracutaneous platelet activating factor (Paf-acether) in man. Br J Derm 112: 285-290.

Barnes PJ (1986). Asthma as an axon reflex. Lancet i: 242-245.

Barnes PJ, Grandordy BM, Page CP, Rhoden KJ, Robertson DN (1987). The effect of platelet activating factor on pulmonary beta-adrenoceptors. Br J Pharmacol 90: 709-715.

Barnes PJ, Chung KF, Page CP (In press) Platelet activating factor as a mediator of allergic inflammation and asthma. J Allergy Clin Immunol.

Beer HJ (1985). Wirkungen des "platelet activating factor" (PAF) auf die thrombozyten des menschen. MD Thesis, University of Zurich.

Camussi G, Pawlowski I, Tetta C, Roffinello C, Alberton M, Brentjens J, Andres G (1983). Acute lung inflammation induced in the rabbit by local instillation of 1-0-octadecyl-2-acetyl-sn-glyceryl-3-phosphorylcholine or of native platelet activating factor. Am J Pathol 112: 78-88.

Capron A, Dessaint JP, Capron M, Joseph M, Amiesen JC, Tonnel AB (1986). From parasites to allergy: a second receptor for IgE. Immunol Today 7: 15-18.

Cartier A, Thomson NC, Frith PA, Roberts R, Hargreave FE (1982). Allergen-induced increase in bronchial responsiveness to histamine: relationship to the late asthmatic response and change in airway calibre. J Allergy Clin Immunol 70: 170-177.

Christman BW, Lefferts PL, Snapper JR (1987). Effect of platelet activating factor on aerosol histamine responsiveness in awake sheep. Am Rev Resp Dis 135: 1267-1270.

Chung KF, Aizawa H, Leikauf GD, Ueki IF, Evans TW, Nadel JA (1986). Airway hyperresponsiveness induced by platelet activating factor: role of thromboxane generation. J Pharmacol Exp Ther 236: 580-584.

Chung KF, Dent G, McCusker M, Guinot Ph, Page CP, Barnes

PJ (1987). Effect of a gingkolide mixture (BN 52063) in antagonising skin and platelet responses to platelet activating factor. Lancet i: 248-251.

Coyle A, Sjoerdsma K, Page C, Brown L, Metzger W (1987). Modification of the late asthmatic response and bronchial hyperreactivity by BN 52021, a platelet activating factor antagonist. Clin Res 35: A214.

Cuss FM, Dixon CMS, Barnes PJ (1986). Effects of inhaled platelet activating factor on pulmonary function and bronchial responsiveness in man. Lancet ii: 189-192.

de Monchy JGR, Kauffman HF, Venge P, Koeter GH, Jansen HM, Suiter J, de Vries K (1985). Bronchalveolar eosinophilia during allergen-induced late asthmatic reactions. Am Rev Resp Dis 131: 373-376.

Dunhill MS (1960). The pathology of asthma, with special reference to changes in the bronchial mucosa. J Clin Pathol 13: 27-33.

Durham SR, Kay AB (1985). Eosinophils, bronchial hyperreactivity and late phase asthmatic reactions. Clin Allergy 15: 411-418.

Evans TW, Chung KF, Rogers DF, Barnes PJ (In press) Effects of platelet activating factor on airway vascular permeability: possible mechanisms. J Appl Physiol.

Fabbri LM (1985). Airway inflammation and asthma. Prog Biochem Pharmacol. 20: 18-25.

Frigas E, Gleich GJ (1986). The eosinophil and the pathophysiology of asthma. J Allergy Clin Immunol 77: 527-537.

Gresele P, Ribaldi E, Grasselli S, Todisco T, Nenci GG (1987). Evidence for platelet activation in allergic asthma. In "Page CP, Menz G, Schmitz-Schumann M" (eds), Platelets, PAF and asthma, Basle, Birkhauser Verlag (In press).

Henson PM, Pinckard RN (1977). Basophil-derived platelet activating factor (PAF) as an in-vivo mediator of acute allergic reactions: Demonstration of specific desensitisation of platelets to PAF during IgE-induced anaphylaxis in the rabbit. J Immunol 119: 2179-2184.

Hargreave FE, Dolovich J, O'Byrne PM, Ramsdale EH, Daniel EE (1986). The origin of airway hyperresponsiveness. J Allergy Clin Immunol 75: 825-832.

Henocq E, Vargaftig BB (1986). Accumulation of eosinophils in response to intracutaneous Paf-acether and allergens in man. Lancet i: 1378-1379.

Hogg JC (1985). The pathology of asthma. In Weiss EB, Segal MS, Stein M (eds): "Bronchial asthma, mechanisms and therapeutics", Boston: Little Brown and Co, pp 209-217.

Laitinen LA, Heino M, Laitinen A, Kava T, Haahtela T (1985). Damage of airway epithelium and bronchial reactivity in patients with asthma. Am Rev Resp Dis 131: 599-606.

Lellouch-Tubiana A, Lefort J, Pirotzky E, Vargaftig BB, Pfister A (1985). Ultrastructural evidence for extravascular platelet recruitment in the lung upon intravenous injection of platelet activating factor in the guinea-pig. Br J Exp Pathol 66: 345-356.

Lellouch-Tubiana A, Lefort J, Pfister A, Vargaftig BB (1987a). Interactions between granulocytes and platelets with the guinea-pig lung in passive anaphylactic shock. Correlations with Paf-acether induced lesions. Int Arch Allergy Appl Immunol (In press).

Lellouch-Tubiana A, Lefort J, Simon MT, Pfister A, Da Lage C, Vargaftig BB (1987b). Comparison of the eosinophilic effect of Paf-acether and antigen in vivo: Role of Paf-acether antagonists and platelets. J Lipid Med (In press).

Mazzoni L, Morley J, Page CP, Sanjar S (1985). Induction of airway hyperreactivity by platelet activating factor in the guinea-pig. J Physiol 365: 107P.

Metzger WJ, Hunninghake GW, Richerson HB (1985). Late asthmatic responses: Inquiry into mechanisms and significance. Clin Rev Allergy 3: 145-161.

Morley J, Sanjar S, Page CP (1984). The platelet in asthma. Lancet ii: 1142-1144.

Morley J, Page CP, Mazzoni L, Sanjar S, Bretz U (1985).

Platelet involvement in hyper-reactivity induced by platelet activating factor (PAF, AGEPC). Ann Allergy 55: 329.

Nakamura T, Morita Y, Kuriyama M, Ishihara K, Ito K, Miyamoto T (1987). Platelet activating factor in late asthmatic responses. Int Arch Allergy Appl Immunol 82: 57-61.

O'Donnell SR, Barnett CJK (1987). Microvascular leakage to platelet activating factor in guinea-pig trachea and bronchi. Eur J Pharmacol 138: 385-396.

Page CP, Touvay C, Villain B, Coyle AJ, Braquet P (1987). Effect of the selective PAF antagonist BN 52021 on antigen-induced bronchial hyperreactivity in the guinea-pig. Am Rev Resp Dis 135: A161.

Roberts NM, Page CP, Chung KF, Barnes PJ (In press) Effect of BN 52063, a selective PAF antagonist on antigen-induced cutaneous responses in atopic subjects. Clin Sci.

Robertson DN, Page CP (In press) Effect of platelet agonists on intrathoracic platelet accumulation and airway reactivity. Br J Pharmacol.

Smal MA, Baldo BA, Harle DG, Redmond JW (In press) Production of antibodies to PAF and their use in a quantitative immunoassay for PAF. Clin Exp Physiol Pharmacol.

Steiger J, Subramanian N, Bray MA (in press) PAF is a potent stimulator of porcine tracheal mucus secretion. Clin Exp Physiol Pharmacol.

Thompson PJ, Hanson JH, Bilani H, Turner-Warwick M, Morley J (1984). Platelets, platelet activating factor and asthma. Am Rev Resp Dis 129: A3.

Vargaftig BB, Lefort J, Chignard M, Benveniste J (1980). Platelet activating factor induces a platelet dependent bronchoconstriction unrelated to the formation of prostaglandin derivatives. Eur J Pharmacol 65: 185-192.

DISCUSSION

Pare: Did you administer PAF to your guinea-pigs by aerosol?

Page: No, in these studies PAF was administered I.V.. But M. Fitzgerald in London (Wellcome Research Laboratories) has shown that PAF administered either by the aerosol or I.V. route increases the airway responsiveness to inhaled spasmogens in the guinea-pig.

O'Byrne: The effects of PAF are inhibited by thromboxane synthetase inhibitors in dogs. Have these studies been repeated in your model?

Page: We cannot inhibit the hyperresponsiveness induced by I.V. PAF with either indomethacin or thromboxane synthetase inhibitors. We haven't looked at these agents against aerosol PAF.

Williams: Do you know what the mediators are in the acute phase in rabbits? Have you tried to block the acute bronchoconstriction?

Page: No we haven't. G. Larsen has shown that DSCG and steroids will inhibit the response. Whether this is due to inhibition of mediator release from an inflammatory cell I don't know.

Mitchell: Do you have any information about the vaso-vagal reflex effects of PAF?

Page: The effects of I.V. PAF are not inhibited by bilateral vagotomy, but this may not rule out local reflex effects.

Paterson: The increase in maximal response was greater than any change in potency you observed. Do you think that you're increasing the number of histamine receptors or receptor coupling?

Page: We have measured histamine and cholinergic binding sites after aerosol or I.V. PAF. There is no change in the number of binding sites in vitro or their ability to couple despite the increased responsiveness in vivo. We have looked at β-adrenergic receptors and also found no change in receptor number, but we've not looked at α-adrenergic receptors.

Mechanisms in Asthma: Pharmacology,
Physiology, and Management, pages 81–90

EFFECT OF PAF-ACETHER IN NON-HUMAN PRIMATES.

B. ARNOUX, A. DENJEAN* and J. BENVENISTE.

INSERM U 200, 32 rue des Carnets and
* Laboratoire d'Explorations Fonctionnelles,
Clamart 92140, FRANCE.

INTRODUCTION

Paf-acether, a putative mediator of immediate hypersensitivity, was originally described as a product released from immunized rabbit basophils following specific antigenic stimulation, and named Platelet-activating Factor (Benveniste et al., 1972). The elucidation of the chemical structure as a 1-O-alkyl-2-acetyl-glycero phosphocholine explains the present name of this phospholipid mediator as paf-acether (Benveniste et al., 1979) or AGEPC (Demopoulos et al, 1979). Intravenous administration of this mediator induced an immediate bronchoconstriction into guinea pigs (Vargaftig et al., 1980), or rabbit (Mc Manus et al, 1981), and intravascular (blood cells and pressure) changes when it was injected to baboons (Mc Manus et al., 1981).

Paf-acether, which is released by inflammatory cells (Benveniste and Arnoux, 1983), is also released by alveolar macrophages from atopic subjects via an IgE-dependent mechanism (Arnoux et al., 1987). It was suggested that paf-acether might be involved in the pathogenesis of allergic asthma. This led us to investigate in a non human primate, the baboon, the respiratory and blood effects of intratracheal deposition of paf-acether. In addition, we used different drugs to demonstrate the specificity of the observed paf-acether effects. The efficiency of anti-asthma drugs was also tested on this model.

MATERIALS and METHODS

Baboons (Papio-papio, 11.8 $\pm$ 1.5 kg, mean $\pm$ SEM) without respiratory disease, were anesthetized for capture, and an endotracheal tube was placed. Before curarization, animals were premedicated with diazepam as previously described (Denjean et al., 1983). Instrumental ventilation at constant volume and frequency was adjusted to maintain end tidal PCO_2 within normal limits. After a stabilisation period of 20 min, animals were challenged either by intratracheal administration, at the carina level, of saline solution, paf-acether or lyso paf-acether (60 ug/kg in 200 ul of saline solution), or by aerosol of histamine or acetylcholine (4% w/v). Measurement of lung function before and after stimulation was performed by the analysis of total pulmonary resistance (Rl), dynamic compliance (Cl dyn), and peak inspiratory pressure (PIp). In the same time, systemic blood cells were analysed every 6 sec for 20 min after challenge. The specificity of the lung reaction was established by animal treatment with aspirin (80 mg/kg), atropine (0.2 mg/kg) or pyribenzamine (5mg/kg). To determine a possible relationship between lung function modifications and platelet pulmonary sequestration, a group of animals received radiolabelled platelets. Platelets were radiolabelled with ^{111}Indium oxine according to Page and Morley (1982). The circulating platelets were monitored continuously with two external probes. Three animals received two consecutive paf-acether challenges within 25 min period, and their lung function and platelet repartition were analysed. Alveolar eosinophilia after stimulation was studied by bronchoalveolar lavages, 10 min before and 1 hour after stimulation. In the same experiments, the anti asthma drugs DSCG, Nedocromil and ketotifen, were administered as indicated and the lung modifications, alveolar eosinophilia and pulmonary platelet sequestration were evaluated.

RESULTS

Intratracheal deposition of paf-acether induced a rapid increase of pulmonary resistance and a decrease of dynamic compliance. These lung function modifications were concomittant with an increase in peak inspiratory pressure (PIp, Table 1), which returned to base line over about 25 - 30 min. Challenge with lyso paf-acether did not induce any modifications of the lung parameters. PIp (5.9 $\pm$ 1.2 cm

H_2O, baseline), increased after histamine (8.4 ± 0.5) as well as acetylcholine (9.8 ± 1.4) deposition. Paf-acether lung modifications were associated with a fall in Pa_{O2} (10.1 ± 0.4 vs 6.3 ± 0.6 kPa, time 0 vs 10 min after challenge) and systemic platelets (216 ± 18 vs 139 ± 12 $x10^{-3}$/ml). A transient neutropenia was detectable at the same time. An increase of heart rate 184 ± 8 vs 136 ± 2 beats/min at time 0 was detected after paf-acether challenge.

Table 1. Lung functions after challenge.

	Time (min)	Saline	Lyso paf-acether	Paf-acether
Rl	0	5.4 ± 1.1	5.4 ± 0.9	5.3 ± 1.0
	10	5.6 ± 1.2	5.7 ± 1.1	12.9 ± 0.6**
CL dyn	0	51.0 ± 4.0	53.0 ± 4.0	52.0 ± 2.0
	10	51.0 ± 5.0	52.0 ± 3.0	47.0 ± 2.0*
PIp	0	5.9 ± 1.0	5.8 ± 0.7	5.7 ± 0.6
	10	5.9 ± 1.2	6.0 ± 0.8	9.7 ± 1.2*

Rl Total pulmonary resistance (cm H_2O/l/sec), CL dyn dynamic compliance (ml/cm H_2O), PIp peak Inspiratory pressure (cm H_2O). Results are expressed as mean ± SEM, n = 6, *$P<0.05$, **$P<0.001$, one way analysis of variance.

Pretreatment with aspirin had no effects on paf-acether-induced lung and blood cell modifications (Table 2).

Table 2. Absence of effect of aspirin treatment on paf-acether challenge.

	Time 0	1 min	10 min
PIp	9.5 ± 4.2	14.5 ± 3.8**	16.1 ± 3.7**
Platelets($x10^{-3}$)	220 ± 24	160 ± 30**	120 ± 15**

Same legend as in Table 1. Aspirin (80 mg/kg) was injected i.v. 20 min before challenge.

Local anesthesia as well as atropine also failed to inhibit the modifications caused by paf-acether challenge. However albuterol (40 mg/kg i.v., 2 minutes after challenge; Ventoline, Glaxo, Paris) caused a marked reversion of PIp to the baseline, and an increase in heart rate (Results not shown).

Pretreatment of the animal by DSCG, nedocromil or pyribenzamine was unefficient in affecting paf-acether -induced changes. By contrast, the treatment with ketotifen (Sandoz R) suppressed the paf-acether-PIp increase, as it blocked the histamine bronchoconstriction. Moreover the pure histamine H_1 antagonist pyribenzamine had no effect on paf-acether-bronchoconstriction (table 3).

The analysis of radiolabelled platelets, shows a transitory two or three-fold increase of ^{111}In-platelets in the thoracic region. Peak pulmonary platelet accumulation reached its maximum 87 seconds after paf-acether challenge, and returned to the baseline within 120 seconds. In the same time, a drop of systemic platelets was detected. In the presence of ketotifen, same platelets repartition were detected.

Table 3 Effect of pharmacological treatment on lung parameters

Challenge §	n	PIp	Time of peak rise PIp	Time of peak rise Thor. pla.
Paf-acether	6	9.7 ± 0.6*	20 ± 7	87 ± 23
Keto/paf-acether	4	5.9 ± 0.4	0	103 ± 18
Pyri/paf-acether	4	9.5 ± 0.4*	21 ± 9	ND
Histamine	4	8.4 ± 0.5*	50 ± 12	0
Keto/histamine	3	6.0 ± 0.5	0	0
Pyri/histamine	3	5.9 ± 0.9	0	ND
Saline sol.	3	5.9 ± 1.2	0	0

§ Keto, ketotifen 1mg/kg or Pyri, pyribenzamine (5mg/kg) injected i.v., 20 min before challenge. PIp value of peak inspiratory pressure at 10 min after challenge. Time of peak rise of PIp and thoracic platelet accumulation (Thor. pla.) are in seconds.

Four differents animals were challenged twice at 25 min interval, with paf-acether (same dose 60 ug/kg). The PIp increased with the same amplitude as before and the peak rise was at 22 ± 8 and 19 ± 9 sec after the first and second challenge respectively. However, platelet thoracic accumulation observed during the first challenge (103 ± 80 sec), was not detected after the second stimulation.

The bronchoalveolar cell population was analysed one hour after stimulation. Five minutes before animal preparation, a first bronchoalveolar lavage was performed with 50 ml of saline solution. A second lavage was performed 1 hour after challenge, with saline solution, histamine, lyso paf-acether or paf-acether. To check the specificity of the modification two groups of animals were treated with ketotifen or pyribenzamine, as in table 3. No significant difference was observed between the bronchoalveolar cellularity in the different groups and between first and second lavage, 188 ± 44 and 166 ± 28 (x 10^{-3} cells/ml of lavage). Total cell number recovered was identical in alveolar macrophages, lymphocytes and polymorphonuclear cells. A significant difference in the percentage of eosinophils present in the second BAL was observed when animals were challenged with either lyso paf-acether or paf-acether (Table 4). Ketotifen treatment had a significant inhibitory effect on the eosinophil accumulation (Table 4).

Table 4. Alveolar eosinophilia following intratracheal stimulation, effect of pyribenzamine and ketotifen treatment.

Challenge	Treatment	% Eosinophil BAL 1	% Eosinophil BAL 2
Paf-acether	none	9 ± 2	25 ± 8 **
Paf-acether	Ketotifen	4 ± 3	7 ± 4
Paf-acether	Pyribenzamine	2 ± 1	13 ± 3 *
Lyso paf-acether	none	4 ± 2	14 ± 3 *
Histamine	none	9 ± 4	11 ± 5
saline sol.	none	4 ± 1	5 ± 1

BAL 1: bronchoalveolar lavage 5 min before challenge, BAL 2: lavage 1 hour after challenge. Mean ± SEM, * $P < 0.02$, ** $P < 0.05$ one-way analysis of variance

on the differences between BAL 1 and BAL 2 after square root transformation of the data.

DISCUSSION

The instillation of paf-acether into the trachea caused an acute and reversible airflow obstruction, as suggested by the rise of total pulmonary resistance, peak inspiratory pressure and a decrease of dynamic compliance in our experimental conditions. This acute and reversible paf-acether-induced bronchoconstriction, and reversible, bears some similitude with acute asthma. It is associated with hypoxemia, reversed immediately by $beta_2$ mimetic agent as it was reported in asthma (Pride, 1977). These results ruled out some mechanisms of paf-acether-induced bronchoconstriction. The bronchomotor effect is neither mediated nor modulated by a vagal reflex or by cyclooxygenase metabolites. Identical results were reported in the guinea pig (Vargaftig et al., 1980 and 1981). A relationship between paf-acether -bronchoconstriction and platelets (activation and/or aggregation) was postulated in different experimental models. Were described a platelet-dependent bronchoconstriction in guinea pigs (Vargaftig et al, 1980), platelet aggregation in rabbits (Mc Manus et al, 1980) and a trapping of blood platelets in lung microvasculature in guinea pigs (Page et al, 1982). The suggestion of a platelet sequestration in the micro vasculature associated with the increase of PIp was based on the significant increase of the ventilated unperfused lung zones that we described (Denjean et al, 1983). The radiolabeled platelet accumulation in the thoracic region described in this study is in agreement with this hypothesis. However the kinetics of PIp and lung platelet accumulation exhibit a significant time difference, indicating that massive lung platelet sequestration is not indispensable for the bronchomotor effect of paf-acether. Such discordance in time to reach the maximal PIp and platelet lung accumulation was reported in the guinea pig (Page et al, 1984). A dissociation between PIp and platelet accumulation was also observed in two consecutive paf-acether challenges and when ketotifen was used. Thus the dissociation between paf-acether-induced bronchoconstriction and platelet aggregation and accumulation in the lung must be considered. Yet activated platelets might influence lung motricity without being physically trapped in the lung vasculature.

The potential role of paf-acether pathway in the pathogenesis of asthma is reinforced by the specific ability of this phospholipid and, quite surprissing of its precursor/metabolite lyso paf-acether to induce an alveolar eosinophilia. The chemotactic effect of paf-acether was described in Boyden chamber and the mediator has been proposed as the more potent chemotactic factor for eosinophils (Wardlaw et al, 1987 and Sigal et al, 1987).

The absence of effect of pyribenzamine treatment on the paf-acether-induced variations in PIp and eosinophilia, suggests that the beneficial effect of ketotifen on paf-acether- broncho constriction is not secondary to its anti-histaminic property (Martin and Römer, 1978). The anti-eosinophilia action of the drug may contribute to the therapeutic efficacy of ketotifen as prophylactic anti-asthma drug.

The present report have demonstrated that instillation of paf-acether into the air space can induce an immediate and reversible bronchoconstriction, followed by a non necessary lung platelet accumulation and a late alveolar eosinophilia. As paf-acether is able to mimic the major characteristics of asthma including a non specific hyperreactivity (Cuss et al, 1986), it may therefore be rewarding to focus attention on paf-acether and alveolar macrophages, eosinophils and platelet activation as underlying determinants of asthma.

REFERENCES

Arnoux B, Joseph M, Simöes M.H, Tonnel A.B, Duroux P, Capron A, Benveniste J, (1987). Antigenic release of paf-acether and b-glucuronidase from alveolar macrophages of asthmstics. Bull. Eur. Physiopathol. Resp. 23: 119-124.

Benveniste J, Henson PM, Cochrane CG, (1972). Leukocyte dependent histamine release from rabbit platelets: The role of IgE, basophils and a platelet-activating factor. J.Exp Med 136: 1356-1377.

Benveniste J, Tencé M, Varenne P, Bidault J, Boullet C, Polonsky J, (1979). Semi-synthése et structure proposée du facteur activant les plaquettes (PAF): PAF-acéther, un alkyl éther analogue de la phosphatidylcholine. C R Acad Sci (Paris) 1979; 289: 1037-1040.

Benveniste J and Arnoux B, (Eds, 1983) Platelet-Activating factor and Structurally-related ether-lipids. INSERM Symposium N° 23, Elsevier Science Publications

Cuss F.M., Dixon C.M.S. & P.J. Barnes, (1986). Effects of inhaled platelet activating factor on pulmonary function and bronchial responsiveness in man. The Lancet 26: 189

Demopolous CA, Pinckard RN, Hanahan DJ, (1979). Platelet-activating factor: Evidence for 1-O-alkyl-2-acetyl-sn-glyceryl-3-phosphorylcholine as the active component (a new class of lipid chemical mediators). J. Biol. Chem. 254: 9355-9358.

Denjean A, Arnoux B, Masse R, Lockhart A, Benveniste J, (1983). Acute effect of intratracheal administration of platelet-activating factor in baboons. J Appl Physiol 55: 799-804.

Martin U, Römer D, (1978). The Pharmacological properties of a new, orally active antianaphylactic compound: Ketotifen, a benzocycloheptathiophene. Drug Res. 28: 770 - 782.

Mc Manus LM, Hanahan RN, Demoupoulos CA, Pinckard RN, (1980). Pathobiology of the intravenous infusion of acetyl glyceryl ether phosphorylcholine (AGEPC), a synthetic platelet-activating factor (PAF), in the rabbit. J Immunol 2919-2929.

Mc Manus LM, Pinckard RN, Fitzpatrick FA, O'Rouke RA, Crawford MH, Hanaham DJ, (1981). Acetyl glyceryl ether phosphorylcholine : Intravascular alteration following intravenous infusion in the baboon. Lab Invest 45: 303-307.

Page CP, Paul W, Basram GS, Morley J, (1982). Platelet activation in asthma. N Engl J Med 307: 252-252.

Page CP, Paul W, Morley J, (1984). Platelet and bronchospasm. Int Arch Allergy Appl Immunol 1984; 46: 62-63.

Pride NB, (1977). Physiology. In Asthma, edited by T.J.M. Clark and S. Godfrey. London: Chapman and Hall: 11-55.

Sigal CE, Valone FH, Holtzman J, Goetzl EJ, (1987). Preferential human eosinophil chemotactic activity of the platelet-activating factor (PAF) 1-O-Hexadecyl-2-acetyl-sn-glyceryl-3-phosphocholine (AGEPC). J.Clin. Immunol. 7: 179 - 184 - 192.

Vargaftig BB, Lefort J, Chignard M, Benveniste J, (1980). Platelet-activating factor induces a platelet dependent bronchoconstriction unrelated to the formation of prostaglandin derivatives. Eur J Pharmacol 65: 185-192.
Vargaftig BB, Lefort J, Wal F, Chignard M, (1981). Role of the metabolites of arachidonate in platelet-dependent and independent experimental bronchoconstriction. Bull Eur Physio Pathol Resp 17: 723-736.
Wardlaw AJ, Moqbel R, Cromwell O, Kay AB, (1986). Platelet-activating factor A potent chemotactic and chemokinetic factor for human eosinophils. J.Clin.Invest. 78: 1701 - 1706.

DISCUSSION

O'Byrne: Cockcroft has shown that ketotifen has no effect against allergen-induced responses in humans. Is ketotifen a good PAF antagonist?

Benveniste: It's very weak. When ketotifen works it is after several weeks' administration and not on an acute basis. I think the mechanism of its effect is via inhibition of eosinophil activity.

Seale: Have you looked at the effects of β-agonists on PAF and lyso-PAF release from alveolar macrophages, given their inhibitory effects on mediator release from mast cells?

Benveniste: These cells were taken from asthmatic patients and nearly all of them were taking β-agonists. We haven't looked at this specifically because it's difficult to find patients not on β-agonists.

Kerrebijn: What happens when PAF is given to patients without platelets?

Benveniste: Has P. Barnes done this?

Barnes: Well if there are absolutely no platelets, patients die. I feel that platelets may not be important in human asthma. Vargaftig has shown that the bronchoconstrictor effect of PAF given by inhalation is completely independent of platelets, but when PAF is given I.V. you do need platelets. I think this is important when you consider that we think of asthma as release of mediators in the lumen of the airway. If I could make a comment on ketotifen. We have completed a study giving it in doses recommended by the company and found that it is without effect on the acute bronchoconstriction to PAF and the subsequent airway hyper-responsiveness. The dose you were giving to baboons would be equivalent to 70 mg in a human and since 2 mg puts most people to sleep, it may be irrelevant.

Benveniste: I agree, I never said ketotifen was a good treatment for asthma or a good PAF antagonist. However, it works well in this system.

Page: If you selectively deplete platelets from guinea-pigs that have been sensitized and challenged with antigen or PAF, there is a significant diminuition of the eosinophil infiltration, suggesting that platelets may be acting as an intermediary in recruiting eosinophils after PAF or antigen.

N. Barnes: The PAF antagonists are very different molecules from PAF itself. What do you think the PAF receptor is like?

Benveniste: Very little direct information is available about the PAF receptor.

Mechanisms in Asthma: Pharmacology,
Physiology, and Management, pages 91-98

THROMBOXANE A_2 AND AIRWAY RESPONSIVENESS TO ACETYLCHOLINE AEROSOL IN THE CONSCIOUS PRIMATE

Gordon L. Letts and Cyril S. McFarlane

Department of Pharmacology, Merck Frosst Canada Inc., P.O. Box 1005, Pointe Claire-Dorval, Québec, H9R 4P8

INTRODUCTION

Recent studies in the dog suggest that Thromboxane A_2 (TxA_2) induces airway hyperresponsiveness. The specific implication of TxA_2, which is a highly potent but labile cyclooxygenase metabolite of arachidonic acid is based on several observations. Firstly, chemically stable analogues of TxA_2, U-46619 and U44069, have been shown to enhance the contractile responses to electrical field stimulation of tracheal tissues in vitro (Chung, K.F. et al., 1985) and of tracheal contractions following vagal stimulation in situ (Munoz, N.M. et al., 1986). Secondly, the potentiated responses to acetylcholine following challenge of the airways with antigen (Chung, K.F. et al., 1986a), LTB_4 (O'Byrne, P.M. et al., 1985), ozone (Aizawa, H. et al., 1985), or PAF (Chung, K.F. et al., 1986b) are inhibited by a selective thromboxane synthase inhibitor, OKY-046.

In these experiments we investigated if an enhanced airway responsiveness to acetylcholine aerosol following inhalation of U-44069 could be demonstrated in the conscious primate. Further, we were interested if the induced hyperresponsiveness to acetylcholine could be affected by treatment with a potent and selective TxA_2 receptor antagonist, thereby providing further evidence for the specific involvement of TxA_2 in airway hyperresponsiveness.

METHODS

The measurement of pulmonary function in the primate has been described earlier (McFarlane, C.S. et al., 1984). In the present study six trained squirrel monkeys (13,15,44,45,49,50) were used. Briefly, the animals were trained to breathe into a face mask, thereby permitting the direct inhalation of either acetylcholine, saline (control) or U44069 aerosol. On each occasion the animals were exposed for a 5 min period. Cumulative dose responses to acetylcholine (0.1 to 30 mg/ml) were determined at 30 min intervals. In the airway hyperresponsiveness studies, exposure to acetylcholine aerosol was between 45 and 75 min after inhalation of U44069 (1 mg/ml) and 15 min after saline aerosol (control). In studies with TxA_2 receptor antagonists, either L-655,240 (Hall et al., 1987) (1 mg/ml) or AH-23848 (De Bono, D.P. et al., 1986) (1 mg/ml) was aerosolized 60 min post U44069 inhalation. In separate experiments, the ability of L-655,240 (1 mg/ml; 15 min before) to inhibit responses to acetylcholine aerosol (10 mg/ml) in normal monkeys was determined.

RESULTS

Responses to individual doses of acetylcholine aerosol in the conscious monkey is illustrated in Fig. 1 and its dose response relationship is shown in Fig. 2. The mean EC_{100} (dose of acetylcholine aerosol required to increase airway resistance by 100%) is 4.3 ± 2.0 mg/ml.

Aerosolization of U44069 (0.1 to 1.0 mg/ml) produced changes in pulmonary function lasting from 15 to 45 min in duration. The peak changes in airway resistance and dynamic compliance are shown in the table.

The responsiveness of the monkey to acetylcholine aerosol 60 min after inhalation of U44069 (1 mg/ml) and when baseline values had returned is also shown in Fig. 2. As illustrated, there were highly significant decreases in the EC_{100} (0.0005 ± .... mg/ml; for acetylcholine, n = , t-test) and increases in airway resistance maximal response (139.3 ± 32.4) VS 192.2 ± 23.6, $p < 0.001$, $n = 6$, t-test). Of these, 2 monkeys had airway resistance values > 260 percent of control. Saline aerosol immediately preceding exposure to acetylcholine did not induce any change in the monitored variables.

TABLE 1. Responses to U-44069 Aerosol in the Monkey

Dose U-44069 (mg/ml)	Changes in Airway Resistance	Changes in Dynamic Compliance
0.1	151.7 ± 39.1	-36.3 ± 3.3
0.3	209.0 ± 40.5	-39.6 ± 4.4
1.0	126.7 ± 33.4	-37.2 ± 5.2

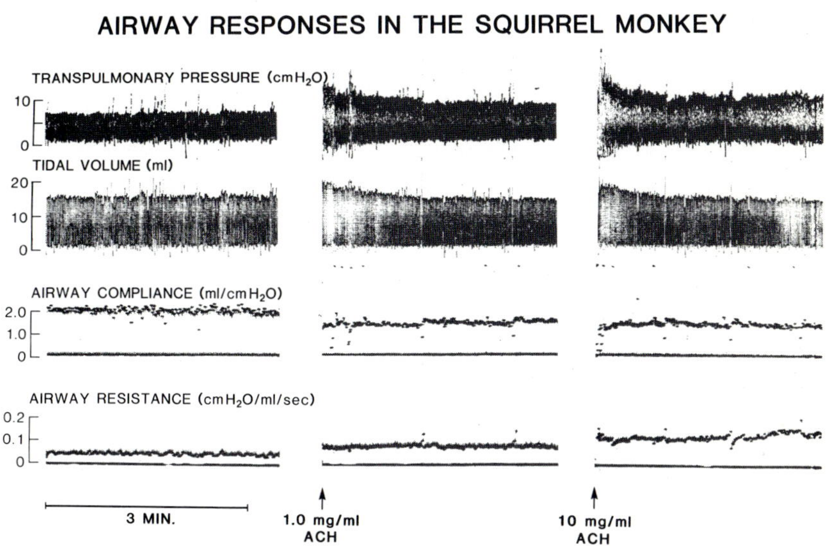

FIGURE 1.

The effects of L-655,240 (1 mg/ml, n = 3) and AH23848 (1 mg/ml, n = 1) on the potentiated acetylcholine aerosol response is shown in Fig. 3. L-655,240 totally and rapidly (< 10 min) reversed the enhanced responses to acetylcholine (0.0001 mg/ml dose). In one experiment only, AH23848 showed minimal activity. In separate experiments the same dose of L-655,240 did not inhibit airway responses to acetylcholine aerosol alone (10 mg/ml) in normal animals.

FIGURE 2.

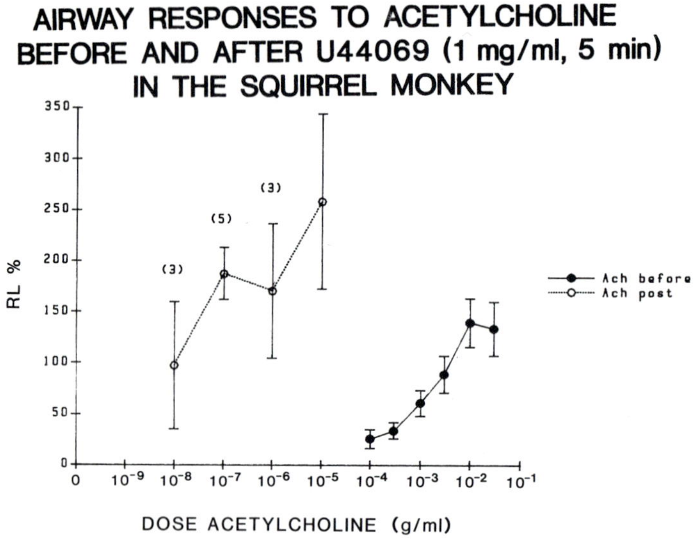

FIGURE 3.

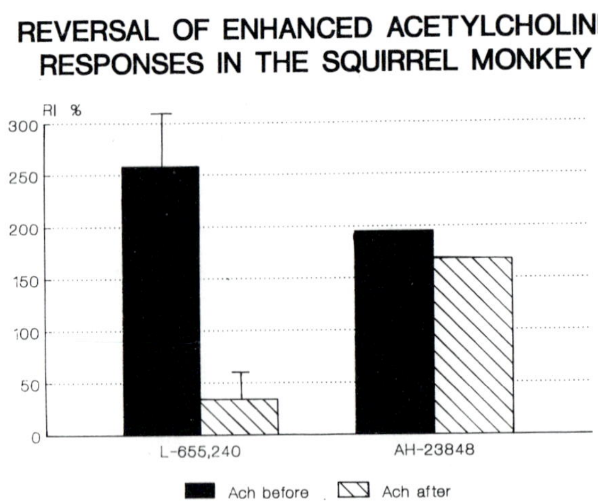

DISCUSSION

In these experiments we have demonstrated that in the conscious primate the airway responsiveness to acetylcholine aerosol is greatly increased following inhalation of the stable TxA_2 mimic, U44069. The hyperresponsiveness to acetylcholine aerosol involved significant changes in sensitivity (dose) and airway resistance (response).

In addition, these studies have shown that airway hyperresponsiveness to acetylcholine can be reversed by inhalation of the selective TxA_2 receptor antagonist L-655,240. It should be noted that L-655,240 itself does not inhibit the responses to acetylcholine in non-hyperresponsive monkeys or anesthetized guinea pigs (Hall et al., 1987).

The mechanism of action of the induced airway hyperresponsiveness to acetylcholine aerosol, and its reversal by L-655,240, is not clear. A number of potential actions could be involved, including actions of TxA_2 on parasympathetic ennervation, selective activation of calcium pools in airway smooth muscle, release of additional mediators, etc. Also, whether TxA_2 induces airway hyperresponsiveness to other spasmogens such as histamine, leukotrienes, prostaglandin D_2, tachykinins, etc is unknown.

In summary, these experiments support the involvement of TxA_2 in the development of airway hyperresponsiveness. They show a potentiated acetylcholine aerosol response following inhalation of a TxA_2 mimic in the conscious primate and its reversal by a potent, selective TxA_2 receptor antagonist.

REFERENCES

Chung K.F., Evans T.W, Graf P.D., Nadel J.A. (1985). Modulation of cholinergic neurotransmission in canine airways by thromboxane mimietic U46619. European J. Pharmacol. 117:373-375.

Munoz N.M., Shioya T., Murphy T.M., Primack S., Dame C., Sands M.F., Leff A.R. (1986). Potentiation of vagal contractile response by thromboxane mimetic U46619. J. Appl. Physiol. 61(3):1173-1179.

Chung K.F., Aizawa H., Becker A.B., Frick O., Gold W.M., Nadel J.A. (1986a). Inhibition of antigen-induced airway hyperresponsiveness by a thromboxane synthase inhibitor (OKY 046) in allergic dogs. Am. Rev. Respir. Dis. 134:258-261.

O'Byrne P.M., Leikauf G.D., Aizawa H., Bethel R.A., Ueki I.F., Holtzman M.J., Nadel J.A. (1985). Leukotriene B_4 induces airway hyperresponsiveness in dogs. J. Appl. Physiol. 59(6):1941-1946.

Aizawa K.F., Chung K.F., Leikauf G.D., Ueki I., Bethel R.A., O'Byrne P.M., Hirose T., Nadel J.A. (1985). Significance of thromboxane generation in ozone induced airway hyperresponsiveness in dogs. J. Appl. Physiol. 59(6):1918-1923.

Chung K.F., Aizawa H., Leikauf G.D., Ueki I.F., Evans T.W., Nadel J.W. (1986b). Airway hyperresponsiveness induced by platelet-activating factor: Role of thromboxane generation. J. Pharmacol and Exptl. Therapeutics. 236:580-584.

McFarlane C.S., Piechuta H., Hall R.A., Ford-Hutchinson A.W. (1984). Effects of a contractile prostaglandin antagonist (L-640,035) upon allergen-induced bronchoconstriction in hyperreactive rats and conscious squirrel monkeys. Prostaglandins 28:173-182.

Hall R.A., Gillard J., Guindon Y., Letts G., Champion E., Ethier D., Evans J., Ford-Hutchinson A.W., Fortin R., Jones T.R., Lord A., Morton, H.E., Rokach J., Yoakim C. (1987). Pharmacology of L-655,240 (3-[1-(4-chlorobenzyl)-5-fluoro-3-methyl-indol-2-yl]2,2-dimethyl-propanoic acid); a potent, selective thromboxane/prostaglandin endoperoxide antagonist. European J. Pharmacol. 135:193-201.

De Bono D.P., Lumley P., Been M., Keery R., Incese, et al., (1986). Effect of the specific thromboxane receptor blocking drug AH23848 in patients with angina pectoris. British Heart Journal 56:509-517.

DISCUSSION

Barnes: I think this is a very interesting study. In a sense R. Fuller and I have done this study in man already because we've used PGD_2, which activates TxA_2 receptors and shown that histamine and acetylcholine responsiveness is increased.

Letts: Have you tried a TxA_2 receptor antagonist?

Barnes: No.

Fuller: What is the mechanism of acetylcholine bronchoconstriction in your model? In man it not only has a direct action but works through a reflex since it induces cough and irritation.

Letts: We haven't investigated the mechanism of action of acetylcholine, however the animals often become agitated while breathing the aerosol. This is in contrast to some of the other spasmogens we've used. My suspicion is that this interaction is through ganglionic transmission and we've just started some experiments with indomethacin to try and determine what is happening.

Piper: In view of the fact that we've seen an interaction between leukotrienes and cyclooxygenase products, have you investigated leukotrienes in the squirrel monkeys and this antagonist?

Letts: No, that's not been done but we will be doing it in the future. These are labour-intensive studies and will take some time to complete.

Thompson: You seem to have a plateau effect with acetylcholine similar to that observed in humans. Is it the case that further doses of acetylcholine will not produce a greater response?

Letts: Yes, that's true. It's also true for histamine, LTD_4 and U46619.

Thompson: Does this mean that these monkeys and man are different to all other animals we use?

Letts: I don't know that you can correlate this model with

human asthma. When we used L649923, a leukotriene antagonist which showed good activity in the primate model, it had little activity in man.

Pare: You express your results as % change in resistance from baseline. What was the baseline resistance after the thromboxane analogue?

Letts: After aerosolization of the thromboxane analogue, we made sure that the resistance returned to the pre-acetylcholine challenge level.

Mechanisms in Asthma: Pharmacology, Physiology, and Management, pages 99–108

A ROLE FOR INFLAMMATORY MEDIATORS IN AIRWAY HYPER-RESPONSIVENESS

Carol L. Armour, Judith L. Black and Peter R.A. Johnson

Department of Pharmacology, University of Sydney, N.S.W. 2006, Australia

INTRODUCTION

Inflammation has been implicated in the altered airway responsiveness which is a feature of asthma. A variety of inflammatory stimuli have been used to induce airway hyper-responsiveness experimentally and these include ozone (Holtzman et al., 1979, 1983), respiratory infection (Ouellette and Reed, 1965; Empey et al., 1976; Walters, 1983), cigarette smoke (Hulbert et al., 1985), C_{5a} des Arg (Berend et al., 1986; Irvin et al., 1986) and water (Black et al., 1985). It has been proposed that the mechanism of this induced hyperresponsiveness is via release of cyclo-oxygenase products of arachidonic acid since indomethacin inhibits these inflammation-induced responses (Walters, 1983; O'Byrne et al., 1984b; Berend et al., 1986). This would indicate that either a prostaglandin (PG) or thromboxane A_2 (TxA_2) released from inflammatory cells may induce an increase in airway responsiveness. In vivo, administration of prostaglandins increases airway responsiveness to histamine and methacholine in both asthmatic (Fuller et al., 1986) and normal subjects (Walters et al., 1981).

The way in which PGs or TxA_2 may produce this alteration in responsiveness is not known although a number of mechanisms have been proposed. These include: 1) An increase in permeability of the airway epithelium resulting in an increased access of inhaled agonists to the smooth muscle. 2) Altered neural control of the airways. 3) An alteration in the smooth muscle sensitivity.

1. AIRWAY PERMEABILITY

Whereas there is some evidence that an alteration in the permeability of the epithelial barrier may explain changes in responsiveness (Holroyde, 1986), it cannot account for all the changes observed in asthma (Elwood et al., 1983).

2. NEURAL CONTROL OF THE AIRWAYS

It is possible that altered airway responsiveness induced by cyclooxygenase products is due to an alteration in neural control of the airways. A neural mechanism has been proposed previously (O'Byrne et al., 1984a; Leff et al., 1985) and it has been suggested that the effects of $PGF_{2\alpha}$ in vivo were localised to the autonomic ganglion (O'Byrne et al., 1984a). We thus decided to test whether PGs could alter neural control of the airways in vitro and whether the site of this alteration was located on the autonomic ganglion. Such an investigation requires the presence of an intact nerve supply and clearly this is not possible in human isolated airway tissue. However, it is possible to study this in a rabbit isolated airway preparation with an intact vagus nerve (Armour et al., 1987a). The vagus nerve is dissected away from the trachea to the branch of the recurrent laryngeal nerve. The distal portion of the vagus is removed. Electrical stimulation of the proximal portion of the vagus nerve stimulates the parasympathetic fibres preganglionically with a resultant contraction of the trachea. This response is suppressed by hexamethonium which inhibits at the parasympathetic ganglion. Electrical field stimulation of the trachea induces tracheal contraction by stimulation of the postganglionic fibres. The responses to both pre- and postganglionic stimulation are inhibited by atropine (10^{-7} M) and tetrodotoxin (10^{-5} M) indicating that tracheal contraction is induced by the release of acetylcholine from parasympathetic fibres. When a reproducible contraction is obtained, $PGF_{2\alpha}$ 10^{-6} M is added. This induces a significant ($p < 0.05$) potentiation of both the pre- and postganglionic stimulation to 149.2±15.9% and 139.0±8.5% ($n = 3$) of control values respectively (Armour et al., 1987a).

The fact that both forms of stimulation were potentiated would seem to indicate that $PGF_{2\alpha}$ potentiates at a site distal to the parasympathetic ganglion. In order to confirm this we then studied isolated bronchial rings from rabbit airways field stimulated to induce a contraction. This contraction was also inhibited by prior administration of atropine (10^{-6} M) and tetrodotoxin (3×10^{-5} M), indicating that release of acetylcholine from postganglionic fibres was responsible for the field stimulation-induced contraction (Fig. 1). $PGF_{2\alpha}$, 10^{-6} M, significantly potentiated the response to field stimulation to 144±5% (n = 4) of the

Figure 1. Contractile responses induced by electrical field stimulation (10-40V, 12-16Hz for 20 sec) of A: rabbit bronchi, B: human bronchi. Stimulation was repeated until a stable contraction height was observed. Tetrodotoxin, 3×10^{-5} M, or atropine, 10^{-6} M, inhibited these responses. In human bronchi raising the tone itself with carbachol, 5×10^{-8} M did not potentiate field stimulation responses.

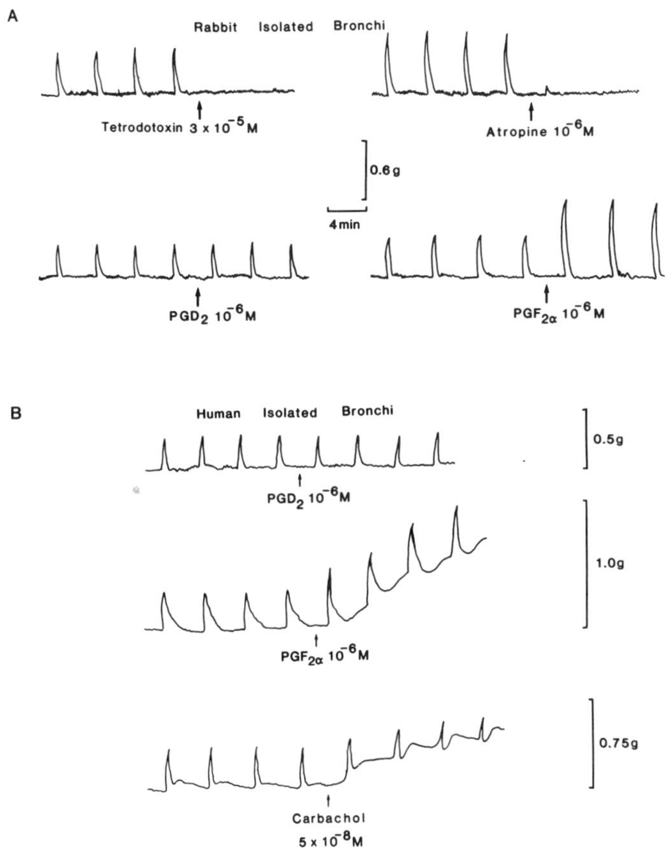

control response (Fig. 1). There was no effect of PGD_2 (10^{-6} M) on the contraction (Fig. 1). This same result was obtained on field stimulated human isolated bronchi. $PGF_{2\alpha}$, 10^{-6} M, produced a significant potentiation to 131±1.7% (n = 4) of control and PGD_2 had no effect (Fig. 1). The potentiation observed with $PGF_{2\alpha}$ was not merely due to an additive effect of 2 contractile agonists, since addition of an equiactive concentration of carbachol rather than $PGF_{2\alpha}$ did not potentiate the stimulation-induced response (Fig. 1). The site of the PG-induced potentiation would seem to be localized either to the parasympathetic postganglionic fibre or to the smooth muscle.

3. SMOOTH MUSCLE SENSITIVITY

In order to determine more closely the site of action of PGs we then studied their effects on smooth muscle sensitivity. Initially cumulative responses to histamine or carbachol were obtained on rabbit bronchial tissue in vitro. The responses were compared in the presence or absence of 10^{-8} M $PGF_{2\alpha}$ or PGD_2. PGs were added 30 min before commencing the cumulative concentration responses to histamine or carbachol. Neither PG induced an alteration in smooth muscle sensitivity. These results would seem to suggest that the mechanism of the PG-induced alteration in responsiveness observed in vivo was not via an increase in smooth muscle sensitivity and that the site of action of $PGF_{2\alpha}$ on field stimulation responses was the postganglionic fibre. However, when we examined previous in vivo studies in greater detail, we found that PGs had been administered immediately before histamine (Walters et al., 1981; Fuller et al., 1986) or methacholine (Fuller et al., 1986). So it would seem that the time period used for incubation with $PGF_{2\alpha}$ is critical. Due to the nature of the field stimulation responses in both the isolated vagus nerve-tracheal preparation and the isolated bronchi from rabbits and humans, $PGF_{2\alpha}$ was added only ½-2 min prior to field stimulation. When the effects of $PGF_{2\alpha}$ or PGD_2 were studied on smooth muscle sensitivity using cumulative contractions to histamine and carbachol, we had incubated tissues with the PG for 30 min before commencing the agonist response. If timing is critical any effect of $PGF_{2\alpha}$ may thus have been missed.

We therefore decided to study the effects of $PGF_{2\alpha}$

on bolus rather than cumulatively added doses of histamine and carbachol. Reproducible contractions to repeated administration of the agonist were first obtained. $PGF_{2\alpha}$, 10^{-6} M, was then added prior to the agonist and the contraction induced by the combined addition was then observed (Fig. 2). $PGF_{2\alpha}$ produced a significant potentiation of the histamine response to 146±7% (n = 3) of control values but not that of carbachol (118±8%, n = 5). So the effects of $PGF_{2\alpha}$ may be

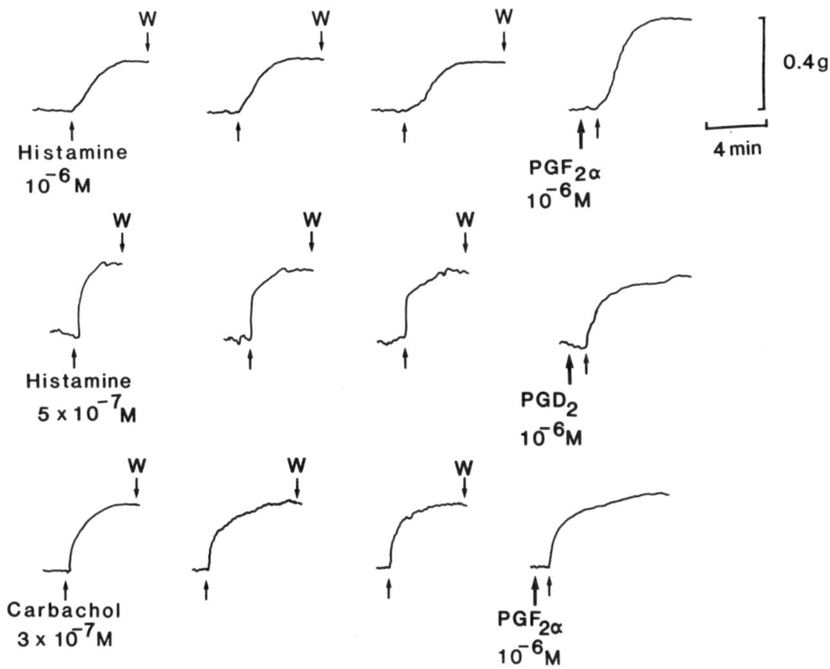

Figure 2. Results from a single experiment in which contractile responses of rabbit bronchi were induced by bolus doses of histamine or carbachol. When contraction height was reproducible $PGF_{2\alpha}$, 10^{-6} M or PGD_2, 10^{-6} M was added. W = washout.

mediated by an alteration in smooth muscle sensitivity although the result obtained with carbachol is difficult to explain. The difference in results obtained for histamine and carbachol requires further investigation.

MECHANISMS

In our studies, the potentiation response was always extremely short-lived (2-8 min). In addition, the fact that the potentiation response could not be repeated suggests that $PGF_{2\alpha}$ may release another mediator which is responsible for the observed potentiation. Since the response is so short-lasting and PGs must be administered either at the same time or just prior to the agonist under investigation, the proposed secondary mediator must have a short half-life.

We propose that this secondary mediator is TxA_2. It has an extremely short half-life (t1/2 = 30 sec at 37°C) and is rapidly metabolized to an inactive metabolite, thromboxane B_2. TxA_2 is released from a variety of cells including platelets (Hamberg et al., 1975), macrophages, eosinophils and neutrophils (Morley et al., 1979). In the in vivo studies in which inflammation-induced airway hyperresponsivness was inhibited by indomethacin (Walters, 1983; O'Byrne et al., 1984b; Berend et al., 1986) not only was prostaglandin formation inhibited but so was that of TxA_2. The thromboxane synthetase inhibitor, OKY-046, inhibits ozone (Aizawa et al., 1985) and LTB_4-induced hyperresponsiveness in dogs (O'Byrne et al., 1985) suggesting that TxA_2 may be involved in airway hyperresponsiveness.

In order to test whether TxA_2 could alter smooth muscle sensitivity, we studied the effects of a stable TxA_2 analogue, U46619, on cumulative responses to histamine and carbachol in rabbit isolated bronchi. The sensitivity to these contractile agonists was compared in the presence and absence of U46619. Tissues were incubated with a concentration of 10^{-8} M U46619 for 30 min. Cumulative response curves to both histamine and carbachol were significantly potentiated in the presence of the TxA_2 analogue (Fig. 3).

SUMMARY

We have demonstrated that $PGF_{2\alpha}$ potentiates airway contraction in vitro and suggested that this response may be mediated by TxA_2. We have localized the site of action of $PGF_{2\alpha}$ to a point distal to the parasympathetic ganglion and

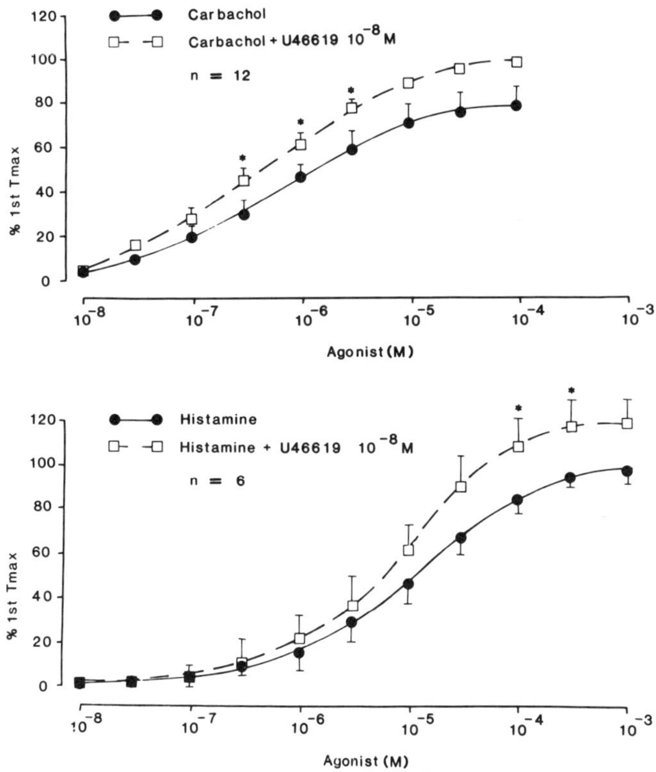

Figure 3. The effect of U46619, 10^{-8} M, on the contractile responses induced by carbachol or histamine on rabbit isolated bronchi. n = number of rabbits. * = point significantly different from control value, $p < 0.05$, Student's paired t-test.

shown that it is a specific effect since PGD_2 produces no similar potentiation. The mechanism of the potentiation may be by a direct alteration in smooth muscle sensitivity induced by TxA_2 (Fig. 4). In our previous studies we have been able to induce hyperresponsiveness in vivo (Berend et al., 1986) but no increased responsiveness in vitro (Armour et al., 1987b). In vivo airway hyperresponsiveness may depend on the presence of a mediator like TxA_2 which has a short half-life, is produced by continual stimulation of inflammatory cells and which is "washed out" in vitro once the source of stimulation is removed. The fact that we can demonstrate an increase in sensitivity in vitro using $PGF_{2\alpha}$ or a TxA_2 analogue, combined with the fact that both mediators are released from a variety of inflammatory cells suggests that one or both of these agents may mediate part of the increased responsiveness observed in asthma.

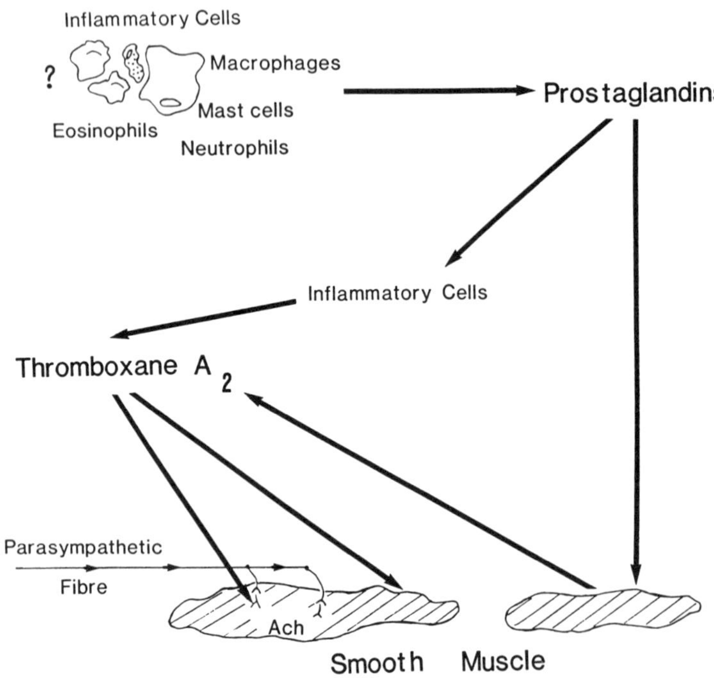

Figure 4. Hypothesis to explain the way in which prostaglandins and/or thromboxane A_2 may alter smooth muscle responsivness.

ACKNOWLEDGEMENTS

This work was supported by the National Health and Medical Research Council of Australia.

REFERENCES

Aizawa H, Chung KF, Leikouf GD, Veki I, Bethel RA, O'Byrne PM, Hirose T, Nadel JA (1985). Significance of thromboxane generation in ozone-induced airway hyperresponsiveness in dogs. J Appl Physiol 59:1918-1923.

Armour CL, Black JL, Johnson PRA, Marthan R (1987a). Enhancement of cholinergic transmission by prostaglandin $F_{2\alpha}$ in the rabbit trachea. Am Rev Respir Dis 135:A180.

Armour CL, Black JL, Vincenc KS, Johnson PRA, Ward H, Berend N (1987b). Airway responses in vitro following C_{5a} des Arg-induced hyperresponsiveness in vivo in rabbits. Clin Exp Pharmacol Physiol 14:7-14.

Berend N, Armour CL, Black JL (1986). Indomethacin inhibits the increased airway responsiveness to histamine following inhalation of C_{5a} des Arg in rabbits. Agents and Actions 18:468-472.

Black JL, Schoeffel RE, Sundrum R, Berend N, Anderson SD (1985). Increased responsiveness to methacholine and histamine after challenge with ultrasonically nebulized water in asthmatic subjects. Thorax 40:427-432.

Elwood RK, Kennedy S, Belzberg A, Hogg JC, Pare PD (1983). Respiratory mucosal permeability in asthma. Am Rev Respir Dis 128:523-527.

Empey DW, Laitinen LA, Jacobs L, Gold WM, Nadel JA (1976). Mechanisms of bronchial hyperreactivity in normal subjects after upper respiratory tract infection. Am Rev Respir Dis 113:131-139.

Fuller RW, Dixon CMS, Dollery CT, Barnes PJ (1986). Prostaglandin D_2 potentiates airway responsiveness to histamine and methacholine. Am Rev Respir Dis 133:252-254.

Hamberg M, Svensson J, Samuelsson B (1975). Thromboxanes: a new group of biologically active compounds derived from prostaglandin endoperoxidases. Proc Natl Acad Sci USA 72: 2994-2998.

Holroyde MC (1986). The influence of epithelium on the responsiveness of guinea-pig isolated trachea. Br J Pharmac 87:501-507.

Holtzman MJ, Cunningham JH, Sheller JR, Irsigler GB, Nadel JA, Boushey HA (1979). Effect of ozone on bronchial reactivity in atopic and nonatopic subjects. Am Rev Respir Dis 120: 1059-1067.

Holtzman MJ, Fabbri LM, O'Byrne PM, Gold BD, Aizawa H, Walters EH, Alpert SE, Nadel JA (1983). Importance of airway inflammation for hyperresponsiveness induced by ozone. Am Rev Respir Dis 127:686-690.

Hulbert WM, McLean T, Hogg JC (1985). The effect of acute airway inflammation on bronchial reactivity in guinea-pigs. Am Rev Respir Dis 132:7-11.

Irvin CG, Berend N, Henson PM (1986). Airways hyperreactivity and inflammation produced by aerosolization of human C_{5a} des Arg. Am Rev Respir Dis 134:777-783.

Leff AR, Munoz NM, Tallet J, Cavigelli M, David AC (1985). Augmentation of parasympathetic contraction in tracheal and bronchial airways by $PGF_{2\alpha}$ in situ. J Appl Physiol 58: 1558-1564.

Morley J, Bray MA, Jones RW, Nugteren DH, van Dorp DA (1979). Prostaglandin and thromboxane production by human and guinea-pig macrophages and leucocytes. Prostaglandins 17: 730-736.

O'Byrne PM, Aizawa H, Bethel RA, Chung KF, Nadel JA, Holtzman MJ (1984a). Prostaglandin $F_{2\alpha}$ increases responsiveness of pulmonary airways in dogs. Prostaglandins 28:537-543.

O'Byrne PM, Walters EH, Aizawa H, Fabbri LM, Holtzman MJ, Nadel JA (1984b). Indomethacin inhibits the airway hyperresponsiveness but not the neutrophil influx induced by ozone in dogs. Am Rev Respir Dis 130:220-224.

O'Byrne PM, Leikauf GD, Aizawa H, Bethel RA, Veki IF, Holtzman MJ, Nadel JA (1985). Leukotriene B_4 induces airway hyperresponsiveness in dogs. J Appl Physiol 59:1941-1946.

Ouellette JJ, Reed CE (1965). Increased response of asthmatic subjects to methacholine after influenza vaccine. J Allergy 36:558-563.

Walters EH (1983). Effect of inhibition of prostaglandin synthesis on induced bronchial hyperresponsiveness. Thorax 38:195-199.

Walters EH, Parrish RW, Bevan C, Smith AP (1981). Induction of bronchial hypersensitivity: evidence for a role for prostaglandins. Thorax 36:571-574.

Neuropeptides, Purines, and Neural Control

Mechanisms in Asthma: Pharmacology,
Physiology, and Management, pages 111–121

NEUROPEPTIDES IN HUMAN AIRWAYS

Peter J Barnes

Department of Clinical Pharmacology, Cardiothoracic Institute, Brompton Hospital, London SW3, U.K.

INTRODUCTION

Many neuropeptides have now been identified in the respiratory tract (Polak and Bloom, 1986). Their precise physiological role in airways remains uncertain, but the potent effects of these neuropeptides on various aspects of airway function suggest that they may be involved in controlling airway tone, vasculature and secretions (Barnes, 1987a). It is possible that defective function of peptidergic nerves might be involved in airway disease, and particularly asthma (Barnes, 1987b).

AIRWAY NANC NERVES

Neural control of airways is more complex than previously recognised and, in addition to classical cholinergic and adrenergic pathways, neural mechanisms which are neither adrenergic nor cholinergic have been described (Barnes, 1986). There is increasing evidence that neuropeptides may be the neurotransmitters of these NANC nerves. Both excitatory and inhibitory NANC mechanisms have been described in airways, but the physiological significance of these pathways will remain uncertain until specific blockers become available. In human airways NANC inhibitory nerves are the only inhibitory nervous pathway, since direct adrenergic innervation of airway smooth muscle is lacking.

VIP

Vasoactive intestinal peptide (VIP), a 28 amino acid peptide originally discovered as a vasoactive substance in lung extracts, potently relaxes airway smooth muscle _in vitro_ (Said, 1982). VIP is the neuropeptide which is most abundant in human lung; in human airways VIP-immunoreactive nerve fibres are associated with airway smooth muscle (particularly in large airways), submucosal glands, bronchial vessels and cholinergic ganglia (Laitinen et al, 1985). VIP relaxes human bronchi _in vitro_ and is about 50 x more potent than isoprenaline, making it the most potent endogenous bronchodilator so far discovered (Palmer et al, 1986a). _In vivo_, inhaled VIP is rather disappointing, since it has no bronchodilator effect and provides only weak protection against histamine-induced bronchoconstriction (Barnes and Dixon, 1984), probably because little of the nebulised peptide can reach receptors in airway smooth muscle. Even when given by infusion VIP has no bronchodilator effect in normal subjects who are able to bronchodilate with isoprenaline, probably because the cardiovascular effects of the peptide prevent administration of a high enough dose (Palmer et al, 1986b).

VIP is a likely candidate for the neurotransmitter of NANC inhibitory nerves since, in animal airways, it mimics the electrophysiological changes produced by NANC nerve stimulation, it is released into the muscle bath when these nerves are stimulated electrically (Said, 1982), and when tolerance is induced by exposure to high concentrations of VIP, then NANC inhibitory nerve effects (but not sympathetic inhibitory effects) are reduced. Histochemical studies show that VIP-immunoreactive nerves diminish in the smaller airways and are virtually absent from bronchioles. Interestingly, non-adrenergic relaxation is almost absent in small airways and these airways fail to relax with VIP, although they are relaxed by isoprenaline (Palmer et al, 1986a). All this evidence points towards VIP as a neurotransmitter of NANC inhibitory nerves but certain proof must await the development of specific blockers.

In animals, VIP is also a potent stimulant of mucus secretion from airway glands (Peatfield et al, 1983), and ion transport in airway epithelium (Nathanson et al, 1983), suggesting that VIP-ergic nerves may also regulate airway secretions. VIP is a potent vasodilator and, in the bronchial circulation, might play an important role in regulation of airway perfusion. Mapping of VIP-receptors in human lung by autoradiography confirms the presence of receptors on airway glands, epithelium and vascular smooth muscle, and also demonstrates the presence of receptors on smooth muscle of bronchi but not bronchioles (Carstairs and Barnes, 1986a).

Ultrastructural studies suggest that VIP may be present in cholinergic nerves in the airways, and may therefore function as a co-transmitter with acetylcholine (Laitinen et al, 1985). VIP may modulate release of acetylcholine, or may modify its effects. VIP reduces the contractile effect of exogenous acetylcholine on airway smooth muscle in vitro and may then act as a braking mechanism to cholinergic bronchoconstriction (Barnes, 1987b). It is possible that VIP is co-released only under certain patterns of neural activation, such as high frequency firing, acting as a protective mechanism. Another possible physiological role for VIP could involve regulation of bronchial blood flow. If cholinergic nerve activity causes bronchoconstriction, release of VIP from activated cholinergic nerves may have an effect on adjacent bronchial vessels, which are very sensitive to VIP (Laitinen et al, 1987), so that bronchial blood flow increases as smooth muscle contracts, thus supplying oxygen to active smooth muscle cells.

Peptide Histidine Isoleucine (PHI) is a 27 amino acid with marked structural similarities to VIP and coded by the same gene (Tatemoto, 1984). In humans there is a terminal methionine and the peptide is therefore termed peptide histidine methionine (PHM). PHI/PHM is present in the same nerves as VIP and has rather similar effects. PHM is equipotent to VIP as a relaxant of airway smooth muscle (Palmer et al, 1986a), although is less potent as a vasodilator than VIP, suggesting that it might act on separate receptors.

Whether any abnormality in NANC inhibitory nerves or VIP might contribute to bronchial hyperresponsiveness is uncertain. A defect in inhibiting control of airway smooth muscle would certainly account for some of the features of hyperresponsiveness. A primary defect in NANC innervation seems unlikely, since there is no abnormality in gastrointestinal sphincters or motility in asthmatic patients which would be expected in a generalised defect of this system. However, it is possible that a functional defect might develop as a result of airway inflammation, which appears to be related to the bronchial hyperresponsiveness which is so characterstic of asthma. Inflammatory cells identified in the asthmatic airway, such as neutrophils, eosinophils and mast cells may release a variety of peptidases which would rapidly break down VIP and PHM. This would be like taking the brake off cholinergic nerves, thereby leading to exaggerated cholinergic bronchoconstrictor responses in the larger airways (Barnes, 1987b). While this is unlikely to be the cause of asthma it may be a contributory factor in the bronchial hyperresponsiveness associated with airway inflammation.

SENSORY NEUROPEPTIDES

Substance P (SP) is localised to unmyelinated sensory nerves (C-fibres) in airways and has several actions which suggest that it may take part in the inflammatory response of asthma (Barnes, 1987b). In addition to contraction of airway smooth muscle, SP also potently stimulates airway mucus secretion, and increases airway microvascular permeability and exudation of plasma into the airway lumen. SP also degranulates mast cells of the skin, although this has not been demonstrated conclusively in lung, and may have chemotactic effects on inflammatory cells. Non-cholinergic bronchoconstrictor nerves have been demonstrated in guinea-pigs. These nerves are antagonised by SP antagonists, suggesting that SP may be the excitatory neurotransmitter (Andersson and Grundstrom, 1983). These studies raise the possibility that SP might be released from sensory nerve endings by retrograde activation, as in an axon reflex.

Capsaicin, the hot extract of pepper, releases SP from unmyelinated sensory nerve endings and, in rats and guinea-pigs, causes acute bronchoconstriction and airway microvascular leakiness (Saria et al, 1983). Chronic treatment with capsaicin leads to depletion of SP-immunoreactivity and is associated with a reduced bronchoconstrictor response to allergen in sensitised animals (Saria et al, 1983) and prevents irritants, such as cigarette smoke or mechanical stimulation of the airway from airway microvascular leakage (Lundberg and Saria,

1983). While these effects of SP innervation are seen in rodents, the relevance of these findings to human airways is less certain. Reports of SP innervation of human airways are conflicting, but human lungs obtained at surgery are usually from older smokers in whom SP content may be reduced. Nevertheless, SP and capsaicin cause contraction of human airways in vitro (Lundberg et al, 1983), and capsaicin causes bronchoconstriction, albeit transiently, when inhaled (Fuller et al, 1985). Autoradiographic studies suggest that SP receptors are localised to smooth muscle of all airways (Carstairs and Barnes, 1986b), and SP may therefore regulate tone in small airways.

Recently, two peptides (tachykinins) related in structure to SP, neurokinin A and neurokinin B have been identified to lung (Hua et al, 1985). NKA is coded by the same gene as SP but has a different spectrum of effects, suggesting the existence of separate receptors (NK-2 receptors). NKA is far more potent that SP in contracting human airway smooth muscle, whereas SP is more potent than NKA in causing vasodilatation and microvascular leakage (via NK-1 receptors). NKB may act via a third type of receptor (NK-3 receptor) which may be neuronal.

Another peptide which has recently been localised to sensory nerves is calcitonin gene-related peptide (CGRP), which may also be co-stored with SP. CGRP is a potent vasodilator and contracts human airways in vitro (Palmer et al, 1987). It may potentiate microvascular leakage caused by SP because of its vasodilator action.

Because sensory neuropeptides, such as SP, neurokinins and CGRP produce many of the features of asthma it is tempting to speculate that they may be involved in its pathogenesis, and the idea of neurogenic inflammatory mechanisms in asthma is attractive (Barnes, 1986b). Damage to airway epithelium (possibly as a result of toxic eosinophil products) may occur even in relatively mild asthmatics, exposing afferent nerve endings. These nerve endings may then be stimulated by inflammatory mediators. Bradykinin, an inflammatory peptide formed by enzymatic cleavage from a plasma precursor, is likely to be formed in the asthmatic airway by the action of enzymes released from inflammatory cells on exudated plasma. Bradykinin selectively stimulates C-fibre endings and may release sensory neuropeptides. Bradykinin is a potent bronchoconstrictor in asthmatics and acts indirectly, possibly by stimulating sensory nerve endings (Fuller et al, 1987). This may result in the retrograde release of sensory neuropeptides such as SP, neurokinins and CGRP from collaterals, via an axon reflex. This could result in bronchoconstriction, mucus hypersecretion and microvascular leakage leading to oedema of the airway wall and extravasation of plasma in the lumen. Local reflexes may thus spread the inflammation through the airways from pathway sites of epithelial damage.

OTHER NEUROPEPTIDES

Several other neuropeptides have been identified in human airway nerves (Polak and Bloom, 1986), but their physiological role is far from certain (Barnes, 1987a).

Neuropeptide Y is colocalised with noradrenaline in adrenergic nerves of the lung (Sheppard et al, 1984). It may play a role in regulating bronchial blood flow and airway ganglia, rather than airway smooth muscle directly, since sympathetic nerves do not directly supply airway smooth muscle in humans. Recent studies suggest that NPY modulates cholinergic nerves in guinea-pig airways (Stretton and Barnes, 1987).

Galanin appears to be colocalised with VIP in airway nerves but has little known direct effect on airway smooth muscle. It may have a neuromodulatory role (Ekblad et al, 1985). Cholecystokinin, somatostatin and gastrin-releasing peptide (mammalian bombesin) have also been found in lung but the function and precise localization of these neuropeptides has not yet been elucidated.

CLINICAL IMPLICATIONS

The presence of so many neuropeptides in airways (and many more may be discussed) raises questions about their physiological role. It seems most likely that they may act as subtle regulators under physiological conditions, but in inflammatory diseases of the airways, such as asthma, they may have a pathogenetic role. Specific antagonists are needed to elucidate the contribution of these potent neuropeptides in human diseases such as asthma.

It is certainly possible that pharmacological agents which interact with neuropeptides may be developed for the treatment of such diseases in the future. Analogues of VIP may be developed as bronchodilators in the future, although such drugs may have problems of acess to the relevant receptors. Non-peptide analogues may be more successful, although would be less effective on peripheral airways than beta-agonists.

Tachykinin antagonists are currently non-specific and of low potency, but again neuropeptide antagonists may be discovered in the future. The recent discovery of highly potent and specific non-peptide antagonists for cholecystokinin raises hope that other non-peptide antagonists of peptide receptors will be developed.

Drugs which modify the release of neuropeptides may also be of value, and the demonstration that the alpha-2 adrenoceptor agonist, clonidine, inhibits NANC excitatory nerves in airways (Grundstrom and Andersson, 1985) is an indication that it may be possible to selectively inhibit these neural pathways. Opioids also selectively inhibit NANC bronchoconstrictor pathways via u-opioid receptors (Frossard and Barnes, 1987). Cromoglycate may also have an action on neuropeptide release from sensory nerves, and indirect evidence in support of this is the observation that cromoglycate is an effective inhibitor of bradykinin-induced bronchoconstriction (Fuller et al, 1987).

Acknowledgement

I thank Madeleine Wray for the careful preparation of this manuscript.

REFERENCES

Andersson RGG, Grundstrom N (1983). The excitatory non-cholinergic, non-adrenergic nervous system of the guinea-pig airways. Eur J Respir Dis 64: 141-157.

Barnes PJ (1986a). Neural control of human airways in health and disease. Am Rev Respir Dis 134: 1289-1314.

Barnes PJ (1986b). Asthma as an axon reflex. Lancet 1: 242-245.

Barnes PJ (1987a). Neuropeptides in the lung: localization, function and pathophysiologic implications. J Allergy Clin Immunol 79: 285-295.

Barnes PJ (1987b). Airway neuropeptides and asthma. Trends Pharm Sci 8: 24-27.

Barnes PJ, Dixon CMS (1984). The effect of inhaled vasoactive intestinal peptide on bronchial hyperreactivity in man. Am Rev Respir Dis 130: 162-166.

Carstairs JR, Barnes PJ (1986). Visualization of vasoactive intestinal peptide receptors in human and guinea pig lung. J Pharmacol Exp Ther 239: 249-255.

Carstairs JR, Barnes PJ (1986). Autoradiographic mapping of substance P receptors in lung. Eur J Pharmacol 127: 295-296.

Ekblad E, Hakanson R, Sundler F, Wahlestedt C (1985). Galanin: neuromodulatory and direct contractile effects on smooth muscle preparations. Br J Pharmacol 86: 241-246.

Frossard N, Barnes PJ (1987). Opiates modulate the non-adrenergic non-cholinergic contraction in airways in vitro. Clin Resp Physiol 23: 313.

Fuller RW, Dixon CMS, Barnes PJ (1985). The bronchoconstrictor response to inhaled capsaicin in humans. J Appl Physiol 85: 1080-1084.

Fuller RW, Dixon CMS, Cuss FMC, Barnes PJ (1987). Bradykinin-induced bronchoconstriction in man: mode of action. Am Rev Respir Dis 135: 176-180.

Grundstrom N, Andersson RGG (1985). In vivo demonstration of &2-adrenoceptor mediated inhibition of the excitatory non-cholinergic neurotransmission in guinea-pig airways. Naunyn-Schmiedeberg's Arch. Pharmacol 328: 236-240.

Hua X-Y, Theodorsson-Norheim E, Brodin E, Lundberg JM, Hokfelt T (1985). Multiple tachykinins (neurokinin A, neuropeptide K and substance P) in capsaicin-sensitive sensory neurons in the guinea-pig. Regul Pept 13: 1-19.

Laitinen A, Partanen M, Hervonen A, Peto-Huikko M, Laitinen LA (1985). VIP-like immunoreactive nerves in human respiratory tract. Light and electron micrsoscopic study. Histochemistry 82: 313-319.

Laitinen LA, Laitinen A, Widdicombe JG (1987). Effects of inflammatory and other mediators on airway vascular beds. Am Rev Respir Dis 135: 567-570.

Lundberg JM, Martling C-R, Saria A (1983). Substance P and capsaicin-induced contraction of human bronchi. Acta Physiol Scand 119: 49-53.

Lundberg JM, Saria A (1983). Capsaicin-induced desensitization of the airway mucosa to cigarette smoke, mechanical and chemical irritants. Nature 302: 251-253.

Nathanson I, Widdicombe JH, Barnes PJ (1983). Effect of vasoactive intestinal peptide on ion transport across dog tracheal epithelium. J Appl Physiol 55: 1844-1848.

Palmer JB, Cuss FMC, Barnes PJ (1986a). VIP and PHM and their role in non-adrenergic inhibitory responses in isolated human airways. J Appl Physiol 61: 1322-1328.

Palmer JBD, Cuss FMC, Warren JB, Barnes PJ (1986b). The effect of infused vasoactive intestinal peptide on airway function in normal subjects. Thorax 41: 663-666.

Palmer JBD, Cuss FMC, Mulderry PK, Ghatei MA, Springall DR, Cadieux A, Bloom SR, Polak JM, Barnes PJ (1987). Calcitonin gene-related peptide is localised to human airway nerves and potently constricts human airway smooth muscle. Br J Pharmacol 91: 95-101.

Peatfield AC, Barnes PJ, Bratcher C, Nadel JA, Davis B (1983). Vasoactive intestinal peptide stimulates tracheal submucosal gland secretion in ferret. Am Rev Respir Dis 128: 89-93.

Polak JM, Bloom SR (1986). Regulatory peptides of the gastrointestinal and respiratory tracts. Arch int Pharmacodyn 280 (Suppl): 16-49.

Said SI (1982). Vasoactive peptides in the lung, with special reference to vasoactive intestinal peptide. Exp

Lung Res 3: 343-348.

Saria A, Lundberg JM, Skofitsch G, Lembeck F (1983). Vascular protein leakage in various tissues induced by substance P, capsaicin, bradykinin, serotonin, histamine and by antigen challenge. Naunyn-Schmiedeberg's Arch. Pharmacol 324: 212-218.

Sheppard MN, Polak JM, Allen JM, Bloom SR (1984). Neuropeptide tyrosine (NYP): a newly discovered peptide is present in the mammalian respiratory tract. Thorax 39: 326-330.

Stretton D, Barnes PJ (1987). Neuropeptide tyrosine modulates cholinergic nerves in guinea-pig trachea. Br J Pharmacol (in press).

Tatemoto K (1984). PHI - a new brain-gut peptide. Peptides 5: 151-154.

DISCUSSION

Church: Could I reinforce some comments you made on the mast cell with peptides? We've done work in this area. Yes, the mast cells do have peptide receptors, but they do not follow the pattern of activation you described for smooth muscle. VIP and substance P, a bronchodilator and a bronchoconstrictor, have virtually the same effect on mast cells. They stimulate skin mast cells to produce an extremely rapid release of histamine with no accompanying prostaglandin. This doesn't happen in lung mast cells, only in those from skin. We've never found any receptors for peptides on lung mast cells.

Barnes: I found your comments very interesting, that you can differentiate lung and skin peptides. I regard this as a non-physiological phenomenon, an effect of substance P which is like the effect of morphine, because they're basic molecules. In the skin, we've tried to look at this by giving capsaicin intradermally, which is extremely unpleasant. This does not lead to histamine release in human skin, suggesting that the endogenous release of neuropeptides is not able to degranulate mast cells.

Fuller: If your hypothesis is correct, how can you explain the lack of sensitivity of asthmatics to inhaled capsaicin?

Barnes: It seems more likely that bradykinin is a relevant stimulant for the nerves that might be involved in asthma. From animal studies we know that bradykinin will release sensory neuropeptides, and that blockers of substance P can attenuate bradykinin's effects in many systems. In your study, you showed bradykinin is a potent bronchoconstrictor in asthmatics although never in normal people, yet it can't contract human airway smooth muscle in vitro even in the presence of inhibitors, suggesting that it is working indirectly.

Mechanisms in Asthma: Pharmacology,
Physiology, and Management, pages 123–130

MODULATION OF TACHYKININS AND BRADYKININ BY ENKEPHALINASE

Jay A. Nadel and D. Benjamin Borson

Cardiovascular Research Institute and Depts of Medicine and Physiology, University of California San Francisco, S.F., California, 94143, U.S.A.

Recently, a novel class of molecules, the neuropeptides has been described. Among these neuropeptides, it has been discovered that the "tachykinins" exist in sensory nerves.

The best known of these tachykinins is substance P (SP). There is substantial evidence that SP and other tachykinins may play an important role in neural inflammatory responses in the airways. Thus, SP immunoreactivity occurs in sensory nerves of the lower respiratory tract in the epithelium, airway smooth muscle, and near blood vessels (Lundberg, 1983). SP has potent effects in airways, including contraction of smooth muscle (Lundberg, 1983; Sekizawa, 1987b), stimulation of gland secretion (Borson, 1987), and increased capillary permeability (Lundberg and Saria, 1982). Upon stimulation of the sensory nerves, substance P is released and the various inflammatory effects of substance P are reproduced, effects that are prevented by lung depletion of SP by capsaicin (Lundberg and Saria, 1983).

These findings provide powerful evidence that tachykinins contained in sensory nerves are mediators of multiple airways functions. It was our idea that degradative mechanisms could also be present in airway tissue and could play an important role in modulating these effects of tachykinins, just as acetylcholinesterase modulates the effects of neurally released acetylcholine. Previous studies in the gut indicated that SP is degraded rapidly in the ileum (Growcott and Tarpey, 1982). The mechanism has not been studied, but it is known that several enzymes degrade tachykinins, including angiotensin converting enzyme (Cascieri, 1984), acetylcholinesterase (Chubb, 1980), serine proteases (Hanson and Lovenberg, 1980), and enkephalinase (Skidgel, 1984). In the present report, we will provide evidence that enkephalinase (dipeptidyl carboxypeptidase), a membrane-bound peptidase located in specific airway cells, by cleaving tachykinins, modulates their actions.

To study mucus secretion, we mounted segments of ferret trachea in Ussing-type chambers, added 0.167 mCi $Na_2{}^{35}SO_4$ to the mucosal side, and we sampled on the luminal side at 15 min intervals. Then we dialyzed and counted the $^{35}SO_4$-labelled macromolecules as a reflection of secretion, as described in detail elsewhere (Borson, 1987). Substance P increased the flux of bound SO_4 in a concentration-dependent fashion. Addition of multiple enzyme inhibitors including captopril, teprotide, leupeptin, aprotinin, bacitracin, BSA, and bestatin had no effect on SP-induced secretions, but thiorphan and phosphoramidon (inhibitors of enkephalinase) potentiated the effects of SP in a dose-dependent fashion (Borson, 1987).

Enkephalinase cleaves SP between the 9 and 10 positions producing the fragment SP^{1-9} (Skidgel, 1984), which we have shown to be inactive in stimulating gland secretion (Borson, 1987). These studies suggest that enkephalinase is present in submucosal glands, and we confirmed this in two ways. First, we showed that significant enkephalinase-like activity exists in airway submucosal glands (Borson, 1986). Second, immunofluorescent studies with enkephalinase antibody performed in our laboratory has demonstrated the presence of enkephalinase in submucosal glands. These findings indicate that enkephalinase present in airways modulates tachykinin-induced secretion. Our results provide no evidence that other peptidases normally play a role in cleaving (and thus modulating) tachykinin effects in these tissues.

We also examined the role of peptidases in modulating tachykinin-induced airway smooth muscle contraction. We removed transverse rings (8 mm long) from ferret tracheas, mounted them in glass chambers, attached them to strain gauges to measure isometric tension and placed the rings between two rectangular platinum electrodes for electrical field stimulation. For details of methods, see Sekizawa (1987b). Substance P alone causes an increased muscle tension, but only at concentrations of $5x10^{-6}$M. Addition of the enkephalinase inhibitor, leucine-thiorphan (l-thiorphan, 10^{-5}M), did not affect resting tension, but it did shift the SP concentration-response relationship to lower concentrations by approximately one log unit (Sekizawa, 1987b). The SP antagonist (D-Pro^2,D-$Trp^{7,9}$-SP) (10^{-6}M) markedly inhibited the contraction produced by SP in the presence of l-thiorphan.

The potentiation of SP-induced contractions by the enkephalinase inhibitor, l-thiorphan, plus the lack of effects of other proteinase inhibitors (eg. captopril, bestatin, and leupeptin) suggests that enkephalinase present in airways modulates SP-induced smooth muscle effects. The main product of enkephalinase cleavage of SP, SP^{1-9} (10^{-6}M) had no effect on smooth muscle tension, indicating that enkephalinase cleavage of SP produces a peptide fragment that is inactive on airway smooth muscle. Thus, enkephalinase-like activity appears to modulate SP effects in smooth muscle. Similar to gland secretion, we found enkephalinase-like activity in the smooth muscle (as assessed by artificial substrates) (Borson, 1986). Further definitive evidence that enkephalinase is present in airway smooth muscle was provided by immunocytochemical localization with an enkephalinase antibody (Sekizawa, 1987a).

We also compared the effects of tissue enkephalinase on the smooth muscle contractile responses to 3 tachykinins in ferrets; substance P (SP), neurokinin A (NKA) and neurokinin B (NKB). All three tachykinins alone contracted smooth muscle, but only at concentrations of 10^{-6}M or greater for NKA and 10^{-5}M for SP and NKB (Sekizawa, 1987a). The rank order of potency was NKA>SP>NKB. L-thiorphan shifted the concentration-response curves to NKB, NKA, and SP to lower concentrations by approximately 4 log units for NKB, 2.5 log units for NKA, and 1 log unit for SP (Sekizawa, 1987a). In the presence of l-thiorphan, the rank order of potency was NKA=NKB>SP. Thus, enkephalinase present in airways has strikingly different effects on the three tachykinins. These differences could be due to different rate constants of cleavage of the substrates, or it could be due to geometric factors such as accessibility of the specific tachykinin to the active cleavage site of the enzyme as it exists in the target cell (muscle) membrane. Regardless of the mechanism, tissue enkephalinase has profoundly different effects on tachykinins NKA, NKB and SP.

In the past, tachykinin receptor classification has been based on rank orders of agonist potency in tissues. Our findings suggest that tachykinin-induced effects may reflect both peptide-receptor affinities and also the rate of degradation of the peptides.

We also studied the effect of tissue enkephalinase on muscle contraction induced by electrical field stimulation (EFS), a stimulus that releases acetylcholine from the vagus nerves. Substance P alone, in concentrations that had no effect on resting tension ($5x10^{-11}$M), augmented the responses to EFS in ferret tracheal smooth muscle. In the presence of SP, inhibition of tissue enkephalinase activity by l-thiorphan produced dose-related increases in the responses to EFS, effects that were abolished by atropine (Sekizawa, 1987b). These studies indicate that tissue enkephalinase modulates SP-induced presynaptic effects.

To examine the role of endogenous enkephalinase in neurotransmission, we examined the effect of l-thiorphan on the response to EFS in the absence of added SP. L-thiorphan potentiated the response to EFS in a concentration-dependent fashion, an effect not found with the addition of other enzyme inhibitors (Sekizawa, 1987b). The SP antagonist D-Pro^2,D-Trp^{7,9}-SP inhibited the increase in the response to EFS induced by l-thiorphan. These studies (Sekizawa, 1987b) provide evidence that an endogenous peptide, probably a tachykinin, mediates a component of the contractile response to neural stimulation, and they suggest that tissue enkephalinase modulates this neural response.

Enkephalinase was first found in renal tissue (Kerr and Kenny, 1974), but no physiologic role of the enzyme has been found in this organ. The enzyme was later discovered in the central nervous system, and it has been suggested that it modulates opioid actions (Malfroy, 1978). Our results suggest an entirely different role for enkephalinase. We suggest that endogenous enkephalinase modulates actions of tachykinins and other peptides such as bradykinin (Borson, 1987). Previous reports have shown enkephalinase to be present in peripheral tissues (Llorens, 1981) including lungs (Johnson, 1985). In airways, we have demonstrated enkephalinase-like activity (Borson, 1986) and immunocytochemical localization of the enzyme (Sekizawa, 1987a) in tracheal epithelium, smooth muscle, vagus nerves and submucosal glands. We also have evidence that enkephalinase exists and plays a functional role in modulation of tachykinin effects in gut smooth muscle (Djokic, Borson, and Nadel, personal communication) and we suggest that the enzyme may exist in other sites where tachykinin receptors are located.

The presence of enkephalinase in loci where tachykinins are released (sensory nerves) and in effector cells where tachykinins have their effects (e.g. epithelium, smooth muscle, glands, blood vessels, neutrophils) provides enkephalinase with the unique opportunity to degrade these inflammatory peptides at critical loci. We also predict that up- or down-regulation of enkephalinase activity in specific tissues will modify the extent of neural inflammatory responses. In addition to their effects on tachykinins, other peptides are cleaved by enkephalinase (Almenoff and Orlowski, 1983; Malfroy and Schwartz, 1985; Matsas, 1984). The key locations of the enzyme may allow it to modulate inflammatory and other physiologic responses to many peptides.

AKNOWLEDGEMENTS: These studies were supported in part by NIH Program Project Grant HL-24136.

REFERENCES

Almenoff J, Orlowski M (1983). Membrane-bound kidney neutral metalloendopeptidase: interaction with synthetic substrates, natural peptides, and inhibitors. Biochemistry 22:590-599.

Borson DB, Malfroy B, Gold M, Ramachandran J, Nadel JA (1986). Tachykinins inhibit enkephalinase activity from tracheas and lungs of ferrets. Physiologist 29:174.

Borson DB, Malfroy B, Gold M, Ramachandran J, Nadel JA (1987). Enkephalinase inhibitors potentiate substance P-induced secretion of $^{35}SO_4$-macromolecules from ferret trachea. Exp Lung Res 12:21-36.

Cascieri MA, Bull HG, Mumford RA, Patchett NA, Thornberry NA, Liang T (1984). Carboxy-terminal tripeptidyl hydrolysis of substance P by purified rabbit lung angiotensin-converting enzyme and the potentiation of substance P activity in vivo by captopril and MK-422. Pharmacol 25:287-293.

Chubb IW, Hodgson AJ, White GH (1980). Acetylcholinesterase hydrolyzes substance P. Neurosciences 5:2065-2072.

Growcott JW, Tarpey AV (1982). Effects of substance P-(1-9) nonapeptide amide on inactivation of substance P in vitro. Eur J Pharm 84:107-109.

Hanson GR, Lovenberg W (1980). Elevation of substance P-like immunoreactivity in rat central nervous system by protease inhibitors. J Neurochem 35:1370-1374.

Johnson AR, Ashton J, Schulz WW, Erdos EG (1985). Neutral metalloendopeptidase in human lung tissue and cultured cells. Am Rev Respir Dis 132:564-568.

Kerr MA, Kenny AJ (1974). The purification and specificity of a neutral endopeptidase from rabbit kidney brush border. Biochem J 137:477-488.

Llorens C, Schwartz J-C (1981). Enkephalinase activity in rat peripheral organs. Eur J Respir Dis 69:113-116.

Lundberg JM, Hokfelt J, Martling C-R, Saria A, Cuello S (1984). Substance P-immunoreactive sensory nerves in the lower respiratory tract of various animals including man. Cell Tis Res 235:251-261.

Lundberg JM, Martling CR, Saria A (1983). Substance P and capsaicin-induced contraction of human bronchi. Acta Physiol Scand 119:49-53.

Lundberg JM, Saria A (1982). Capsaicin-sensitive vagal neurons involved in control of vascular permeability in rat trachea. Acta Physiol Scand 115:521-523.

Lundberg JM, Saria A (1983). Capsaicin-induced desensitization of airway mucosa to cigarette smoke, mechanical and chemical irritants. Nature 302:251-253.

Malfroy B, Schwartz J-C (1985). Comparison of dipeptidyl carboxypeptidase and endopeptidase activities in the three enkephalin-hydrolysing metallopeptidases: "angiotensin-converting enzyme", thermolysin and "enkephalinase". Biochem Biophys Res Commun 130:372-378.

Malfroy B, Swerts JP, Guyon A, Rogues BP, Schwartz J-C (1978). High affinity enkephalin degrading peptidase in mouse brain and its enhanced activity following morphine. Nature 276:523-526.

Matsas, R, Kenny AJ, Turner AJ (1984). The metabolism of neuropeptides; the hydrolysis of peptides, including enkephalins, tachykinins and their analogues, by endopeptidase-24.11. Biochem J 233:433-440.

Sekizawa K, Tamaoki J, Graf PD, Basbaum CB, Borson DB, Nadel JA (1987a). Enkephalinase inhibitor potentiates mammalian tachykinin-induced contraction in ferret trachea. J Pharmacol Exp Ther (in press).

Sekizawa K, Tamaoki J, Nadel JA, Borson DB (1987b). Enkephalinase inhibitor potentiates substance P- and electrically induced contraction in ferret trachea. J Appl Physiol (in press).

Skidgel RA, Engelbrecht A, Johnson AR, Erdos EG (1984). Hydrolysis of substance P and neurotensin by converting enzyme and neutral endoproteinase. Peptides 5:769-776.

DISCUSSION

Williams: Do you think you could have situations where enkephalinase is inactivated, for instance by superoxide generation in an inflammatory situation, and then the effects of neuropeptides could be much enhanced?

Nadel: It's a key question: what modulates enkephalinase, and are there the enzymes that break it down? Serine proteases break it down, aminopeptidases cleave it rapidly and inactivate it. I originally did the studies with virus, hoping, and I think I might be right, that the virus takes the enkephalinase pathway. This material has to have a very specific and complicated pathway. Viruses don't do things on their own, they go in and take other people's pathways. So I was hoping it would inhibit the insertion of the enkephalinase into the membrane of the epithelium, and that still may be the mechanism. It's just that I chose the wrong virus. I also think there are materials like morphine that may up- or down-regulate it, neuropeptides themselves may up- or down-regulate it. Your question suggests the possibility that inflammatory proteases or free radicals may also cleave it. I think it's possible in the case of free radicals, and it's certain in the case of some peptidases.

Black: If asthmatics have damaged epithelium and they therefore have perhaps less of the enkephalinases around, why aren't they more sensitive to inhaled substance P?

Nadel: The response to inhaled substance P from the luminal surface will depend on the ability to cleave the neuropeptide as it exists on the luminal surface. There is a whole series of peptidases that will cleave substance P, and in asthma almost all those probably exist. Tryptase cleaves it, serum proteinases cleave it, kininase-2 cleaves it. So that there are many ways of breaking down substance P on the epithelial surface, particularly in the presence of inflammation. One of the dilemmas we have is that we don't deliver any peptide the way it's released. I'm hoping that somebody is going to reveal exactly where all these neuropeptides are. Where they're not, they may still be there, but they're broken down; that might be the case for NK B. So I think there is a dilemma, you can't extrapolate too far from a negative experiment. My own prediction is that if there's a wild inflammatory reaction and you don't get an effect of tachykinin, it would be very difficult to inhibit whatever's cleaving it, because there may be multiple enzymes.

Benveniste: Not knowing the field well, I find some difficulty to interpret some of what you showed. For example, what is the specificity of thiorphan to enkephalinase?

Nadel: What I said was that phosphoramidon does not block any other of the known enzymes, and I'll list the ones that it doesn't: serine proteases, acetylcholinesterases, aminopeptidases, kinase, tryptase, trypsin, so it's selective.

Benveniste: In your hands, it doesn't have any effect by itself on the mucus production?

Nadel: No, it does not have an effect.

Benveniste: And in the hypersensitivity that you show, it will not work with any other agonist?

Nadel: No, histamine, acetylcholine, serotonin, they are not influenced by it.

Mechanisms in Asthma: Pharmacology,
Physiology, and Management, pages 131–148

NEUROCHEMICALS IN THE INFANT LUNG

Louise Plowman, Tethys Scheibner
and Colin E. Sullivan

Department of Thoracic Medicine,
University of Sydney, Australia, 2006.
From the David Read Laboratory

INTRODUCTION

Although lung innervation has been extensively investigated no underlying concept has yet emerged, which allows the correlation of anatomy, physiology and pharmacology. With the advent of sensitive and specific immunocytochemical techniques the issue of lung innervation can now be readdressed. These techniques allow the visualization of specific neurochemicals contained within neural tissue such as found in the lung.

Particularly significant is lung development. Recent reports suggest that neurochemicals released by intrinsic lung neural tissue may play a trophic role during development (Cutz et al., 1984). Abnormal levels of neurochemicals have also been implicated in pathological states such as respiratory distress syndrome (Ghatei et al., 1983).

In this study we chose to focus on neurochemical distribution in the infant lung obtained from babies dying of sudden infant death syndrome (SIDS). Most infants dying in the first year of life are victims of SIDS. Although we are not attempting to address the causes of SIDS, these infants were the source of our tissue due to the difficulty of obtaining adequate non-SIDS lung samples. Clearly our findings might include abnormalities related to the unknown cause of death in these infants.

Using the latest immunocytochemical techniques we examined the distribution and morphlology of Substance P (SP), Vasoactive Intestinal Peptide (VIP), Bombesin (BN) and Serotonin (5HT) immunoreactive neural structures in the infant lung.

METHODS

Collection

Lungs from 17 infants were collected at autopsy from the Sydney City Morgue, Australia. Coroner's findings indicated that the death in all infants was consistent with SIDS. The age of the infants ranged from 1 to 16 weeks (mean = 9 $\pm$ 4) and 12 were male.

Fixation

The time between death and autopsy was 5 to 96 hours (mean = 40 $\pm$ 25). Lung tissue (excluding first generation airways) was quickly blocked and fixed in 4% phosphate buffered paraformaldehyde (pH 7.6) at 4°C using a technique developed to increase penetration of fixative. Tissue, immersed in fixative, was placed in a cooled vacuum embedder maintained at a pressure of -25 mm Hg for 20 to 30 mins. Following this procedure the tissue was immmersion fixed in 4% phosphate buffered paraformaldehyde for 3-4 weeks at 4°C, and then transferred to 25% phosphate buffered sucrose at 4°C for at least a further 3 weeks.

Reaction

Tissue blocks were frozen in liquid nitrogen, and cut using a cryostat at a thickness of 20μm. In tissue blocks from most infants adjacent sections were collected and reacted to reveal SP, VIP and BN immunoreactivity. In a further 2 infants tissue was also reacted for 5HT immunoreactivity. Tissue sections were reacted on slides using the avidin-biotin-peroxidase complex technique of Hsu et al. (1981). Briefly, this technique involves incubation of the tissue with primary antibodies directed against SP (monoclonal; Sera-Lab), VIP (polyclonal; INC), BN (polyclonal; Sera-Lab) and 5HT (monoclonal; Sera-Lab) for 18-24 h at 4°C in a humid chamber. All antibodies were diluted in phosphate buffered saline containing 0.1% Triton (PBS-Triton; pH 7.4) at the following dilutions; SP, 1:500, VIP, 1:2000, BN, 1:1500, 5HT, 1:500. Slides were then rinsed with PBS-Triton and secondary anti-IgG biotinylated antibodies applied to the tissue at a concentration of 1 in 50 for 1 h at room temperature. Slides were again rinsed with PBS-Triton and then incubated for 1 h at room temperature with avidin-peroxidase conjugate at the dilution recommended by the manufacturer (Vector Laboratories). Following the final incubation the tissue was rinsed in Tris buffer (Sigma; pH 7.6) containing 0.1% Nickel Ammonium Sulphate. The Tris-Nickel buffer was allowed to remain on the tissue for a further 20-30 mins to enhance the reaction product. In the final step sections were reacted with a solution of 5 mg diaminobenzidine hydrochloride (Sigma) and 1-2μl of H_2O_2 (Boehringer) in 10 mls of Tris-Nickel buffer. After 5-10 mins the reaction was stopped with a Tris-Nickel buffer rinse. The majority of sections were lightly counterstained with Toluidine Blue. All sections were dehydrated through graded alcohols and coverslipped from xylene.

RESULTS

General Results

All infant lung tissue examined contained SP, VIP, BN and 5HT reaction product. The density and distribution of labelling was consistent between individuals except for SP-like immunoreactivity. In two infants the density of SP labelling was considerably greater than that found in the majority of infant lung tissue, determined at a qualitative level. However the distribution pattern was similar in all infants.

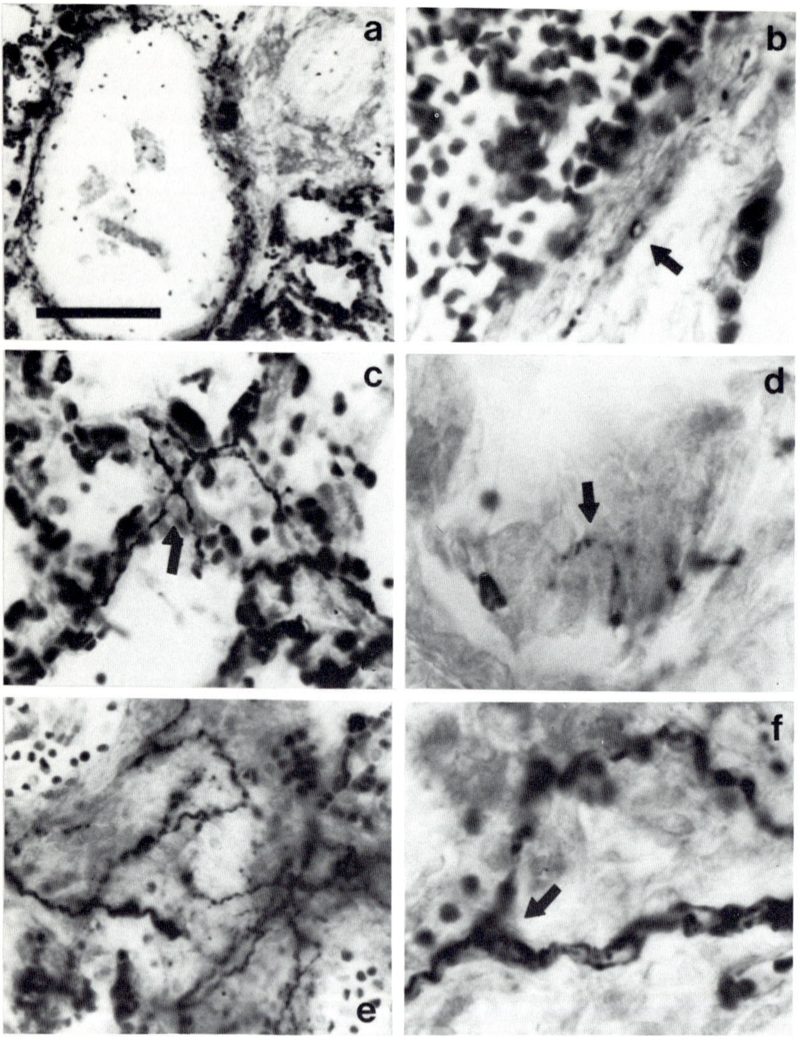

Figure 1. a) Low power view of bronchiole (left) and adjacent blood vessel (right). Note extensive SP labelling around the bronchiole. b) A single SP-IR fiber (arrow) in a blood vessel wall. c) An SP-IR fiber network (arrow) in alveolar walls. d) Fine SP-IR varicose fibers in columnar epithelium. e) Extensive SP-IR fiber network near airway bifurcation. f) SP-IR fiber bundle collateralizing (arrow). Scale bar = 50 μm in a and e, and 25 μm in b,c,d and f.

Substance P

Fiber labelling: SP fiber labelling was extensive in the bronchial walls (1A) but was relatively sparce in blood vessel walls (1B).

In the bronchi, SP immunoreactive (SP-IR) fibers were found amongst the columnar epithelial cells (1D), and extended throughout the lamina propria, airway smooth muscle and submucosa. Labelled fibers were also observed within seromucous glands. The density of fibers in the bronchi was greatest in the lamina propria and the submucosa, often forming extensive fascicles comprising of ten or more fibers (1F). These fascicles were particularly prominent at airway bifurcations (1E). Extensive fiber labelling was also found in the remainder of the airways including terminal bronchioles and the walls of the alveoli (1C).

A characteristic feature of fiber labelling throughout the airways was the complex pattern of collateralization. Parent fibers often gave rise to numerous branches which could be traced into several adjacent bronchi, bronchioles or alveolar walls (1C and 1E). In some instances entire fiber bundles would collateralize (1F).

Sparce fiber labelling was also observed in walls of medium sized blood vessels (arterioles and venules). Typically, single fibers were found within the muscle layer (1B).

Regardless of their location, SP-IR fibers were fine and bore numerous small to large varicosities (diameter 0.5 to 2.5μm).

Cell labelling: SP-IR cells were found in three locations. Within ganglia (presumably autonomic), below the epithelium within airways, and in the walls of alveoli.

In ganglia which contained reaction product most ganglion cells displayed SP immunoreactivity (2A,C). In addition, a number of small cells were SP-IR (2C-arrow). Associated with the labelled ganglia were SP-IR fibers and terminals (2A). These SP fibers formed part of fiber bundles continuous with the ganglia. Some of these fibers were seen to arise from the labelled ganglion cells. Labelled terminals were closely associated with both immunoreactive (arrow 2A) and non-immunoreactive ganglion cells.

SP-IR ganglia were consistently located in the connective tissue surrounding pulmonary arteries. In adjacent sections, reacted to reveal VIP-, BN- or 5HT-immunoreactivity no reaction product was observed.

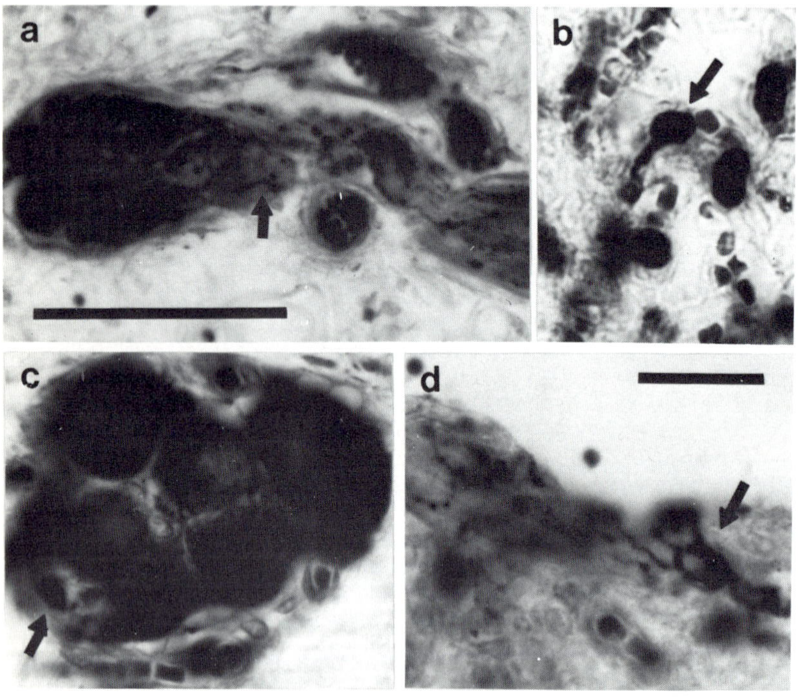

Figure 2. a) SP-IR ganglion in blood vessel connective tissue. Note SP-IR fibers and terminals (arrow) near SP-IR ganglion cells. Also shown is a fiber bundle (right) containing SP-IR fibers. b) SP-IR cell body and process in alveolar wall. c) High magnification photomicrograph of another SP-IR ganglion. Arrow indicates a small labelled cell. d) SP-IR subepithelial cell with extensive processes projecting towards the airway lumen. Both scale bars = 25 μm; b,c and d are at the same magnification.

Within airway (2D) and alveolar walls (2B) numerous cells were SP immunoreactive. Labelled cell diameters ranged from 9 to 25 μm. Those cells found in the bronchial walls were multipolar with fiber networks extending for up to 150 μm from the cell body (2D). Cells found in alveolar walls were predominantly bipolar (2B), and their processes could not be traced far from the cell body.

Some SP-IR cell bodies in bronchial walls were innervated by fibers containing SP. These fibers formed a network around the labelled cell bodies giving rise to numerous varicosities and apparent terminals as illustrated in the 3-dimensional camera lucida reconstruction in figure 3.

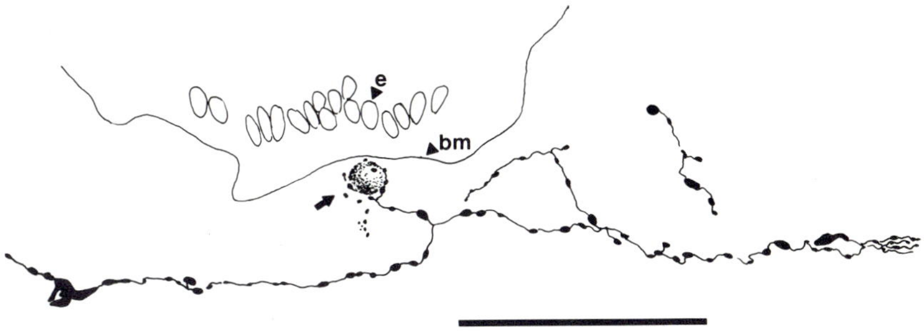

Figure 3. Camera lucida drawing showing the spatial relationship between an SP-IR subepithelial cell (arrow) and a varicose, SP-IR fiber network. e - epithelium, bm - basement membrane. Scale bar = 50 μm.

Vasoactive Intestinal Peptide

VIP labelling was localized within bronchial walls and ganglia. In the bronchial walls VIP immunoreactivity was found in most ciliated epithelial cells such that the entire airway lumen was labelled. However, labelling did not extend to the basement membrane of the epithelium (4B). In addition, fine varicose fibers were observed between columnar epithelial cells and in the basement membrane.

Reaction product in ganglia was in small cells (arrow C, 4A) and in fibers enclosing and running between non-immunoreactive ganglion cells (arrow F, 4B).

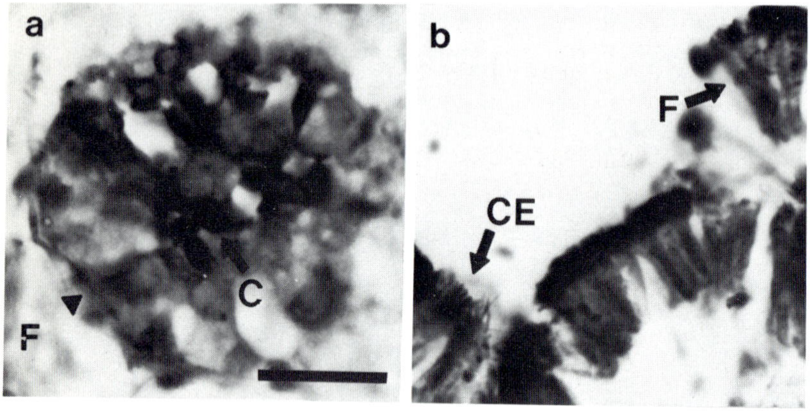

Figure 4. a) Photomicrograph showing VIP-IR structures in a ganglion. Both fibèrs (F) and small cells (C) are labelled. b) Section of labelled airway epithelium. VIP-IR is found in ciliated epithelial cells (CE) and fibers (F). Scale bar = 25 μm.

Bombesin and Serotonin

BN- and 5HT-immunoreactivity was restricted to non-ciliated bronchial epithelial cells of similar morphology. Although some of these cells were typically columnar, others were round or bipolar and oriented obliquely to the non-immunoreactive epithelium (5A). Immunoreactive cells were either found in clusters (5B, 5HT) or separately (5A, BN). Cells found separately often extended processes across as many as 20 surrounding non-immunoreactive epithelial cells. Conversely, clustered BN and 5HT immunoreactive (BN-IR, 5HT-IR) cells rarely extended their processes beyond several surrounding non-immunoreactive cells. Instead their processes were directed towards other immunoreactive cells in the cluster (5B,C). In all sections examined we found more BN- than 5HT-IR cells, regardless of airway generation.

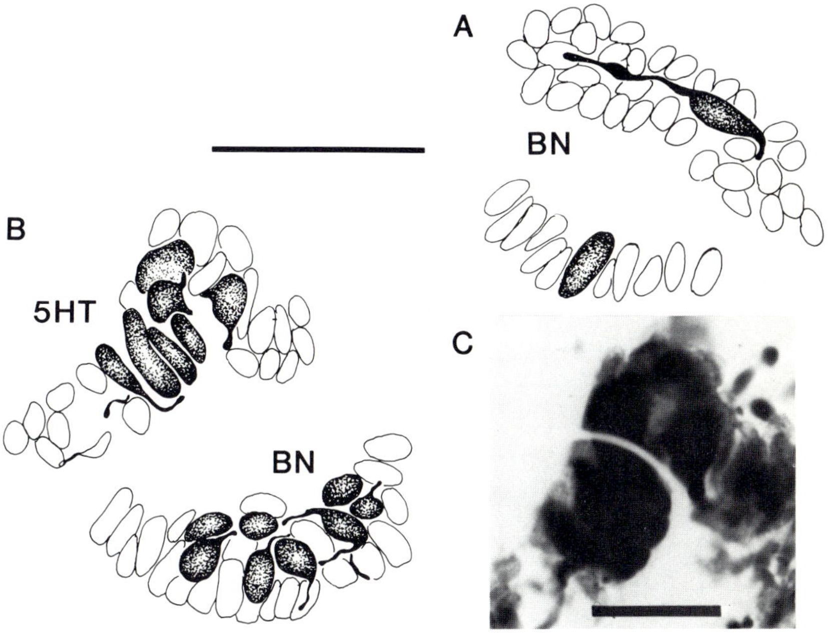

Figure 5. a) Camera lucida drawing of BN-IR solitary epithelial cells, many of which extend processes across surrounding epithelial cells. b) BN- and 5HT-IR epithelial cell clusters. Processes remain within the cluster. c) Photomicrograph of the 5HT-IR cell cluster illustrated in b. Scale bar = 50 μm in a and b and 25 μm in c.

DISCUSSION

General Discussion

In the present study we have examined SP-, VIP-, BN- and 5HT-immunoreactivity in the infant lung. This study differs from previous reports where the majority of studies have focused on adult non-human tissue (Lundberg et al., 1984, Wharton et al., 1978,1979). Because our studies are on infants with the diagnosis of SIDS, it is possible that our findings do not reflect normal lungs. However, there is no support for the hypothesis that the lungs are primarily involved in these deaths.

The interpretation of immunocytochemical data must take into account several potential sources of error. These include the possible cross-reactivity of the primary antibody, and post-mortem changes in the levels of the neurochemicals under investigation. The antibodies used in this study were obtained commercially and have either been characterized or tested, by the manufacturer, with tissue known to contain the antigen against which they have been raised.

It is conceivable that the differences in distribution of the four neurochemicals examined in this study may be due to differential rates of neurochemical decay. Findings which argue against this conclusion are that regardless of time between death and autopsy the distribution of each neurochemical was consistent in all individuals. Further, Helme (1986) has shown that between 2 and 48 hours after death SP levels remain relatively stable. The post mortem stability of VIP, BN and 5HT levels has however not been reported. Therefore, in this study, comparison of neurochemical distribution is restricted to a qualitative level.

The important findings of this study are that each of the transmitters examined have a unique distribution within infant lung tissue. SP immunoreactivity is localized in extensive fiber networks, particularly in the airways, in fibers and cells of autonomic ganglia and in small, subepithelial airway nerve cells. VIP immunoreactivity is found in ciliated epithelial cells, nerve fibers associated with epithelium, and in autonomic ganglia. BN and 5HT immunoreactivity is restricted to non-ciliated epithelial cells with BN labelled cells being more extensive.

The following are important new findings. SP immunoreactivity in infant lung is found in subepithelial airway and alveolar cells and in ganglion cells, observations which have not previously been reported. On the basis of their morphology epithelial cells which contain either BN or 5HT appear to fall into two categories. This finding is discussed in greater detail below.

The Airway Nerve Cell System

Our results clearly demonstrate that the entire lungs of infant humans have a complex network of neurons and fibers which appears, in a general sense, to be as complex and as extensive as the enteric nervous system. In the enteric nervous system of animals there is now extensive knowledge which demonstrates subpopulations of neurons on the basis of neurochemical co-localization and connectivity (Furness and Costa, 1987). In our preliminary work, a similar complex pattern is emerging, and with the four neurochemicals we have examined, two distinct morphological and neurochemical sets of cell groups have emerged.

The first cell group is found in the airway epithelium and is at least BN- and 5HT-IR but not SP-IR. This group can further be divided into two subgroups; (1) clustered cells which extend processes mainly to other immunoreactive cells within the cluster, and (2) solitary cells which are typically bipolar, are oriented obliquely to the epithelium and extend processes to numerous surrounding epithelial cells. The second cell group is subepithelial and is SP-IR but not BN-, 5HT- or VIP-IR. Such cells have not previously been described.

Our evidence suggests that group 1 and group 2 cells are interconnected via reciprocal processes as illustrated in the schematic diagram in figure 6. SP-containing fibers are present in the epithelium and in many instances it is clear that these are processes of SP-IR group 2 cells. Secondly, some group 1 cells extend their processes in subepithelial parts of the airway walls.

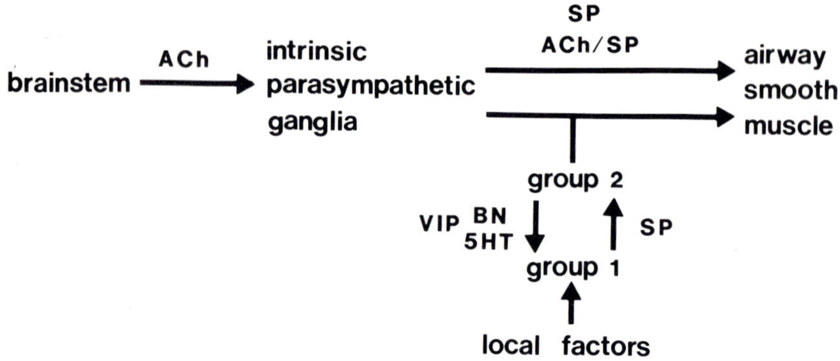

Figure 6. Schematic diagram of proposed interaction between the autonomic system and local airway nerve cells.

The group 1 and group 2 cell system appears to interact locally with the classical parasympathetic innervation of airway smooth muscle. This is based on evidence that group 2 cells are innervated by collaterals of SP-IR fibers (see fig 3) which probably originate from intrinsic parasympathetic ganglia. We have shown that most cells in such ganglia contain SP (see fig 2A,B), and further, appear to be the origin of the fibers innervating the group 2 cells and bronchial smooth muscle. Before proceeding, it is pertinent to discuss, in more detail, our results regarding the fiber connections of these SP-IR parasympathetic ganglia.

As illustrated in figure 2B, SP-IR ganglia are associated with fiber bundles. These fiber bundles consist of some SP-IR fibers but are predominantly non-immunoreactive. However, the majority of cells within any one ganglion contain SP, therefore a large proportion of preganglionic fibers must be SP-IR, presumably cholinergic. It also follows that most postganglionic fibers contain SP co-localized with acetylcholine, since the majority of cell bodies contain SP-immunoreactivity and postganglionic parasympathetics are known to be cholinergic.

The BN- and 5HT-IR epithelial cells which we identified in the airways are undoubtedly the neuroepithelial cells or bodies described extensively in the past (see Lauweryns et al.,

1972,1973). Although neuroepithelial bodies have been implicated in local sensory control between airways and blood vessels (for example as a component of local ventilation-perfusion matching by sensing airway gas composition and regulating regional blood flow) there has been no morphological evidence of how this might be achieved. Our results now provide evidence that these cells have reciprocal connections with the SP-IR subepithelial cells. The subepithelial cells are in turn innervated by SP-IR postganglionic parasympathetic fibers. Thus the group 1 and group 2 cells are part of a local neural network. The remarkable similarity of these cell groups to individual glomeruli of the carotid body is very suggestive that these are sensory receptor-like neurons which have an array of similar sensory functions.

Interaction between Autonomic Innervation and the Airway Nerve Cell System

The function of parasympathetic innervation of the lung is well established in the literature. Parasympathetic stimulation results in airway smooth muscle contraction. Recently, the role of peptides, particularly SP, in the regulation of airway smooth muscle tone has attracted much attention. In vitro, SP induces a dose-dependent contraction of human segmental bronchi (Lundberg et al., 1984). Further, studies in vivo have documented SP release in the lung (Saria et al., 1985). SP is generally thought to be located in non-myelinated afferent nerve fibers and terminals.

One current concept of how these participate in the local regulation of airway and vascular tone is that SP, and other peptides, are released when action potentials destined centrally propagate back through fiber collaterals (ie. axon reflex). The cell bodies of such afferents are located in the extrapulmonary vagal ganglia or the dorsal root ganglia of spinal thoracic nerves (Saria et al., 1985). Although many of the fibers which we have observed in the infant lung are undoubtedly afferents, our findings suggest that SP also affects the parasympathetic system at the postganglionic level. Thus SP alone or co-localized with acetylcholine in postganglionic parasympathetic fibers induces airway smooth muscle contraction. This effect may be modulated by the airway nerve cells in response to local airway stimuli such as hypoxia. A possible mechanism of action involves the stimulation of group 1 cells which we have demonstrated have reciprocal connections with group 2 cells and contain BN and 5HT. Although the physiological role of BN has not been fully elucidated, 5HT is known to be a potent bronchoconstrictor (Szarek et al., 1986) and may exert its effects via this system. Group 1 cells affect group 2 cells which are innervated by collaterals of postganglionic parasympathetic fibers. Thus by this locally mediated mechanism the airway nerve cell system is able to modify smooth muscle tone.

This study raises many questions about the role of different nerve cell types, their neurochemical content and their connectivity in lung control. For instance, what is the role of SP-IR alveolar cells? Are they group 1 or group 2 cells or a separate system? Are the VIP-IR ciliated epithelial cells part of the proposed airway nerve cell system? In vitro studies suggest that VIP reduces airway smooth muscle tone (Morice et al., 1983). Finally, it must be stressed that this study has focused on four of the many neurochemicals known to be present in lung tissue. However, it clearly demonstrates the presence of a highly organized local nervous system in the lungs just as has emerged within the enteric nervous system (Furness and Costa, 1987).

REFERENCES

Cutz,E, Gillan,JE, Track,NS. (1984) Pulmonary endocrine cells in developing human lung and during neonatal adaptation. In: Becker,KL, Gazdar,AF, (eds), The endocrine-lung in health and disease, WB Saunders Co., Philadelphia, pp 210-231.

Furness,J and Costa,M. (1987) The enteric nervous system. Livingston Churchill Press, Lond.

Ghatei,MA, Sheppard,MN, Henzenlogman,S, Blank,MA, Polak,JM, Bloom,SR. (1983) Bombesin and vasoactive intestinal polypeptide in developing lung: Marked changes in acute respiratory distress syndrome. J. Endocrinol. Metab. 57:1226-1232.

Helme,RD. (1986) Effects of autopsy delay on substance P distribution in rat spinal cord. Amer. Neurosci. S53.

Hsu,SM, Raine,L, Fanger,H. (1981) The use of avidin-biotin-peroxidase complex (ABC) in immunoperoxidase techniques: a comparison between ABC and unlabelled antibody (PAP) procedures. J. Histochem. Cytochem. 29: 577.

Lauweryns,JM, Cokelaere,M, Theunynck,P. (1972) Neuroepithelial bodies in the respiratory mucosa of various mammals. A light optical histochemical and ultrastructural investigation. Z. Zellforsch. 135:569-592.

Lauweryns,JM, Cokelaere,M. (1973) Hypoxia sensitive neuroepithelial bodies intrapulmonary secretory neuroreceptors modulated by the CNS. Z. Zellforsch. 145:521-540.

Lundberg,JM, Hökfelt,T, Martling,C-R, Saria,A, Cuello,C. (1984) Substance P-immunoreactive sensory nerves in the lower respiratory tract of various mammals including man. Cell. Tissue Res. 235:251-261.

Morice,A, Unwin,RJ, Sever,PS. (1983) Vasoactive intestinal peptide causes bronchodilation and protects against histamine-induced bronchoconstriction in asthmatic subjects. Lancet ii:1225-1226.

Saria,A, Martling,C-R, Dalsgaard,CJ, Lundberg,JM. (1985) Evidence for substance P-immunoreactive spinal afferents that mediate bronchoconstriction. Acta Physiol. Scand. 125:407-414.

Szarek,JL, Gillespie,MN, Altiere,RJ, Diamond,L. (1986) Reflex activation of the nonadrenergic noncholinergic inhibitory nervous system in feline airways. Am. Rev. Respir. Dis. 133:1159-1162.

Wharton,J, Polak,JM, Bloom,SR, Ghatei,MA, Solcia,E, Brown,MR, Pearse,AGE. (1978) Bombesin-like immunoreactivity in the lung. Nature 273:769-770.

Wharton,J, Polak,JM, Bloom,SR, Will,JA, Pearse,AGE. (1979) Substance P like immunoreactive nerves in the mammalian lung. Invest. Cell. Pathol. 2:3-10.

DISCUSSION

Daniel: I'm concerned about the use of immunoreactivity without appropriate controls, and in particular I'd like to know what controls you have to demonstrate that VIP was really in the epithelial cells as you describe. Did you do absorption and have you tried to isolate these cells and measure VIP?

Scheibner: The antibodies we use are commercially available and their specificity has been tested. In addition to that, we do several controls. One is pre-absorption with VIP to eliminate this labelling, which it does, and secondly, leaving out the primary antibody to ensure that it's not the subsequent stages of the reaction which are producing a non-specific reaction product. We haven't as yet tried to measure the content of VIP.

Daniel: Probably some people would be reluctant to accept VIP and some of these other peptides in that location until that final step is done.

Scheibner: I think regardless of exactly what we're looking at, if it is a neurochemical then this is very important, because we're looking at anatomy, at evidence of some cells, no matter what they contain, within the lung system.

Church: There is a bit of confusion in my mind between your talk with VIP and Peter Barnes' talk. According to Peter, when VIP is inhaled, it causes no bronchodilation, and yet we think of it as a bronchodilator, perhaps, following its endogenous release. Now you say that it is found only in the ciliary part of the epithelium, right out where it would be deposited, where you'd inhale it. I'd like to ask Jay, does the epithelium break down VIP in the same way that it breaks down SP?

Scheibner: Although in the epithelium we only saw it in the ciliated epithelial cells, we also saw VIP in ganglia. It wasn't in the large ganglion cells, it was rather in smaller ganglion cells.

Nadel: No, VIP is not broken down by enkephalinase at physiological concentrations, nor by tryptase.

Coburn: I just wanted to say that we found substance P in

some of the peri-tracheal ganglia as well. We can't see whether they're axons or dendrites because of the nerve density, but it's rather frequent and it's seen in most of the ganglia surrounded by VIP cell bodies.

Sparrow: I thought those were marvellous pictures you've shown, but I feel the same way, that when you've said that the substance P neurones or cell bodies stain cytochemically with substance P, have you actually shown that this antibody, monoclonal is it or polyclonal, is absolutely specific and stains nothing else, if you take out a bit of tissue and run it on a plate and do a TLC on it?

Scheibner: Yes, I assure you. It's a commercially available antibody, it's monoclonal, it's been tested and apparently it reacts with the 5-8 C fragment of substance P itself and it has a low cross-reactivity with eledoisin but no other tachykinin. If you eliminate substance P, if you preabsorb the antibody with substance P, you don't get any labelling.

Kerrebijn: In your abstract you suggest that the substance P fibres are more dense in asthmatic lung than in non-asthmatic lung. My question is, what about chronic bronchitis and cystic fibrosis, diseases in which chronic airway inflammation takes place, in which enkephalins may be broken down more substantially so that it may well be that the substance P-producing system is hypertrophic?

Scheibner: We haven't yet looked at any other tissue, but are in the process.

Nadel: I want to defend the paper. I think it's different from what other people describe, but I think it's spectacular and it meets the criteria (in 1987) as far as I'm concerned, with specific quenching, with a reasonably characterized antibody, and anatomic loci, and I think that the major advantage that Dr Scheibner has is that she has available tissue that's reasonably fresh. In looking at the sections, these cells aren't all sloughed away, as are most tissues that most of us see and use, and I would say that, until proven otherwise, the question for us is to figure out what it means physiologically.

Barnes: I thought it was an extremely interesting presentation and of course it does mean that cutting the vagus nerve or giving a ganglion blocker like hexamethonium can't by any means exclude neural mechanisms in hyperreactivity. If, as you suggest in the abstract, this system is increased in asthma, that there are more of these nerves or they have more of the peptide, that supports the idea that axon reflexes may be important in the human airway. Very few people would actually support that view at present, they say it's found in rodents but not in humans. I think your paper has really revived the idea that nerves could be very important in human asthma.

Mechanisms in Asthma: Pharmacology,
Physiology, and Management, pages 149–157

FACTORS WHICH MODIFY NEURAL CONTROL OF THE AIRWAY

Jennifer Maclagan

Pharmacology Department, Royal Free Hospital
Medical School, Rowland Hill Street, London NW3

The dominant control of airway diameter is considered to be exerted by the parasympathetic nerves which release acetylcholine (Ach) onto the post-junctional muscarinic receptors on the smooth muscle cell. Modulation of the transmitter output from these nerves should be considered as an important mechanism which could alter airway reactivity in vivo. This paper will consider the effect of neurotransmitters, autocoids and neuropeptides on pulmonary parasympathetic neurotransmsission.

The parasympathetic nerves innervating the lung probably originate in the nucleus ambiguus and descend in the vagi to synapse in small ganglia located in an extensive nerve plexus within the airway walls: short postganglionic fibres supply airway smooth muscle, and gland cells (Richardson, 1979; Baker et al, 1982).

GANGLIONIC MODULATION

During spontaneous inspiration the preganglionic nerves supplying airway smooth muscle fire at 25 Hz in synchrony with the burst of impulses in the phrenic nerve. This rhythm may be determined by mechanisms operating within the CNS (Mitchell et al, 1984). Alternatively, the firing rate may be modulated at the ganglionic level by the slow inhibitory post-synaptic potential which is mediated via muscarinic receptors.

α and β-adrenoceptros have been demonstrated in pulmonary parasympathetic ganglia but they are not innervated in all species suggesting that the sympathetic nervous system may not be an important modulator of activity in the parasympathetic ganglia.

Peptidergic neurones may exert an excitatory modulating action on ganglionic transmission in the parasympathetic nerves as removal of the peptide containing fibres by capsaicin pre-treatment reduced the bronchoconstrictor response elicited by pre-ganglionic vagal nerve stimulation in vivo (Martling et al, 1984). This effect was not due to an action on the parasympathetic nerve terminals or on the muscarinic receptors of airway smooth muscle, as contractile responses elicited by transmural stimulation or by exogenous Ach were unaltered ex vivo.

PRE-JUNCTIONAL MODULATION

The final terminals of the post-ganglionic parasympathetic nerves are an important site for modulation of transmission to airway smooth muscle by neurotransmitters, neuropeptides and local hormones.

Muscarinic Receptors

Work in my laboratory has demonstrated the existence of pre-junctional muscarinic receptors on the postganglionic neurones of the pulmonary parasympathetic nerves using the selective muscarinic antagonist gallamine to reveal the presence of the receptors. These receptors have been found in two species, the guinea-pig (Fryer et al, 1984) and the cat (Blaber et al, 1985) but do not appear to be present in rat or rabbit lung (Maclagan et al, 1987b).

These neuronal autoreceptors have an inhibitory function and stimulation with a muscarinic agonist such as Ach or pilocarpine reduces transmitter output (Faulkner et al, 1986). In contrast, blockade of the receptors with gallamine enhances transmitter release resulting in potentiation of the bronchoconstriction induced by vagal nerve stimulation.

The potentiation of vagally induced bronchoconstriction produced by gallamine was dependent on dose and on the frequency of stimulation so that the effect of vagal stimulation in the lung was increased tenfold by a dose of 10mg/kg at a frequency rate of 15Hz. In the heart however the effect of gallamine was unrelated to frequency as the cardiac receptors are located post-junctionally and are not modulating transmitter output (Fryer et al, 1984).

Potentiation of vagally-induced bronchoconstriction induced by gallamine was unrelated to any involvement of the sympathetic nervous system as pretreatment with guanethidine did not affect the results. Neither could the results be explained by an alteration of airway contractility as histamine-induced bronchoconstriction was unaltered by gallamine.

These results suggested that muscarinic receptors exist on the pulmonary parasympathetic nerves and exert an inhibitory effect on transmitter output. The receptors appear to be located on the postganglionic parasympathetic neurones innervating the trachea and bronchioles (prejunctional site) for the effect of gallamine could also be demonstrated when the nerves were excited by DMPP in vivo, or by transmural stimulation in vitro (Faulkner et al, 1986). The latter finding suggests that it should be possible to use this method to show the presence or absence of these receptors in human airway tissues.

Gallamine had little effect on the post-junctional muscarinic receptors in airway smooth muscle shown by lack of effect on the bronchoconstriction induced by intravenous injection of Ach (Fryer et al, 1987a). However, the other muscarinic antagonists such as atropine, pancuronium, pirenzipine (Maclagan et al, 1986) and the antimuscarinic bronchodilator, ipratropium (Fryer et al, 1987b), had post-junctional effects. Despite this effect, potentiation of vagally-induced bronchoconstriction could be demonstrated with all of these drugs.

The degree of potentiation depended on the balance between their pre- and post-junctional antagonist potency so that gallamine caused a six to ten-fold potentiation, pirenzipine and ipratropium doubled the response and the effect of atropine was jest detectable (Fryer et al, 1987a).

Figure 1 shows the location of muscarinic receptors in the autonomic nerves supplying the lungs compiled from results

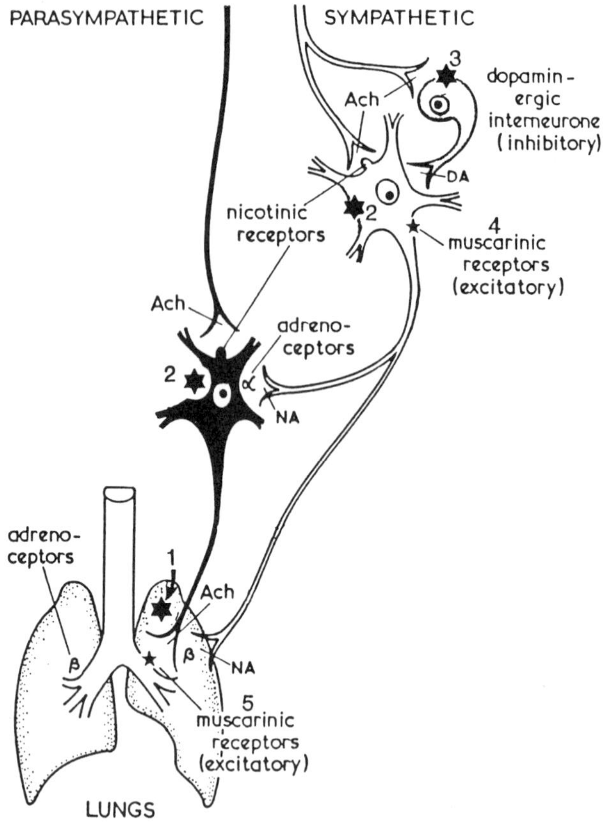

Figure 1: Location of inhibitory (✱) and excitatory muscarinic receptors at five sites in the pulmonary autonomic innervation.

obtained in my laboratory and by extrapolation from results reported for the ganglia innervating other organs. The majority of these muscarinic receptors have an inhibitory effect on the cell bearing them, (large asteriks), and gallamine is an antagonist for many of these receptors. The exceptions to this are the excitatory muscarinic receptors on the sympathetic ganglion cells which mediate the slow EPSP (Ashe & Yarosh, 1984) and the receptors on airway smooth muscle (these receptors are indicated by the small asteriks in the figure).

Gallamine is considered to be a selective antagonist for the cardiac muscarinic receptors which are usually classified as belonging to the M2 subclass. It has also been shown to block the receptors at site 1, 2 and 3 in Fig 1 so these receptors should probably be classified as M2 receptors. Pirnzepine, at low doses, is known to be a selective antagonist for M1 receptors in the CNS and in ganglia so that potentiation of vagally-induced bronchoconstriction obtained with this drug suggests the existence of M1 receptors. The effect of pirenzipine, however, unlike the effects of the other antagonists, was abolished by pre-treatment with propranolol, and this suggests that the M1 receptors must lie in the sympathetic neural pathway and have an excitatory function (Site 4). Thus these receptors would be comparable to the muscarinic receptors demonstrated in the superior cervical ganglia in the rabbit (Ashe & Yarosh, 1984). These results also suggest that under the conditions used in the guinea-pig exiperiments, the sympathetic nerves are exerting a tonic inhibitory influence on the parasympathetic nerve terminals (Maclagan et al, 1987b).

The muscarinic receptors on airway smooth muscle (Site 5) probably belong to a third class, comparable to the receptors on intestinal smooth muscle but there is, at present, no agreement on the nomenclature which should be used to describe these receptors which have been classified as M_3, M_4 or as a subdivision of subtype M_2.

Effect Of Autacoids, Local Hormones And Catecholamines

Many autocoids and local hormones can be released from lung tissue during inflammatory responses or by immunological challenge and some of them modify transmission in the prejunctional terminals of the pulmonary parasympathetic nerves. For example, trachealis muscle contractions elicited by electrical field stimulation are decreased by histamine and 5-HT (McCaig, 1986), and by PGE2 (Walters et al, 1984; Ito and Tajima, 1981). The response to exogenous Ach was unaffected by these substances indicating that the effects were due to an action on prejunctional nerve terminals.

Transmission in these terminals can also be reduced by sympathetic nerve stimulation and β-adrenoceptors are implicated. This indicates that the sympathetic nerves may impinge on the parasympathetic nerve terminals in some species. This possibility is included in Figure 1.

In contrast, potentiation of transmission in the parasympathetic nerve terminals has been reported for the stable thromboxane mimetic U46619 (Chung et al, 1985) and for the tachykinin neuropeptides, especially neurokinins A (Barnes et al, 1987). In the case of the tachykinins, the experimental conditions were critical and the potentiating response increased at submaximal voltages.

Post-Junctional Modulation

Leukotrienes also potentiate nerve-induced responses but in this case the effect is due to a post-junctional action on the smooth muscle cell. Ach-induced contraction was increased but the contractile responses to histamine were unaltered indicating that the process involved is secondary to muscarinic receptor activation (Maclagan et al, 1987a).

CONCLUSIONS

The final terminals of the pulmonary parasympathetic nerves innervating airway smooth muscle appear to be susceptible to attack by neurotransmitters, neuropeptides, local hormones and autacoids. The effects of the inflammatory mediators on the parasympathetic nerve terminals are relatively minor, however, compared with the inhibitory feedback effects of the cholinergic transmitter on prejunctional muscarinic autoreceptors. This suggests that the autoreceptor mechanism plays an important role in modulating parasympathetic neurotransmission, both at rest and during reflex activation of the nerves. Changes in this mechanism could be implicated in the hyperactivity of airway smooth muscle which occurs during inflammation and asthma.

REFERENCES

Ashe JH, Yarosh CA (1984). Differential and selective antagonism of the slow-inhibitory-post-synaptic potential and slow-excitatory-post-synaptic potential by gallamine and pirenzepine in the superior cervical ganglion of the rabbit. Neuropharmacology 23:1321-9.

Baker DG, Basbaum CB, Herbert DA, Mitchell RA (1983). Transmission in airway ganglia of ferrets: inhibition by noradrenaline. Neurosci Lett 41:139-143.

Baker DG, Basbaum CB, Herbert DA, Mitchell RA (1983). Transmission in airway ganglia of ferrets: inhibition by noradrenaline. Neurosci Lett 41:139-143.

Baker DG, Herbert DA, Mitchell RA (1982). Cholinergic neurotransmission in airway ganglia: inhibition by noradrenaline. Physiologist 25:225.

Barnes PJ, Maclagan J, Meldrum LA (1987). Effect of tachykinins on cholinergic neural responses in guinea-pig trachea. Br J Pharmacol 90:138P.

Blaber LC, Fryer AD, Maclagan J (1985). Neuronal muscarinic receptors attenuate vagally-induced contraction of feline bronchial smooth muscle. Br J Pharmac 86:723-728.

Chung KF, Evans TW, Graf PD, Nadel JA (1985). Modulation of cholinergic neurotransmission in canine airways by thromboxane mimetic U46619. Eur J Pharmacol 117:373-5.

Faulkner D, Fryer AD, Maclagan J (1986). Postganglionic muscarinic inhibitory receptors in pulmonary parasympathetic nerves in the guinea-pig. Br J Pharmacol 88:181-7.

Fryer AD, Maclagan J (1984). Muscarinic inhibitory receptors in pulmonary parasympathetic nerves in the guinea-pig. Br J Pharmac 83:973-978.

Fryer AD, Maclagan J (1987a). Pancuronium and gallamine are antagonists for pre- and post-junctional muscarinic receptors in the guinea-pig lung. Naunyn-Schmiedeberg's Arch Pharmacol 335:367-371.

Fryer AD, Maclagan J (1987b). Ipratropium bromide potentiates bronchoconstriction induced by vagal nerve stimulation in the guinea-pig. Eur J Pharmacol 139:187-191.

Ito Y, Tajima K (1981). Spontaneous activity in the trachea of dogs treated with indomethacin: an experimental model for aspirin-related asthma. Br J Pharmacol 73:563-71.

McCaig D (1986). Autonomic responses of the isolated innervated trachea of the guinea-pig: interaction with autonomic drugs, histamine and 5-hydroxytryptamine. Br J Pharmacol 88:239-48.

Maclagan J, Faulkner D (1987 a). Leukotrienes potentiates parasympathetic neurotransmission in guinea-pig trachea by pre- and post-junctional mechanisms. Br J Pharmacol 91:368P.

Maclagan J, Fryer AD, Faulkner D (1987b). Proceedings Xth International Congress of Pharmacology Sydney Australia: P1348.

Martling C, Saria A, Andersson P, Lundberg JM (1984). Capsaicin pre-treatment inhibits vagal cholinergic and non-cholinergic control of pulmonary mechanics in the guinea-pig. Naunyn Schmeidebergs Arch Pharmacol 325:343-8.

Mitchell RA, Baker CB, Basbaum DG, Herbert DA (1984). In vivo recording from tracheal parasympathetic ganglia. Physiologist 26:A37

Richardson JB (1979). Nerve supply to the lungs. Am Rev Respir Dis 119:785-802.

Walters EH, O'Byrne PM, Fabbi LM, Graf PD, Holtzman MJ, Nadel JA. Control of neurotransmission by prostaglandins in canine trachealis smooth muscle. J Appl Physiol 57:129-34

DISCUSSION

Barnes: Encouraged by your work, we've looked at this in human bronchi in vitro, and we can clearly demonstrate these inhibitory muscarinic receptors which are activated by pilocarpine and blocked by gallamine and AFDX116, and they are so powerful they can switch off completely the cholinergic nerve stimulation. We've also been able to demonstrate this in vivo in normal individuals in which pilocarpine is able to shut off sulphur dioxide-induced bronchoconstriction, which is a vagal reflex. We have some preliminary evidence that asthmatics don't have this capacity to shut off acetylcholine, so that could be a defect which could lead to hyperresponsiveness.

Maclagan: I'm delighted you did it in man, especially as you were the first person to say that this was a guinea-pig phenomenon. I should have mentioned that we cannot show these autoreceptors in rabbit nerves nor in the rat, but we can show them in the cat and the guinea-pig; it's very species-dependent.

Paterson: In your experiment where you looked at ipratropium, initially it potentiated and then it blocked, but you explained the reason for that. It clarifies a lot of confusion about treatment using anti-cholinergics. Do you think that this level of vagal bronchoconstriction varies much in your animals? Is the turn-around point variable, suggesting variable vagal tone in different animals?

Maclagan: No it isn't, but my animals have no spontaneous vagal tone as I've cut the vagi. You're thinking of humans where you have reflex activation of the vagi, that is more difficult to work with. Our animals do not vary much because there is no vagal tone, they're very consistent. I know Stephen Holgate thinks that the untoward bronchospasms that have been reported with ipratropium in man are due to the solvent or the preservative, but I think there is room to continue to think that any drug which acts pre-junctionally, if given in a low dose or if the airways are full of mucus, when the drug is given by inhalation, might cause bronchospasms. Homeopathic doses of ipratropium are not a good idea.

de Jongste: We have looked at the effect of leukotriene C_4 on human central airways in vitro with field stimulation, and we did not find potentiation of the cholinergic response, but we did find an inhibition of the non-adrenergic inhibitory component. Do you think that this could also have happened in your preparation, which also has such an inhibitory component, I expect?

Maclagan: I have no evidence in my preparation that I'm exciting the non-adrenergic inhibitory component. All the contractions I get are abolished by atropine, and of course the in vitro preparation of the guinea-pig has no spontaneous tone, so there is nothing to relax. The conditions are quite different.

Mechanisms in Asthma: Pharmacology,
Physiology, and Management, pages 159–166

ADENOSINE IN ASTHMATIC LUNG

Martin K. Church and Stephen T. Holgate

Immunopharmacology Research Group, Centre Block, Southampton General Hospital, Southampton SO9 4XY, U.K.

RELEASE OF ADENOSINE

Adenosine is a naturally occurring purine nucleoside which has a ubiquitous presence in human tissues. The catabolism of high energy adenosine phosphates such as adenosine 5′-tri- and di-phosphates (ATP and ADP) and adenosine-3′,5′-cyclic monophosphate (cyclic AMP) results in the formation of intracellular adenosine-5′-mono-phosphate (AMP). When sufficient oxygen and energy is available AMP is normally reconverted to high energy phosphates as an economical component of the energy cycle. However, in cases of excessive cell stimulation or hypoxia, when oxygen and energy utilization exceeds its supply, AMP is transported to the exterior of the cell where it is metabolized to adenosine by the enzyme 5′-nucleotidase. This extracellular adenosine may then re-enter the cell by a facilitated transport mechanism which may be blocked by dipyridamole, or be metabolized via the purine metabolism pathway to uric acid.

The transient increase in adenosine in the local environment during negative energy or oxygen balance may be perceived by other cells which may then modify their metabolism or function accordingly. This occurs following stimulation of purinoceptors of which the most well characterized are the A_1- and A_2-receptors coupled to adenylate cyclase (Londos *et al.*, 1980). A_1-receptor stimulation inhibits adenylate cyclase activation whilst A_2-receptor stimulation stimulates the enzyme. The release of adenosine during oxygen insufficiency in cardiac muscle induces A_2-receptor mediated dilation of the blood vessels of the heart to increase the supply of oxygen and nutrients to the local environment (Berne, 1980). Similarly, stimulation of A_1-receptors on nerves decreases their firing rate thus protecting them during times of energy deprivation (Phillis, 1979). These observations have given rise to the theory that adenosine is a defensive autacoid which serves to protect tissues against the effects of metabolic deficiency.

Asthma may represent such a case of metabolic distress. Stimulation of cells within the lung for mediator secretion as in the case of mast cells or other inflammatory cells, or contraction, as is the case of bronchial smooth muscle, increases energy and oxygen demand. Conversely the bronchoconstriction which occurs will decrease the oxygen supply and possible the supply of nutrients, particularly to the contracted smooth muscle. It did not surprise us, therefore, to find an increase in circulating adenosine levels in patients following bronchial provocation with either allergen or the bronchoconstrictor agent, methacholine (Mann *et al.*, 1986a). These results are supported by the *in vitro* observations in rat or dog lung tissue, mouse mast cells and human leukocytes that hypoxia or activation with antigen or calcium ionophore results in increased adenosine accumulation in the extracellular fluid (Mentzer *et al.*, 1975; Fredholm, 1981; Marquardt *et al.*, 1984a; Mann *et al.*, 1986b).

ACTIONS OF ADENOSINE IN ASTHMA

Inhalation of adenosine by asthmatic subjects causes a rapid and profound bronchoconstriction which is not evident following inhalation of the related purine nucleoside guanosine or the initial adenosine metabolite, inosine (Cushley *et al.*, 1983). Interestingly, however, adenosine did not cause bronchoconstriction in non-asthmatic non-allergic subjects, but the use of high concentrations of the purine nucleoside was limited by its poor solubility (Cushley *et al.*, 1983). To overcome this practical problem subjects were asked to inhale AMP which is rapidly converted to adenosine by the cell surface enzyme, 5'-nucleotidase. A necessary pre-requisite to this experiment was to compare the effects of inhaled adenosine and AMP and satisfy ourselves that the effects correlated one with the other ($r = 0.83$, $p<0.01$) (Mann *et al.*, 1987a). The effects of inhaled AMP with methacholine in asthmatic subjects, allergic non-asthmatic subjects and in non-asthmatic non-allergic (normal) subjects were then compared (Cushley *et al.*, 1987). We found that methacholine caused bronchoconstriction in all subjects but was approximately 10 times more potent in asthmatics when compared to the other two groups suggesting its activity to be related to non-specific airways hyper-reactivity. A different pattern emerged with AMP. All asthmatic subjects responded with a profound broncho-constriction whereas the non-allergic normals showed little or no response. The allergic non-asthmatic group, however, showed intermediate responsiveness to AMP. This suggests that, unlike methacholine where the degree of bronchial hyper-responsiveness is the sole determinant of sensitivity to the provocant, an additional factor associated with the allergic state also plays a role in determining the sensitivity of subjects to AMP.

INVESTIGATIONS INTO THE MECHANISM OF ADENOSINE INDUCED BRONCHOCONSTRICTION

When considering the mechanisms by which adenosine causes bronchoconstriction, it was first necessary to establish whether it is likely to be a direct interaction of the purine nucleoside with bronchial smooth muscle or whether its effects are mediated through the assistance of an intermediate cell. The observation that its effects were more closely related to the allergic state than to non-specific bronchial hyper-responsiveness suggests that a direct effect on the bronchial musculature is unlikely (Cushley *et al.*, 1987). This is supported by studies on human bronchus where adenosine is only a weak and inconsistent contractile agonist (Church *et al.*, 1986). Furthermore, if asthmatic individuals are subjected to two AMP provocations one hour apart, the second fails to elicit a significant bronchoconstriction (Daxun *et al.*, 1987). This tachyphylaxis, which is not seen in smooth muscle experiments *in vitro*, is a phenomenon similar to the refractory period between two exercise challenges where hyperosmolar activation of luminal mast cells has been suggested as the stimulus for bronchoconstriction (Belcher *et al.*, 1986). Evidence that adenosine-induced bronchoconstriction is not neurally mediated derives from the failure of muscarinic blockade with ipratropium bromide to block bronchoconstriction (Mann *et al.*, 1985).

The hypothesis that adenosine may induce or enhance mast cell mediator secretion is supported by the ability of sodium cromoglycate and nedocromil to inhibit bronchoconstriction (Cushley and Holgate, 1985; Crimi *et al.*, 1986). Also, terfenadine and astemizole, two potent and selective but chemically unrelated H_1-receptor antagonists, inhibit AMP-induced bronchoconstriction by more than 85% (Rafferty *et al.*, 1987). The extent of inhibition by H_1-antagonists, together with the observation that AMP- induced bronchoconstriction is not associated with late asthmatic reactions (Phillips and Holgate, unpublished observations) suggests that the response is due to the selective release of preformed but not newly generated mast cell mediators. This is supported by the *in vitro* studies in rodent cultured mast cells performed by Marquardt *et al.* (1984b).

The precise mechanism by which adenosine exacerbates histamine release from mast cells is not clearly understood. Incubation of mast cells with adenosine or its analogues does not result in histamine release *per se* but is capable of modulating histamine release induced by allergen (Hughes *et al.*, 1984; Church *et al.*, 1986). In human mast cells precincubation of mast cells with adenosine before allergen challenge results in an inhibition of histamine release (Hughes *et al.*, 1984). At least three mechanisms are involved with this effect: these are an A_2-purinoceptor mediated effect on adenylate cyclase (Hughes *et al.*, 1984), an inhibitory effect on adenylate mediated via P-site activation (Hughes and Church, 1986) and an interaction of adenosine with S-adenosylmethionine-dependent methylation reactions (Hughes *et al.*, 1987). When added after challenge i.e. when mediator release has already been initiated, then adenosine enhances mediator release. In human mast cells, unlike rat mast cells (Church *et al.*, 1986), this effect appears to be mediated through the A_2-purinoceptor and adenylate cyclase stimulation (Hughes *et al.*, 1983; 1984). Such a mechanism would be consistent with the observations in man that the cell surface purinoceptor antagonist theophylline (Cushley *et al.*, 1984) inhibits the broncho-constrictor effect of adenosine whereas dipyridamole, an inhibitor of the facilitated uptake of adenosine into cells (Cushley *et al.*, 1986), does not inhibit the action of adenosine.

CONCLUSION

We conclude from our studies that adenosine enhances the release of preformed mediators from luminal mast cells in the bronchi in asthma. The mechanism by which it does this is clearly dependent upon an action by the mast cell adenylate cyclase receptor, however the precise mechanism of this interaction is not yet apparent. The ability of anti-asthmatic drugs such as sodium cromoglycate, nedocromil and theophylline to inhibit the effects of adenosine may contribute to, but not explain in total, their beneficial effects in asthma.

ACKNOWLEDGEMENTS

We would like to thank all our colleagues, particularly Drs. M.J. Cushley and J.S. Mann, whose endeavours have made the preparation of this manuscript possible. This study was supported in part by a grant from the Medical Research Council.

REFERENCES

Belcher NG, Rees PJ, Clark TJH, Lee TH (1986). Asthma precipitated by exercise and hyperosmolar aerosol may have similar mechanisms [Abstract]. J Allergy Clin Immunol 77(Suppl): 163.

Berne RM (1980). The role of adenosine in coronary blood flow. Circ Res 47: 807-813.

Church MK, Featherstone RL, Cushley MJ, Mann JS, Holgate ST (1986). Relationship between adenosine, cyclic nucleotides and xanthines in asthma. J Allergy Clin Immunol 78: 670-676.

Church MK, Hughes PJ, Vardey CJ (1986). Studies on the receptor mediating cyclic AMP-independent enhancement by adenosine of IgE-dependent mediator release from rat mast cells. Br J Pharmacol 87: 233-242.

Crimi N, Palermo F, Oliveri R, Cacopardo B, Vancheri C, Mistretta A (1986). Adenosine-induced bronchoconstriction: comparison between nedocromil and sodium cromoglycate. Eur J Respir Dis 69 (Suppl 147): 158-162.

Cushley MJ, Chan WN, Holgate ST (1987). Airway effects of inhaled adenosine 5'-monophosphate: Relationship to adenosine- and methacholine-induced bronchoconstriction in normal and asthmatic subjects. Am Rev Respir Dis In Press.

Cushley MJ, Holgate ST (1985). Adenosine induced broncho constriction in asthma: role of mast cell mediator release. J Allergy Clin Immunol 75: 272-278.

Cushley MJ, Tallant N, Holgate ST (1986). The effect of single dose intravenous dipyridamole on histamine- and adenosine-induced bronchoconstriction in normal and asthmatic subjects. Eur J Respir Dis 86: 185-192.

Cushley MJ, Tattersfield AE, Holgate ST (1983). Inhaled adenosine and guanosine on airway resistance in normal and asthmatic subjects. Br J Clin Pharmacol 15: 161-165.

Cushley MJ, Tattersfield AE, Holgate ST (1984). Adenosine induced bronchoconstriction in asthma: antagonism by inhaled theophylline. Am Rev Respir Dis 129: 380-384.

Daxun Z, Rafferty P, Richards R, Holgate ST (1987). Airway refractoriness to the bronchoconstrictor effect of inhaled adenosine 5' monosphosphate. Clin Sci 73(Suppl.17): 4P.

Fredholm BB (1981). The release of adenosine from rat lung by antigen and compound 48/80. Acta Physiol Scand 111: 507-508.

Hughes PJ, Benyon RC, Church MK (1987). Adenosine inhibits IgE-dependent histamine secretion from human basophil leukocytes by two independent mechanisms. J Pharmacol Exp Ther In Press.

Hughes PJ, Church MK (1986). Inhibition of immunological and non-immunological histamine release from human basophils by adenosine analogues that act at P-sites. Biochem Pharmacol 35: 1809-1816.

Hughes PJ, Holgate ST, Church MK (1984). Adenosine inhibits and potentiates IgE-dependent histamine release from human lung mast cells by an A2-purinoceptor mediated mechanism. Biochem Pharmacol 33: 3847-3852.

Hughes PJ, Holgate ST, Roath ST, Church MK (1983). The relationship between cyclic AMP changes and histamine release from basophil-enriched human leucocytes. Biochem Pharmacol 32: 2557-2563.

Londos C, Cooper DMF, Wolff J (1980). Subclasses of external adenosine receptors. Proc Natl Acad Sci USA 77: 2551-2554.

Mann JS, Cushley MJ, Holgate ST (1985). Adenosine-induced bronchoconstriction in asthma: role of parasympathetic stimulation and adrenergic inhibition. Am Rev Respir Dis 132: 1-6.

Mann JS, Holgate ST, Renwick AG, Cushley MJ (1986). Airway effects of purine nucleosides and nucleotides and release with bronchial provocation in asthma. J Appl Physiol 61: 1667-1676.

Mann JS, Renwick AG, Holgate ST (1986). Release of adenosine and its metabolites from activated human leucocytes. Clin Sci 70: 461-468.

Marquardt DL, Gruber HE, Wasserman SI (1984). Adenosine release from stimulated mast cells. Proc Natl Acad Sci USA 81: 6192-6196.

Marquardt DL, Walker LL, Wasserman SI (1984). Adenosine receptors on mouse bone marrow-derived mast cells: functional significance and regulation by aminophylline. J Immunol 133: 932-937.

Mentzer RM, Rubio R, Berne RM (1975). Release of adenosine from hypoxic canine lung tissue and its possible role in the pulmonary circulation. Am J Physiol 229: 1625-1631.

Phillis JW (1979). Diazepam potentiation of purinergic depression of central neurones. Can J Physiol Pharmacol 57: 432-435.

Rafferty P, Beasley CR, Holgate ST (1987). The contribution of histamine to bronchoconstriction produced by inhaled allergen and adenosine 5'-monophosphate in asthma. Am Rev Respir Dis In Press.

DISCUSSION

Barnes: In the study looking at effects of adenosine in allergic non-asthmatics, allergic asthmatics and normals, were the allergic non-asthmatics hay fever sufferers? Have you looked at non-allergic asthmatics?

Church: Yes, they had hay fever. Adenosine works in non-allergic asthmatics but not as well. You need a higher provoking dose of adenosine in non-allergic asthmatics.

Barnes: What is your explanation for that? You were suggesting that the allergy rather than the asthma is important for adenosine sensitivity.

Church: That seems to be true, but the question is, is there mast cell involvement in non-allergic asthma too? If this is the case, then we have to extend the "allergy" bracket to asthmatics who may have mediator hypersensitivity, leaky or twitchy mast cells. This has been suggested for exercise-induced asthma, for which there is no known allergy phenomena. Some experiments at the moment suggest that adenosine is cross-tachyphylactic with exercise.

Temple: You just made light of the relevance of histamine release from human mast cells, but you do mention it in your abstract. The problem I have with this is that when you add your adenosine before challenge you get a reduction in release, and when you add it after challenge you get an enhancement of release which was not very great. Also guinea-pigs, rats and man all act differently. I have problems with your histamine release from mast cells.

Church: So do I, this is why I didn't illustrate it in great detail. In vivo I think the evidence with histamine is fairly conclusive, and cromoglycate supports the theory. But in vitro, we are trying to work out the mechanism. At present we are doing experiments in which we're looking at the effect of adrenaline on mast cells, which is downgrading the histamine release in response to antigen, and adenosine is doing some very peculiar things. We think now that there is a modulation of histamine release by a third factor, it's not a direct effect. I agree with you.

O'Byrne: Only about fifty percent or less of allergic asthmatics who get an immediate response get a late response. You showed us that inhaled adenosine gave an immediate response but no late response. Was that done in people who get a late response to allergen?

Church: Yes it was. In our experience, often the late response depends on how much antigen you can get into them and the severity of the immediate response, but I think that's a separate discussion. They were people who gave a late response to antigen, and it was these same people we used.

Mechanisms in Asthma: Pharmacology, Physiology, and Management, pages 167–176

EFFECTS OF INFLAMMATORY MEDIATORS ON NEUROMUSCULAR TRANSMISSION IN CANINE TRACHEA *IN VITRO*

E.E. Daniel, R. Serio, J. Jury, M. Pashley and P. O'Byrne[+]

Departments of Neurosciences and [+]Medicine, McMaster University, Faculty of Health Sciences, Hamilton, Ontario, Canada L8N 3Z5

INTRODUCTION

Exposure to ozone produces acute hyperresponsiveness of canine airway to inhaled bronchoconstrictors such as acetylcholine or histamine (2,7,10) which seems to be mediated by release of attractants for neutrophils and other cell types from the inflamed airways (8,12,13), migration of these and other immune cells into the airway which may be caused by release of platelet activating factor (PAF), or leukotriene B_4 (LTB_4) (1,3,14). If thromboxane A_2 (TxA_2) formation or action are blocked, airway hyper-responsiveness to ozone, PAF or LBT_4 does not occur (1,3,14). Therefore TXA_2 formation may be part of the final common pathway for this response to ozone in dogs. Airway hyperresponsiveness to inhaled acetylcholine *in vivo* is accompanied by a transitory hyperresponsiveness of tracheal muscle *in vitro*, characterized by increased responsiveness to field stimulation of acetylcholine release, but not by a similar increase in responsiveness to exogenous acetylcholine (18).

The objective of this study was to determine which of the immune mediators involved in hyperresponsiveness to ozone might have direct effects on airway smooth muscle which could account for the observed hyperresponsiveness *in vitro*.

METHODS

The production of ozone effects were carried out as described in detail elsewhere (1,3,7,8,12,13,14,18). In brief, dogs were anesthetized with pentobarbital (30 mg/kg). After a baseline total pulmonary resistance (RL) was determined, a dose-response curve to acetylcholine aerosols was obtained and the acetylcholine provocative acetylcholine to increase RL by 5 cm H_2O.L.S above baseline). Dogs were exposed to O_3 at a concentration of 3 ppm for 30 min. Then the dose-response curve to acetylcholine was repeated. Control animals were treated similarly, but received an inhalation of air instead of ozone. Immediately after completion of the second acetylcholine dose-response curve, the animals were killed with an overdose of pentobarbital (65 mg/kg) and the lungs removed for structural (14) and functional studies (5,198.

For electrophysiological study, trachea was removed from dogs large enough to provide a 1.5 mm x 2.5 cm long strip. This was dissected off at room temperature after careful removal of mucosa, in oxygenated Krebs Ringer (KR) Solution (Composition in mM: NaCl, 115.5; $NaHCO_3$, 21.9; NaH_2PO_4, 1.6; $CaCl_2$, 2.5; KCl, 4.2; $MgCl_2$, 1.2; glucose, 11.5 and pH 7.4 when bubbled with 95% O_2 - 5% CO_2). It was mounted in the single or double sucrose gap under 10 mN tension apparatus as previously described (18) and perfused with K.R. at 29°C. Excitatory junction potentials (E.J.P.s) and, in the double sucrose gap, electrotonic potentials (E.P.s) were applied from Ag:AgCl electrodes as previously described (4,5,15). When maximal or submaximal field stimulation (F.S.) of nerves was carried out no more frequently than once every 100 seconds, the E.J.P.s were stable over many hours as previously demonstrated (5). For comparison of effects of ozone, E.J.P. amplitude and duration were compared in response to different voltages and frequencies of F.S.

Chemicals

The following agents (and their sources) were used: U46619, a stable TxA_2 analog (CAYMAN Chemical); SQ 29,548 a TxA_2 receptor antagonists (a gift from Squibb); PAF (Bachem or Sigma), Indomethacin (Sigma) were used. Leukotrienes (LTB_4 and LTD_4) were gifts from Merck-Frosst (Canada), acetylcholine and guanethidine were from Sigma.

RESULTS AND DISCUSSION

Effects of Mediators of Immune Responses on Neural and Myogenic Activities.

LTB_4 and LTD_4 in concentrations from 10^{-11} to 10^{-7}M (n = 6 strips from 5 dogs) had no effect on the E.J.P. generated by submaximal field stimulation or on contractions to field stimulation of strips in the muscle bath (n = 15 strips from 3 dogs). Similarly, they had no effect in the sucrose gap upon responses to 10^{-6}M acetylcholine which was infused for 30 sec. This procedure was chosen to yield a reproducible depolarization to acetylcholine in the same range of amplitudes as the E.J.P. However, the contractile responses to the acetylcholine infusion was much larger than the response to the E.J.P.

Figure 1 illustrates such an experiment with LTD_4; note that the control E.J.P.s were followed by one or two additional membrane oscillations and that the contraction duration approximated that of the total electrical response to F.S. Previous studies have suggested (6) that the E.J.P. and the Ach-depolarization are the responses to the release of intracellular Ca^{2+} by the action of acetylcholine; this Ca_i^{2+} increase seems to activate a Cl^--conductance since it is accompanied by decreased membrane resistances susceptible to replacement of external chloride by a non-permeant anion (a procedure which depolarizes the cell membrane) and the E.J.P. has a reversal potential about 25 mv positive to the resting potential (near the equilibrium potential for chloride ion (E_{Cl}) = 35 mv). Alterations in chloride content of the perfusing medium affected membrane potentials, membrane resistance, E.J.P. amplitude, and acetylcholine depolarization in a manner consistent with this interpretation. The E.J.P., thus, seems to reflect the effect of the increase in intracellular Ca^{2+} to open Cl^- channels. In a medium containing only non-permeant anions, there was a residual E.J.P. and a residual depolarization to acetylcholine (40 to 60% of control). This had a reversal potential 15 to 20 mv positive to the resting potential; it was not abolished by removing Na^+ or Ca^{2+}. It may represent a non-selective cation conductance or a residual outwardly-directed anion gradient. The E.J.P. or secondary membrane potential oscillations and responses to Ach were not affected by

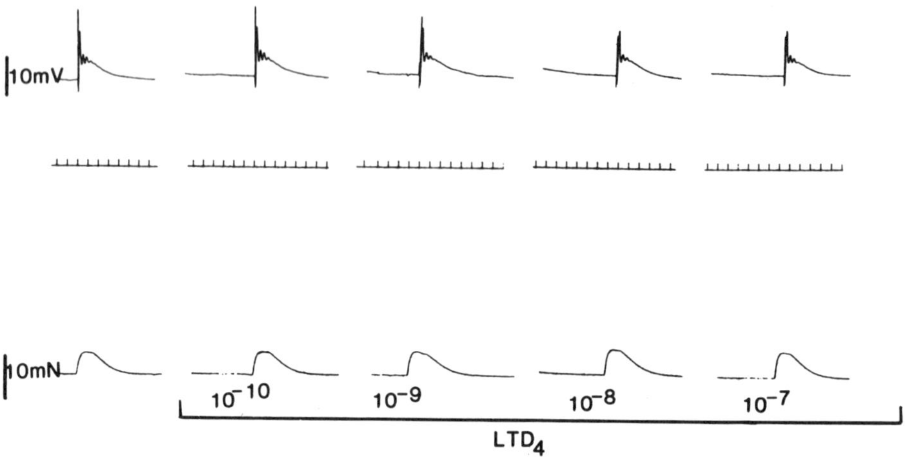

Figure 1. Recordings of excitatory junction potentials (E.J.P.s) and secondary oscillations and associated contractions from canine tracheal muscle strip in the single sucrose gap and effects of LTD_4. Stimuli were applied at 30 pps for 0.3 sec at a just submaximal voltage (18 v). Note the stimulus artifact preceding the E.J.P. There was no significant change in any component of response except a gradual decline in the E.J.P. amplitude which was not reversed by washout of LTD_4 and attributed to the prolonged duration of the experiment. Calibrations at left of each trace; time marker every 10 sec.

organic Ca-channel antagonists even though they were abolished either quickly by Ca-free medium alone (E.J.P.) or gradually along with the contraction by repeated exposure in this medium to Ach (Ach depolarization).

The secondary oscillations after the E.J.P. seen in Fig. 1 were attributed (6) to propagation of effects of delayed and prolonged release of acetylcholine at sites distant from the sucrose Krebs interface; these had reversal potentials 15 to 20 mv positive to the resting potential and were enhanced by depolarization associated with potassium channel blockade by TEA (6). The extent to which the E.J.P., by its depolarizing action, opens voltage-dependent, but organic Ca-channel antagonist independent, Ca channels is unclear. Such an effect was not manifest in reduced contraction to Ca channel blockade. In light of these previous findings, it appears that LTB_4 and LTD_4 have no important effects on acetylcholine release or on any of the response mechanisms to it or on the myogenic properties of the tissue.

In contrast, U46619, the TxA_2 analog, potentiated in a concentration-dependent fashion (10^{-10} to 10^{-7}M), the duration and the amplitude of the contractile response to field stimulation. In the sucrose gap, there was no change in the E.J.P. amplitude or duration (Fig. 2) but the oscillations following the E.J.P. increased in duration along with the contraction. The TxA_2 analog did not potentiate responses to Ach at submaximal concentration of 10^{-10} or 10^{-9}M. Also, the TxB_2 analog caused at higher concentrations such as 10^{-7} M, a small depolarization of the membrane potential (3 to 5 mv at maximum) and a submaximal (about 40% of the Ach maximum) tonic contraction. In the double sucrose gap there was no evidence of altered membrane conductance accompanying the effects of U46619. We attributed (16) these effects to: 1) a direct action on the muscle, possibly a partial release of intracellular Ca^{2+} as the cause of membrane depolarization and submaximal concentration; and 2) an enhanced duration of release of acetylcholine or alternately an enhanced propagation of the E.J.P.s following acetylcholine release from remote sites as the explanation of the increased responses to field stimulation. No evidence was obtained that the responses to the TxA_2 analog were affected by sympathetic nerves or prostaglandin release since guanethidine and indomethacin had no effect on these responses. TxA_2 rather than other possible receptor types were implicated on the responses to U46619 since the specific TxA_2 antagonist (SQ 29,548) competitively inhibited both types of responses (Fig. 2B). It had no effect on its own in strips from control dogs.

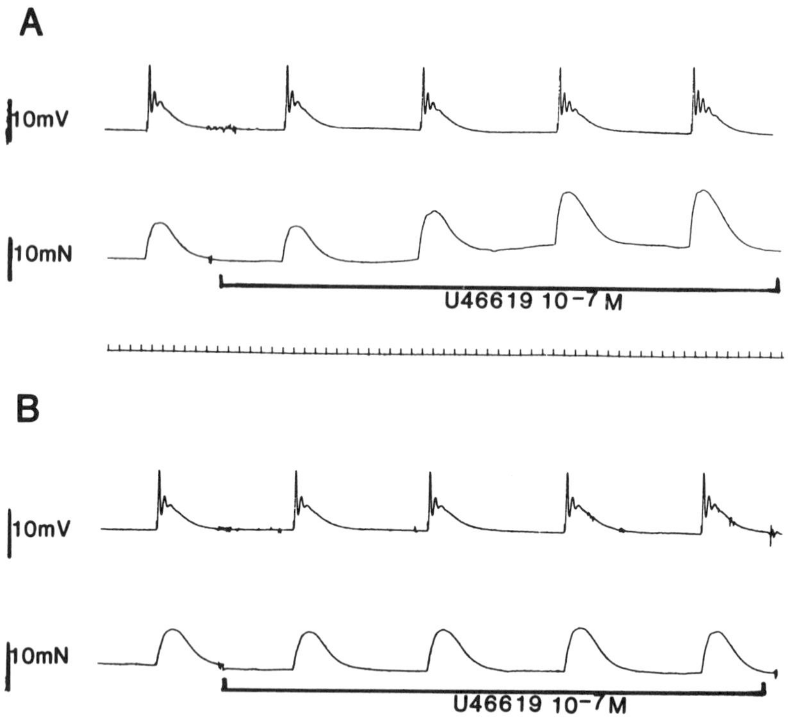

Figure 2. Recordings in the single sucrose gap of E.J.P.s, secondary oscillations and contractions in A before and after exposure to 10^{-7} \m of the thromboxane A_2 analog (U46619) and repetition of these in B after blockade by 10^{-6} M Sq 29,584, a thromboxane receptor antagonist. U46619 effects which wee reversible and repeatable were prevented by the antagonist. These effects consisted of increase and number and duration of secondary oscillations associated with increased amplitude and duration of contraction, slight depolarization (not evident in this tracing) and partial tonic contraction. Calibrations as in Figure 1.

Therefore, TxA_2 is apparently not released under our control conditions. However, TxA_2 clearly had actions which could account for the hyperresponsiveness of the airway in vitro to field stimulation, when it is released by exposure to ozone (1,3).

Platelet-activating factor (PAF) had no direct effects on muscle and no effects on field stimulated responses in the muscle bath (6 experiments with 30 strips). Usually it had no effect in the sucrose gap (13 out of 20 strips), but in the remaining 7 strips it caused slight depolarization, slightly reduced E.J.P. amplitude, no charge in membrane resistance, enhanced and prolonged secondary oscillations and enhanced and prolonged contractions (Fig. 3). The

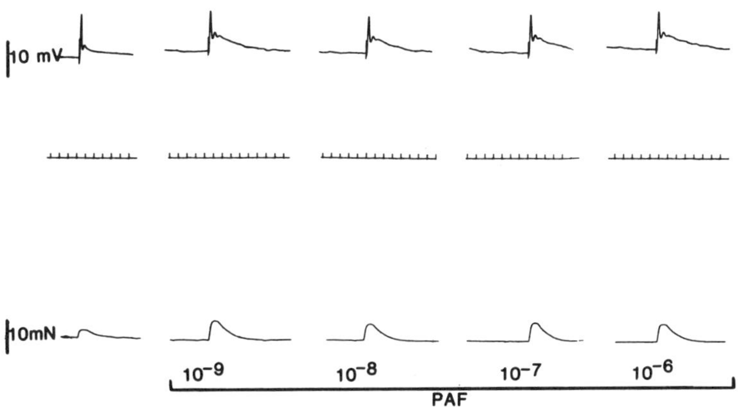

Figure 3. Recordings of E.J.P.s, secondary oscillations and contractions in 1 of the 7 experiments in 20 total in which platelet activating factor has positive effects. These included increased duration of secondary oscillations accompanied by increase amplitude and duration of contractions, resembling responses to U46619 in Figure 2. Calibrations as in Figure 1.

mechanism of these positive effects, when seen, could not be investigated because the responses showed rapid tachyphylaxis and did not recover fully even after a prolonged wait. We were, thus, unable to test whether PAF receptor antagonists blocked these responses or whether TxA_2 release was involved. We could also find no reason why most strips were unresponsive to PAF but a few in the sucrose gap showed a consistent time of effect. Neither the source of the PAF nor the history of the dog seemed to have any relevance. We suggested that in some strips contained in the sucrose gap, immune cells with PAF receptors were retained in blood vessels or tissues and provided a limited source of other mediators such as TxA_2. This implies that PAF does not act directly on the nerve or muscle locally in the airway. This is in seeming contradiction to a recent report using intra-arterial perfusion of the canine trachea (11) which caused dose-dependent contractions reduced by atropine and nearly abolished by an histamine H_2-antagonist or methysergide (putative 5-HT antagonist). The authors interpreted their findings in terms of a direct action of PAF on trachea; however, we suggest that they were direct only in the sense of being local and depended upon the presence of immune cells with PAF receptors and located in the blood supply and in the tissue. These cells, platelets, basophils and mast cells apparently released histamine, 5HT and a TxA_2-like substance.

In summary, our studies showed that TxA_2-related immune mediators apparently acted directly to contract tracheal muscle and prolong the release of acetylcholine. No other mediator tested, including PAF, LTB_4 or LTD_4 had such direct action. We postulated that TxA_2 is involved in hyperresponsiveness to nerve stimulation after ozone as a result of its two actions. A recent report based on muscle bath studies (17) is in essential agreement with ours; it showed that U46619 potentiated field stimulated contractions of canine trachea and this was blocked by SQ 29,548. It did not potentiate acetylcholine contractions. Platelet aggregation was able to release TxA_2 to mimic that response.

CONCLUSIONS

From these studies, we conclude that TxA_2-like immune

mediators have direct myogenic and neurogenic actions on canine tracheal strips, that LTB_4, LTD_4 and PAF do not have such direct actions. We also conclude that TxA_2 could be the mediator of the ozone-induced hyperresponsiveness seen in tracheal strips in vitro, but further tests of this hypothesis are required. The mechanism of action of TxA_2-like agents remains to be determined but possibilities (not mutually exclusive) include increased cell-to-cell coupling, prolonged release of acetylcholine and direct actions to release a limited pool of intracellular Ca^{2+}.

REFERENCES

1. Aizawa, H., K.F. Chung, G.O. Lukauf, I. Ueki, R.A. Bethel, P.M. O'Byrne, J. Hirose and J.A. Nadel. Significance of thromboxane generation in ozone-induced airway responsiveness in dogs. J. Appl. Physiol. 59: 1918-1923, 1985.
2. Boushey, H.A., H.A. Holtzman, J.R. Sheller and J.A. Nadel. State of the art. Bronchial hyperreactivity. Am. Rev. Respir. Dis. 121: 384-413, 1980.
3. Chung, K.F., H. Aizawa, G.D. Leikauf, I.F. Ueki, T.W. Evans and J.A. Nadel. Airway hyperresponsiveness induced by platelet-activating factor: role of thromboxane generation. J. Pharmacol. Exp. Therap. 236: 580-584, 1986.
4. Daniel, E.E., Jager, L.P. and Jury, J. Catecholamines release mediators in the opossum oesophageal circular smooth muscle. J. of Physiol. 382: 489-508, 1987
5. Daniel, E.E., Davis, C. and Sharma, V. Effects of endogenous and exogenous PGE_2 in neurotransmission in canine trachea. Can. J. Physiol. Pharmacol. (in press).
6. Daniel, E.E., F. Inoue, L.P. Jager, J. Jury and R. Serio. Excitatory junction potentials in canine trachealis smooth muscle cells mediated via an increased chloride conductance. Submitted to J. Physiol.
7. Holtzman, M.J., L.M. Fabbri, B.-E. Skoogh, P.M. O'Byrne, E.H. Walters, H. Aizawa and J.A. Nadel. Time course of airway hyperresponsiveness induced by ozone in dogs. J. Appl. Physiol. 55: 1232-1236, 1986.
8. Holtzman, M.J., L.M. Fabbri, P.M. O'Byrne, B.D. Gold, H. Aizawa, E.H. Walters, S.E. Alpert and J.A. Nadel. Importance of airway inflammation for

hyperresponsiveness induced by ozone. Am. Rev. Respir. Dis. 127: 686-690, 1983.

9. Jones, G.L., O'Byrne, P.M., Pashley, M., Serio,R., Jury, J., Lane, C.G. and Daniel, E.E. Airway smooth muscle hyperresponsiveness to acetylcholine in vitro from dogs with airway hyperresponsiveness in vivo. (in preparation).

10. Lee, L.-Y., E.R. Bluker and J.A. Nadel. Effect of ozone on bronchomotor response to inhaled histamine aerosol in dogs. J. Appl. Physiol. 43: 626-631, 1977.

11. Leff, A.R., S.R. White, N.M. Munoz, K.J. Popovich, T. Shioya and N.P. Stimler-Gerard. Parasympathetic involvement in PAF-induced contraction in canine trachealis in vivo. J. Appl. Physiol. 62: 599-605, 1987.

12. O'Byrne, P.M., E.H. Walters, B.D. Gold, H.A. Aizawa, L.M. Fabbri, S.E. Alpert, J.A. Nadel and M.J. Holtzman. Neurophil depletion inhibits airway hyperresponsiveness induced by ozone exposure. Am. Rev. Respir. Dis. 130: 214-219, 1984.

13. O'Byrne, P.M., E.H. Walters, H. Aizawa, L.M. Fabbri, M.J. Holtzman and J.A. Nadel. Indomethacin inhibits the airway hyperresponsiveness but not the neutrophil influx induced by ozone in dogs. Am. Rev. Respir. Dis. 130: 220-224, 1984.

14. O'Byrne, P.M., G.D. Leikauf, H. Aizawa, R.A. Bethel, I.F. Ueki, M.J. Holtzman, and J.A. Nadel. Leukotriene B_4 induced airway hyperresponsiveness in dogs. J. Appl. Physiol. 59, 1941-1946, 1985.

15. Serio, R. and Daniel, E.E. Thromboxanes and other inflammatory modulators of canine trachealis neuromuscular function. Submitted to J. Appl. Physiol.

16. Serio, R. and Daniel, E.E. Electrophysiological analysis of responses to intrinsic nerves in circular muscle of the opossum esophageal muscle. Submitted to Am. J. Physiol.

17. Tamaoki, J., K. Sekizawa, M.L. Osborne, I.F. Ueki, P.D. Graf and J.A. Nadel. Platelet aggregation increases cholinergic neurotransmission in canine airway. J. Appl. Physiol. 62: 2246-2251, 1987.

18. Walters, E.H., P.M. O'Byrne, P.D. Graf, L.M. Fabbri and J.A. Nadel. The responsiveness of airway smooth muscle in vitro from dogs with airway hyperresponsiveness in vivo. Clinical Science 71: 605-611, 1986.

Characteristics of Airway Smooth Muscle

Mechanisms in Asthma: Pharmacology,
Physiology, and Management, pages 179–203

ULTRASTRUCTURE OF AIRWAY SMOOTH MUSCLE

E.E. Daniel

Department of Neurosciences, McMaster University Health Sciences Centre, Hamilton, Ontario, Canada. L8N 3Z5.

with the Collaboration of Drs. C. Hirshman and P. O'Byrne and Technical Assistance of I. Berezin

INTRODUCTION

There are many gaps in our knowledge of airway smooth muscle and the structural relationships of neural, endocrine and immune systems which control or modulate the myogenic activity of the airway. Another major area of uncertainty is the nature of the systems coupling muscle contraction to the mechanical load of airway tissue. In this report, I will focus on neural and immune systems affecting airway smooth muscle by virtue of their proximity to it and consider briefly the connective tissue (elastin and collagen) multilayers of the interstitial space between muscle and mucosa and which may be a barrier to migration of immune cells.

I will emphasize studies on canine airways using ostensibly normal dogs, dogs with genetic hyperresponsiveness and dogs made hyperresponsive by ozone. The objective will be to see if there are structural changes which may relate to or explain airway hyperresponsiveness. For the purposes of this presentation, only qualitative or semiquantitative data will be presented.

Some comparative data will also be presented about human airway and guinea pig airway.

METHODS & MATERIALS

Normal control animals (greyhounds) and hyperresponsive Basenji-greyhound animals with or without sensitization (19a&b) were obtained after fixation from Dr. Carol Hirshman (Oregon Health Sciences University). Similarly, anesthetized animals were treated with ozone or a placebo inhalation according to the protocol described in (37). In each dog, a dose-effect curve to inhaled acetylcholine was determined before and after the ozone or placebo. The dogs were killed with an overdose of pentobarbital. Their lungs were then removed and dissected for electrophysiological, mechanical and structural study. Tissues studied included the trachea and bronchi down through the 5th order.

Tissues were fixed as previously described in detail (10) in 2% glutaraldehyde in 0.1M Na cacodylate buffer containing 1.5 mM Ca Cl_2 and 4.5% sucrose. After 2 to 4 hours, fixation, they were transferred to 0.1M cacodylate buffer (pH 7.4) at 4°C and kept until processed further. They were postfixed with 2% OsO_4 in 0.05M cacodylate buffer for one hour, stained for 90 min en bloc with 2% uranyl acetate, dehydrated in graded alcohols and embedded in Spurr resin. They were stained for 2 minutes on the section with Pb citrate (1%) as described in detail in (10).

Tissues were sectioned so that the smooth muscle bundles and nerves were cross-sectioned. In all the smaller bronchi, 2nd through 5th order, the interstitial region between muscle bundles and mucosa and the mucosa itself were also studied.

In each tissue, two grid squares covered as much as possible with smooth muscle cells were chosen randomly under low magnification for study. Each section was scanned in a Philips 301 TEM for nerves, gap junctions and immune cells at 3300x (and 33,000x on the screen). Each nerve or nerve bundle was photographed, using a 35 mm camera, at 4200x to 5500x; gap junctions were photographed at 7200x until at least ten (if present) were photographed and the remainder were recorded. Then, the grid square was photographed 260x or at 550x for construction of a montage of prints at 15x higher magnification (about 3900x or

8250x). This was used to measure plasma membrane length (ignoring membrane caveolae as previously described (2)). Nerve or gap junction photographs were printed 8x larger (approximately 44000x or 57600x). Corrections were ultimately made for the actual compared to the nominal magnification. Gap junctions were measured and nerve profiles were classified as previously described (2,8) i.e., as containing predominantly small agranular vesicles (often with some large granular vesicles), as containing small granular vesicles (presumably adrenergic) or as containing neurofilaments and neurotubules and less than 3 synaptic vesicles (hence considered to be axons). Only nerve profiles not surrounded by a perineurium, and located within 2.6 μm of smooth muscle cells were considered to innervate the smooth muscle. There were so few nerves with predominantly large granular vesicles or mitochondria (less than 5%) that they were lumped together with axons for the purposes of this presentation.

Data were normalized in terms of the number of nerve profiles or gap junctions per 1000 μm of plasma membrane. Since plasma membrane caveolae were ignored during measurements of plasma membrane length, these numbers are about 45% less than the total membrane area (based on measurements of plasma membrane length in the same cells at high and low magnifications). However, these values reflect the smoothed surface area of the cells considered and provide a basis for comparison; also gap junctions are never found on plasma membrane with caveolae.

The interstitial space between muscle and mucosa was scanned by nerves, immune cells, elastin layers and collagen in 2 or more grid squares. Similarly, the mucosa in two grid squares was scanned for nerves, immune cells, damaged regions, neuroendocrin cells and other cell types.

Some earlier studies of human, canine and guinea pig airways are included here for comparison.

RESULTS AND DISCUSSION

Previous studies (1,9,23) from our laboratory have shown that canine and human trachea have a sparse innervation by nerves which contain mostly small agranular vesicles (putative cholinergic) and some large granular vesicles (putative peptidergic). Innervation by putative adrenergic nerves (with small granular vesicles) was sparse. Functionally, the innervation was primarily cholinergic in canine trachea (8,12,13,23) and cholinergic plus non-adrenergic inhibitory in human trachea (9,15). There were numerous gap junctions between muscle cells and they were also well coupled electrically so that space constants greater than 2 mm long were found in canine airways (9,15). Similar conclusions were drawn from studies of bovine trachea; i.e., the muscle was sparsely innervated mainly by cholinergic nerves (4) and many gap junctions and good cell-to-cell coupling were found (5). In contrast, in guinea pig trachea there was a smaller proportion gap junction membrane and a much denser innervation by varicose nerve profiles which have mostly small agranular vesicles with some large granular vesicles and a few with small granular vesicles (22). Functionally, the guinea pig trachea, like the human, appears to have a cholinergic innervation, an adrenergic and a non-adrenergic inhibitory innervation (see 7,26,39). However, it differs from canine and bovine trachea not only in its possession of a non-adrenergic inhibitory innervation, but also in having spontaneous membrane oscillations (slow waves) whereas the others are quiescent (32). Human trachea was recently reported (21) to have membrane potential oscillations which seem to control active tension as in guinea pig trachea. All trachea studied in this regard (bovine, canine and guinea pig) share the property of strong rectification of depolarizing currents (18,24,25) i.e., they do not pass depolarizing currents as easily as hyperpolarizing ones and as a consequence, they cannot initiate action potentials or other propagated active responses. Rectification is a consequence of voltage or Ca-dependent K^+-currents which when activated lead to outward, hyperpolarizing currents which oppose inward, depolarizing ones (18,24,25). When these K^+ currents are blocked; depolarization initiates propagated Ca^{2+}-dependent action potentials.

Smaller airways have received much less study compared to trachea. We have observed 4th to 7th order (~ 1mm diameter) human bronchi (10). They differed markedly from human trachea: they lacked visible gap junctions and had a dense innervation with nerves containing many small agranular vesicles and some large granular vesicles and a higher proportion than trachea nerves with small granular vesicles. Other studies, too, (31) have indicated clearly the presence of a higher density of adrenergic nerves in smaller human bronchi. To date, it is unclear how these adrenergic nerves function; i.e., as direct inhibitory innervators of smooth muscles or in presynaptic inhibitory control of acetylcholine release. In canine airways, they appear to exert prejunctional inhibition of acetylcholine release (14); however, this was demonstrated only by prolonged exposure to 10^{-4}M tyramine and not by field stimulation of nerves. The absence of detectable gap junctions does not prove the absence of cell-to-cell coupling since gap junctions are rare or absent in a number of well-coupled smooth muscles (see 11).

We have recently studied canine bronchi down to 5th order. The results are summarized in Tables 1 and 2, and illustrated in the following figures. In contrast to human airways, gap junctions persist in canine airways in numbers and in proportions relative to that of plasma membrane in the smaller bronchi as in the larger bronchi (Figure 1 and Table 2). Although one might predict an inverse correlation between the density of gap junctions and the density of nerves, in fact, in smaller bronchi, beginning with the second order bronchi, there was a marked increase in nerve density without a decrease in gap junction density (Table 2). Unlike the trachea, these nerves penetrated within and between muscle bundles but nerve profiles of a nerve were rarely or never found $\leq$ 20 nm from muscle. Furthermore, there was a remarkable increase in the proportion if varicose nerve profiles with small granular vesicles (adrenergic) to 60%. There was also an increase in the occurrences of these nerve varicosities in bundles together with varicosities containing mostly small agranular vesicles (Fig. 2). They provide a structural basis for a hypothetical adrenergic presynaptic control of cholinergic nerves. Since the incidence of varicose nerve profiles containing mostly large granular vesicles was so low as to be negligible, any peptidergic mediators may have also been located in nerve profiles in the few large granular vesicles present in addition to the small agranular ones. However, peptidergic nerve functions of intrinsic nerves have not been established in the tissues.

TABLE 1. Gap Junctions in Canine Airway Smooth Muscle

	n	No/1000 μm PM mean ± SEM	μm GJ/1000 μm mean ± SEM
Trachea	13	2.93 ± 0.60	1.218 ± 0.232
Bronchi			
2°	12	3.28 ± 0.78	1.504 ± 0.407
3°	5	3.45 ± 1.07	1.989 ± 0.630
4°	11	2.47 ± 0.36	1.061 ± 0.164

n refers to the number of grid squares analyzed. No significant differences noted. Data are incomplete. Since each gap junction profile occurs in two cells, the values of length per unit of PM should be multiplied by 2.

TABLE 2. Nerve Density

Nerve Density per 1000 um of Smooth Muscle Plasma Membrane

(mean ± SEM)

TISSUE	n	NERVE TYPE				RATIO
		SAV	SGV	AX	TOTAL	SGV/SAV
Trachea	15	0.78±0.25	0.69±0.34	1.01±0.34	2.47±0.81	0.74±0.46[+]
Bronchi						
2°	13	6.29±1.55	1.75±0.40	9.06±2.13	17.20±4.31	0.36±0.08
3°	6	10.10±2.30	3.82±0.70	14.17±3.37	28.07±5.70	0.43±0.07
4°	11	10.31±2.14	6.77±2.02	16.59±3.62	33.67±7.13	0.60±0.08

[+]The high incidence of SGV in trachea is believed to be a sampling error owing to the presence of one grid square with SGV 7 x the number of SAV. Without this value, the values became 0.30±0.11.

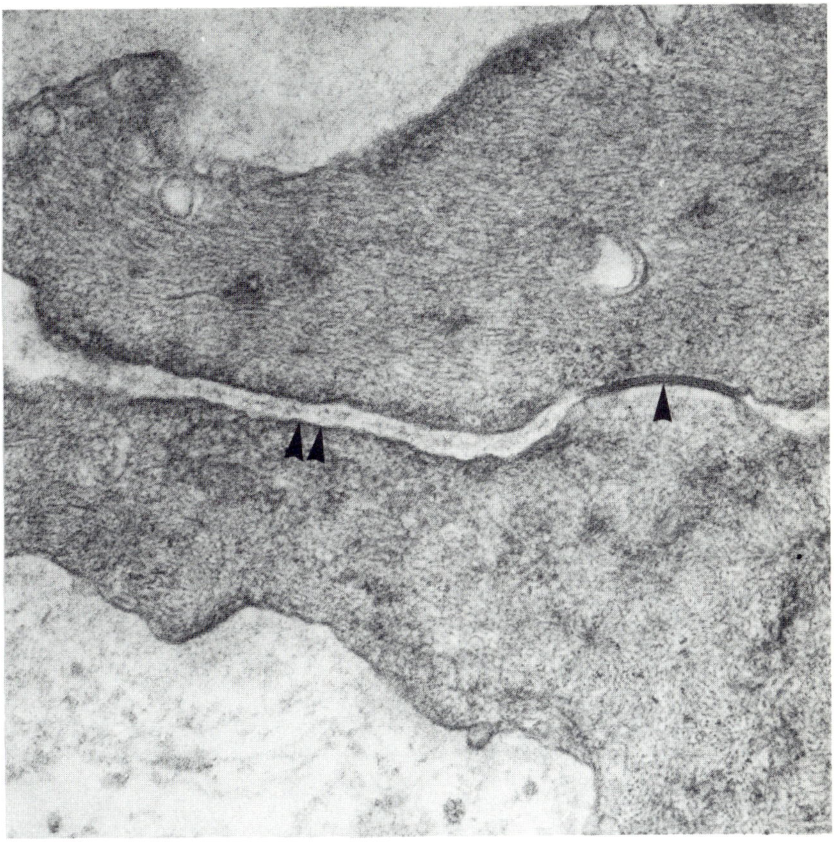

Figure 1. Gap junction in 5th order canine bronchi after ozone treatment. A gap junction (arrowhead) beside an intermediate contact (double arrowheads). The latter are very rare in canine airway muscle. The same structures are found in airways from control animals. Magnification: x 68,850.

If these vesicles contain peptides, the release of peptidergic mediators also may also be subject to presynaptic inhibitory control by adrenergic nerves. Furthermore since these putative adrenergic nerve profiles are usually closer to the cholinergic nerve profiles than to smooth muscle, it seems likely that higher concentrations of adrenergic mediator will be present around nerves than around muscles. If adrenergic pre- and post-synaptic receptors have equal sensitivities to norepinephrine, control will be exerted primarily at the former set of receptors.

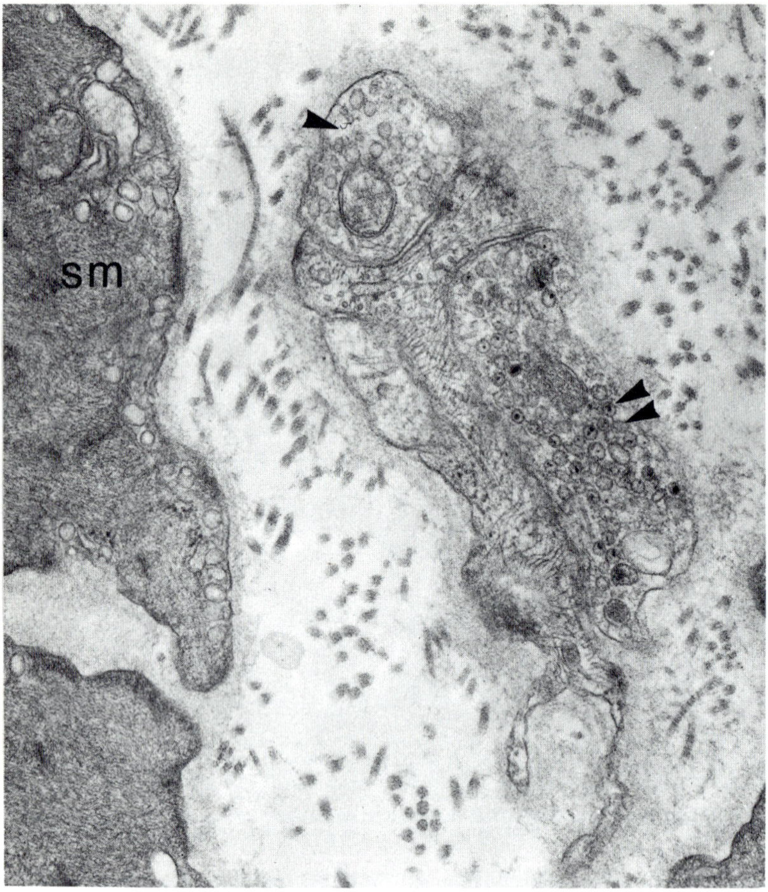

Figure 2: Nerve bundle within a smooth muscle bundle of 5th order canine bronchi after ozone treatment. Note that both putative cholinergic and adrenergic nerve profiles (labelled with single and double arrowheads respectively) are present nearby one another. The same structures are present in control animals. Magnification: x 38,040.

From these structural studies, one would propose that the major direct control of tracheal and bronchial muscle will be cholinergic, but that a much more significant adrenergic function exists in bronchi compared to trachea, that this control is likely to be exerted presynaptically. The limited functional evidence available supports these predictions (14) by suggesting that $beta_1$ adrenoceptors on cholinergic nerves inhibit acetylcholine release and can be activated by norepinephrine released from sympathetic nerves.

The Interstitial Space Between Bronchial Muscle and Mucosa

The region between the smooth muscle bundles and the mucosa of bronchi is occupied by a series of layers or plexus of elastin running perpendicular to the radius of the bronchi (Fig. 3). These are discontinuous and separated by bundles of collagen as well as by blood vessels and some nerves and mast cells. The elastin layers or lamina are in intimate relationship to two cell types or their processes; mast cells and a fibroblast-type cell (Fig. 4). Often, the elastin fibers appear to be continuous with fibers in the cytoplasm of these cells when viewed at higher magnifications. Mast cells are sometimes, but not invariably, associated with nerve bundles within a few microns. The structural arrangements in this region strongly suggest that it will be a barrier to proposed (29,30) migration of neutrophils and other immune cells which enter the region from local blood vessels or move from their locus in this region into and through the mucosa. It is important to point out that mast cells and rarely other immune cells are found primarily in this region in normal animals.

The Mucosa of Bronchi

Canine airway mucosa contains a mixture of cell types (Fig. 5): these include ciliated epithelial cells, goblet cells, basal cells and neuroendocrin-like cells. Nerve profiles were observed very rarely and then always close to the internal basal lamina. Similarly, neuroendocrin cells were noted primarily at the inner face of the mucosa (Fig. 6), although their processes extended toward the epithelium. Mast cells, eosinophils, neutrophils, platelets and macrophages were not observed in mucosa of normal animals.

Changes Associated with Genetic Hyperresponsive Airways and with Ozone-Induced Hyperresponsive Airways

A slightly greater proportion of gap junction membrane per unit of plasma membrane appeared to be present in Basenji-Greyhound hyper-responsive dogs compared to control animals. However, no clear differences in innervation were seen; i.e., no increase or decrease in any class of innervation or change in their relationships. Analysis of

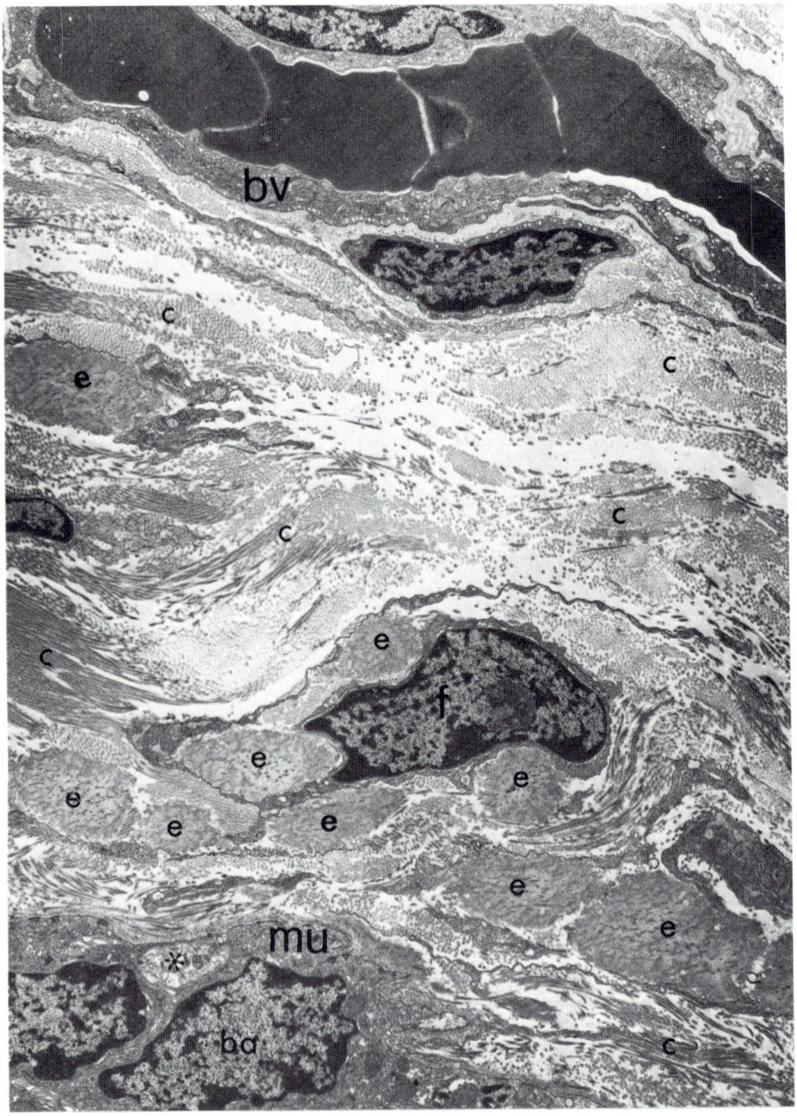

Figure 3. A portion of the interstitial space between the smooth muscle bundles and the mucosa (labelled mu) from 5th order bronchi in a control animal. (Similar in all bronchi). This region contains many blood vessels (one is labelled bv at top) and plane sheets of elastin (labelled e) and bundles of collagen (labelled c). Note fibroblast (f) associated intimately with elastin. Magnification x 7900.

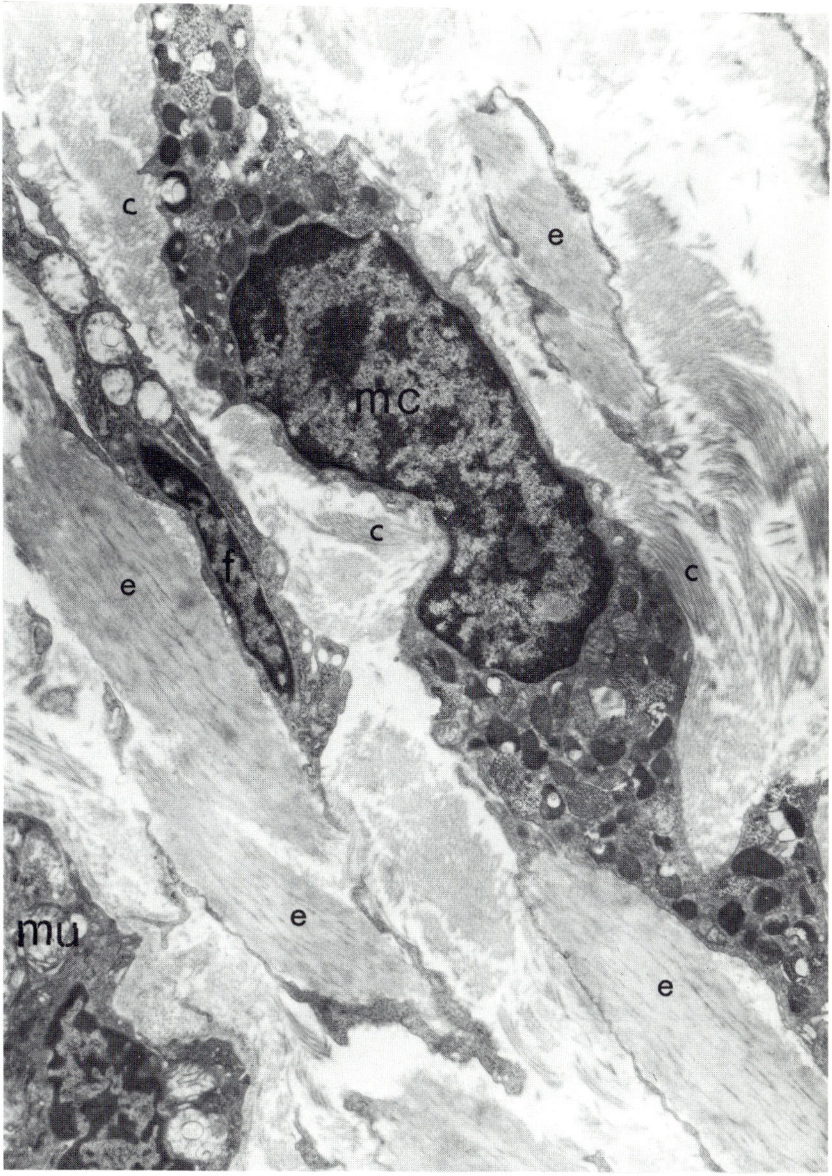

Figure 4. Mast cell (labelled m.c.) and a fibroblast (labelled f) in close proximity to profiles of elastic layer (labelled e) in the interstitial space from 4th order bronchi after ozone treatment. Similar structures were present in control animals. Magnification: x 10,350.

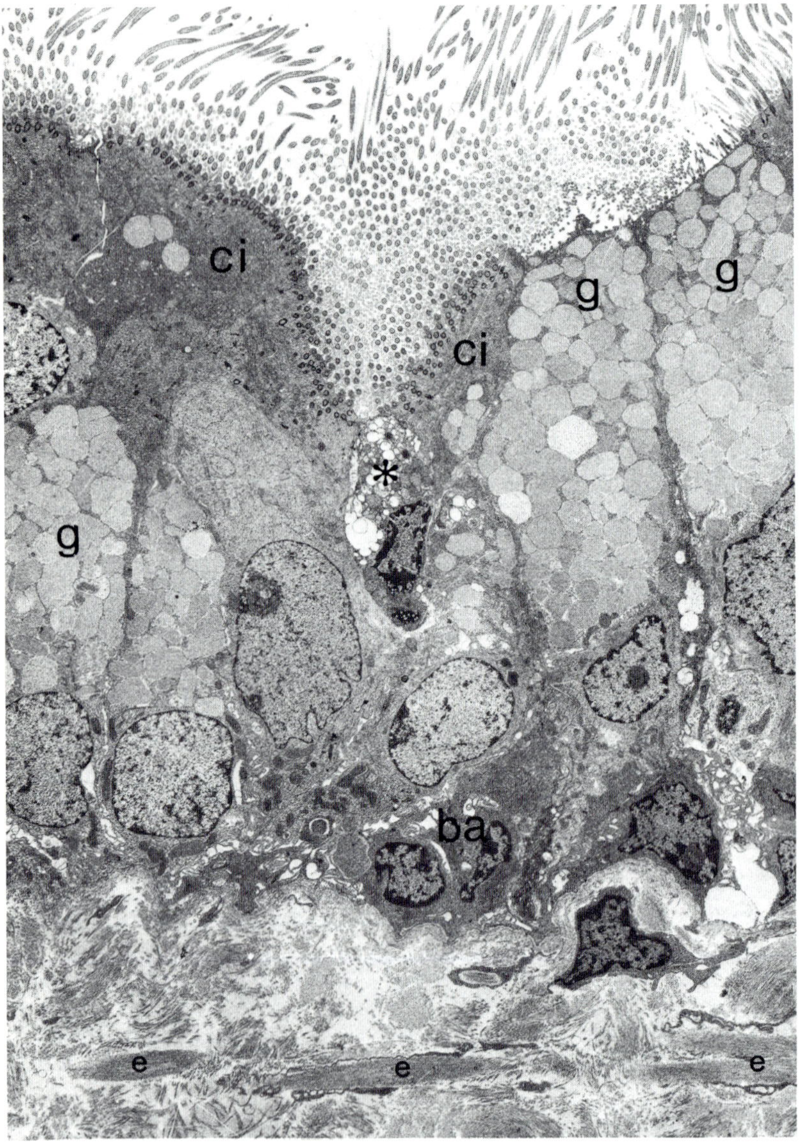

Figure 5. Low power view of ozone-exposed canine mucosa of 3rd order bronchi after ozone treatment. Goblet cells (labelled g), ciliated cells (labelled ci) and basal cells (labelled ba) damaged cell at asterisk. Note elastin (e) in interstitial space. Magnification: x 3400.

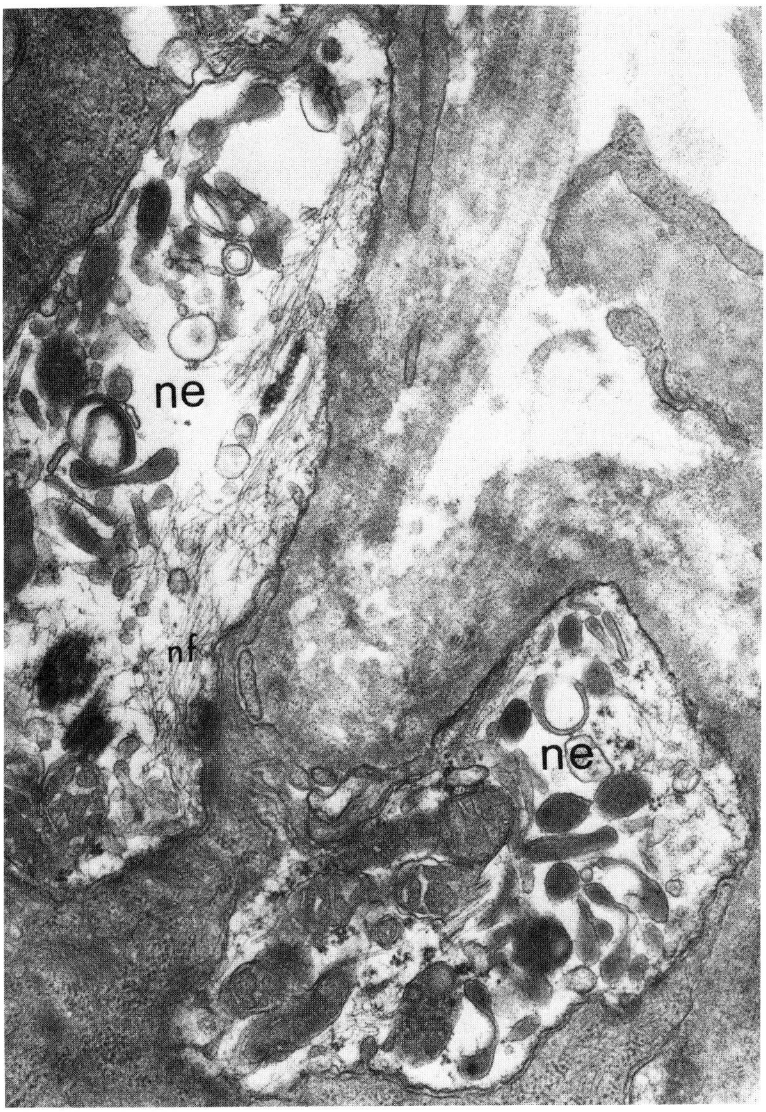

Figure 6. Profiles (labelled ne) interpreted as profiles from neuroendocrin cells, located at the border of the mucosa and the interstitial space from 4th order bronchi in a control dog. Note the profiles large granular vesicles and tubules and the fibers resembling neurofilaments (nf). One cell may contain cilia (near nf). Magnification: x 38,040.

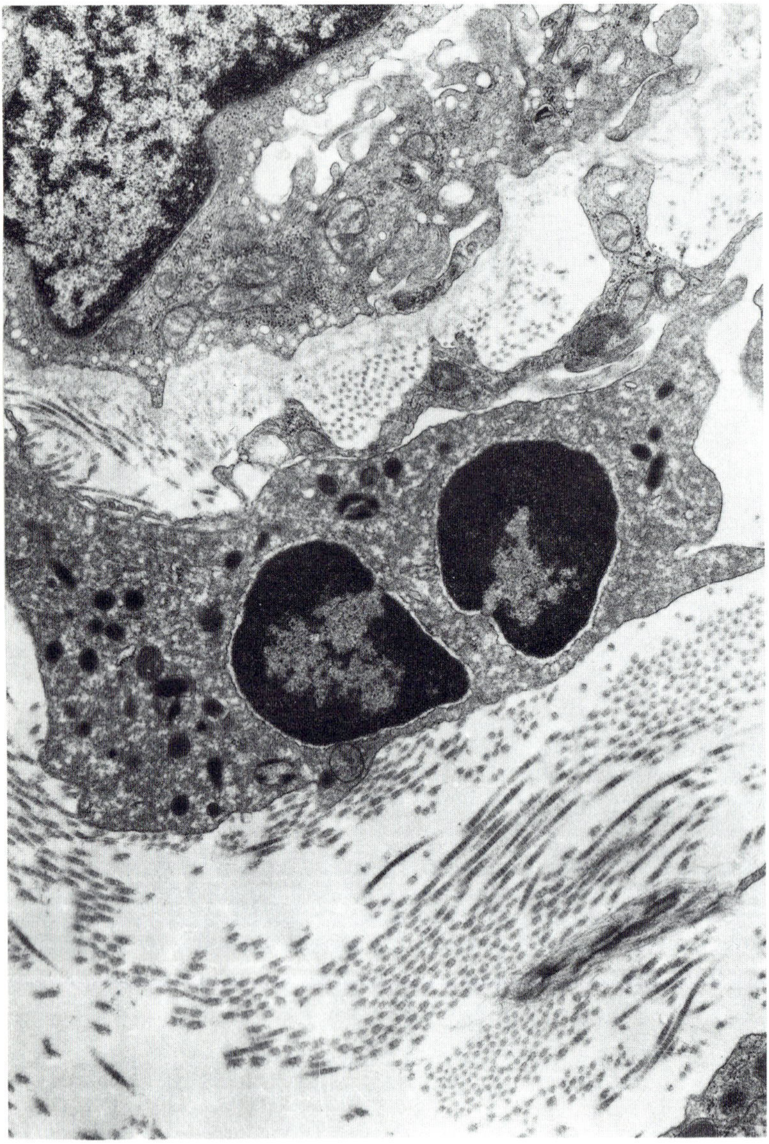

Figure 7. Cell interpreted to be a neutrophil near a blood vessel in the interstitial space of a 5th order bronchi from an ozone-treated dog. Note granules of neutrophil. Magnification: x 17,390.

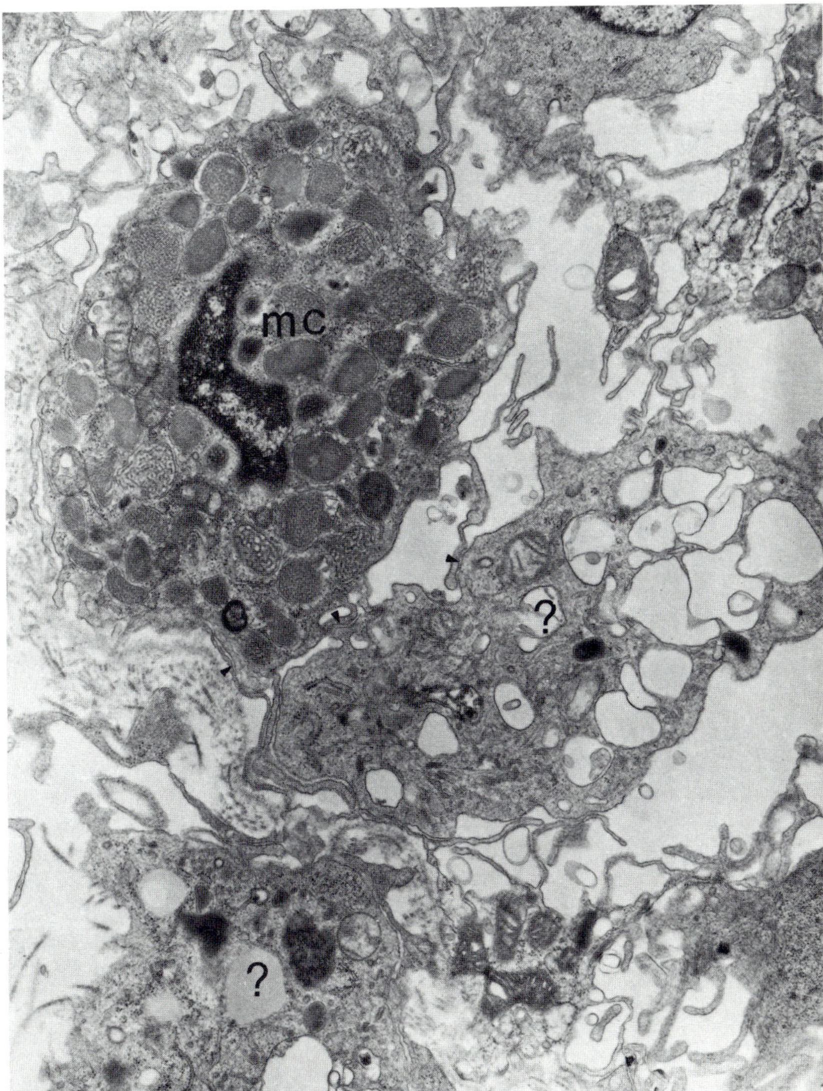

Figure 8. Cell resembling mast cell (labelled mc) invading damaged mucosa near its border with the interstitial space of 5th order bronchi after ozone treatment. Other damaged cells nearby (labelled ?) were not identified with certainty. Note close contacts (arrowheads) between mast cell and one of these cells. Magnification: X 15,750.

gap junctions in ozone-treated dogs is incomplete. However, there was a clear increase in the number of immune cells seen in the interstitial space between smooth muscle bundles and mucosa and in the mucosa itself in ozone-treated animals. In fact, in control animals only mast-cells were regularly observed in the interstitial space in these animals. In contrast, many mast cells, neutrophils as well as other immune cells and platelets were regularly observed in this region (Figure 7 shows a neutrophil). Furthermore, after ozone inhalation, mast cells and other immune cells were found in the process of invading the mucosa (Fig. 8) and occasionally near smooth muscle. It should be noted, too, that neither in Basenji-Greyhound- or ozone-hyperresponsiveness dogs was there any generalized loss of epithelium from the mucosa. There were regions of discrete damage usually to ciliated cells. Figure 5, in fact, is from an ozone-treated animal and shows such discrete damage.

Interpretation and Hypotheses from Structural Findings

The most striking features differentiating canine bronchi from trachea are: 1) the increase of density of innervation close to smooth muscle; 2) the increased number of putative adrenergic nerves and 3) the increased incidence of varicose nerve structures in which "adrenergic" (containing small granular synaptic vesicles) nerve profiles were located very near to "cholinergic" or mixed "cholinergic-peptidergic" (containing small agranular synaptic vesicles or a mixture of these with some large granular vesicles) nerves. The adrenergic nerve profiles were never observed very close (< 20 nm; usually > 100 nm) to smooth muscle, but were often close (20-100 nm) to cholinergic nerve profiles. We conclude that this is a structural arrangement seemingly designed to provide for presynaptic control of release of acetylcholine by inhibitory adrenergic mediators.

Some pharmacological evidence of such control exists by beta adrenoceptors (14). However, evidence of physiological control is lacking. We (L. Janssen and E.E. Daniel, unpublished) have found the 3rd to 5th order airways regularly produce an excitatory junction potential (EJP) on focal stimulation with a single pulse. After adrenergic nerve functions are antagonized by propranolol, functional effects on the size of the E.J.P.s produced by a train of twenty pulses of field stimulation delivered at various frequencies were increased, especially at frequencies of 1 to 2 pps. This suggests that adrenergic control may be exerted during repetitive stimulation at low frequencies in a physiological range. No hyperpolarizations have been observed following stimulation of nerves after atropine and no depolarizations have been seen after atropine and propranolol.

Canine bronchi, unlike human bronchi (39) contain a large number of gap junctions and probably are electrically well coupled. The existence of a system of gap junctions providing for good cell-to-cell coupling along with a high density of nerves is somewhat unusual among smooth muscle tissues (3,6). These airway muscles are likely to be highly reactive to neural control systems compared to trachea since innervation is dense and junction potentials easily propagated.

The guinea pig trachea is another airway which contains a dense innervation and gap junctions (22) and good electrical coupling (32). The dense innervation of guinea pig trachea is stressed because there seems to be misunderstanding of this point on the part of some authorities. It, too, has a mixture of cholinergic excitatory, adrenergic inhibitory and non-adrenergic inhibitory innervation (26,39). Ultrastructural studies (22) confirm the existence of many varicose profiles with mostly small agranular and some large granular and some varicosities with small granular vesicles. There is functional evidence of direct smooth muscle innervation by adrenergic nerves as well as the direct smooth muscle innervation by cholinergic excitatory and non-adrenergic inhibitory nerves (39). Adrenergic inhibition was mediated by beta adrenoceptors. All these airways (guinea pig and others) are normally unable to initiate action potentials because of the strong rectify properties of the activation of potassium channels on depolarization (see above).

The unanswered question from structural studies is how bronchi with many nerves, good cell-to-cell coupling, but no action potentials, and pre-synaptic and post-synaptic inhibitory control of excitation function normally and after inflammation. We hypothesize that such airways are normally highly responsive to excitatory nerve input because of the existence of pharmaco-mechanical coupling of contraction to muscarinic cholinergic receptors leading to release of intracellular Ca^{2+} (13) and because of electrotonic propagation of excitatory junction potentials. We suggest that a major inhibitory control of bronchoconstriction in canine bronchi may be exerted presynaptically by adrenergic nerves at ganglia of the airway and also at axonal levels; a direct inhibitory control be exerted in some cases by adrenergic and non-adrenergic inhibitory systems (guinea pig and human). In trachea, cell-to-cell coupling in such airway might be irrelevant to or even inhibitory to propagation of excitation in trachea because propagation of depolarizing EJPs would not initiate contraction or action potentials and good coupling decreases the current density of the depolarizing electrotonic potential by increasing the area of cell membrane through which it flows. In bronchi, with denser innervation than trachea, improved cell-to-cell coupling may aid in propagation of excitation, but this is not established. In canine trachea, our recent evidence (13) is that EJPs are the result of an intracellular Ca release which also causes contraction and are not the main cause of contraction.

Asthma is characterized by non-specific hyperresponsiveness of the airway and recently it was shown (33,34,35,38) also to be characterized by an increased maximal bronchoconstrictor response. Recent theoretical and experimental analyses of these two pathophysiological features (27,28) have suggested that they may reflect different pathological processes. Increased narrowing may be due to a breakdown of the interdependence between parenchyma and airway wall (unloading of airway muscle) increase in smooth muscle force of contraction and/or reduction in smooth muscle resting length (25c). Decreased loading of airway muscle secondary to papain treatment to soften cartilage was shown to increase baseline resistance and maximal response to intravenous acetylcholine in rabbits (27,28). Increased hypertrophy or hyperplasia of smooth muscle, edema of mucosa or interstitial space hyperemia of the interstitial space, increased mucous secretion, all leading to increased wall thickness, could also cause increased maximum bronchial response (28). It seems doubtful that these changes explain the increased sensitivity of the airways to a variety of stimuli as well as the increased maximum response. They do not account for the increased responsiveness of ozone-treated airway in vitro to field stimulation and exogenous acetylcholine, which we attribute (see elsewhere this volume) to effects of thromboxane A_2 on neural and myogenic control.

Two changes in smooth muscle structure and function would lead to non-specific airway sensitivity to stimuli; 1) improved cell-to-cell coupling and 2) abolition of the voltage dependent K^+ conductance and of rectification, so that propagated action potentials can be initiated, smooth muscle thickening owing to hypertrophy or hyperplasia could. No experiments to date have tested whether these events do or do not occur, but evidence has been obtained that gap junctions of airways are labile under the influence of immune mediators (1). Dose-effect curves to various agonists studied in vitro do not assess either cell-to-cell coupling (since responses are initiated by the agonists acting on every cell) or occurrence of action potentials.

Changes in structure associated with inflammation or associated with genetic hyperresponsiveness of the airways include an apparent increase in the gap junctions of bronchi but quantitative assessment is still incomplete. When acute inflammation is induced by ozone, there is also acute hyper-responsiveness to inhaled acetylcholine in vivo (20) and in vitro (see elsewhere in this volume) or to field stimulation in vitro (37), associated with the movement of a variety of immune cells from the blood stream into the airway (neutrophils, eosinophils, basophils and platelets) and the apparent movement of these and of tissue mast cells or transformed mast cells out of the interstitial space into the mucosa (and later the lumen) (17,20).

Several functional hypotheses based on our structural findings relate to function of these cells and may help explain increased airway narrowing; 1) the connective tissue (elastin and collagen) of the interstitial space seems likely to provide a significant barrier to movement of immune cells to the mucosa; hence it seems likely that immune cells will have the ability to remove these barriers by way of protein degradation. In other words, they are likely to possess, when activated to move, elastase and possibly collagenase. Neutrophils are well known to contain elastase (16,36). It is also possible that mast cells along with fibroblasts secrete these connective tissue proteins in normal airways and inflammation is associated with degradation and then remodelling of the connective tissue. 2) degradation of elastase and collagen depending on the products is likely to lead acutely to edema by exertion of osmotic effects by these products and because of the loss of structural integrity of the interstitial space; 3) bronchoconstriction will be more effective as a result of the increased wall thickness (and decreased viscosity?) of the interstitial space; [What happens in the region external to the smooth muscle layer is also obviously important but not addressed here]; 4) there must be sources of chemotactic substances in the mucosa directing immune cell movement; whether there are also inhibitors of movement and of connective tissue degradation in the interstitial space which must be inactivated or rendered ineffective for immune cell movement is unclear. 5) Since immune cells are frequently found near nerves and nerves and neuroendocrin-like cells are present in the mucosa, they may provide a source of trophic or chemotactic material for some immune cells.

In conclusion, these structural studies provide a basis for hypotheses about normal and abnormal (owing to inflammation) control of airway function. Where very limited functional data exist there is good agreement; where it is absent, these studies suggest some appropriate experiments.

REFERENCES

1. Agrawal, R. and E.E. Daniel. Control of gap junction formation in canine trachea by arachidonic acid metabolites. Am. J. Physiol. 250 (Cell Physiol. 19): C495-C505, 1986.
2. Allescher, H.-D., I. Berezin, J. Jury and E.E. Daniel. Development of a model for electrophysiological evaluation of non-adrenergic, non-cholinergic neurotransmission in lower esophageal sphincter. Submitted to Am. J. Physiol.
3. Burnstock, G. Autonomic innervation and transmission. Br. Med. Bull. 35: 253-262, 1979.
4. Cameron, A.R. and C.T. Kirkpatrick. A study of excitatory neuromuscular transmission in the bovine trachea. J. Physiol.(Lond.) 270: 733-745, 1977.

5. Cameron, A.R., C.G. Bullock and C.T. Kirkpatrick. The ultrastructure of bovine tracheal muscle. J. Ultrastruct. Res. 81: 290-305, 1982.
6. Campbell, G. Autonomic nervous system to effector tissues. In: Smooth Muscle, Ed. By E. Bulbring, A. Brading, A.W. Jones and T. Tomita. Edward Arnold, London, pp. 457-495, 1970.
7. Coburn, R.F. and T. Tomita. Evidence of non-adrenergic inhibitory nerves in the guinea pig trachealis muscle. Am. J. Physiol. 224: 1072-1080, 1973.
8. Daniel, E.E., G.S. Taylor, V.P. Daniel and M.E. Holman. Can non-adrenergic inhibitory varicosities be identified structurally? Can. J. Physiol. Pharmacol. 55(2): 243-250, 1977.
9. Daniel, E.E., C. Davis, T.R. Jones and M.S. Kannan. Control of airway smooth muscle. In: Airway Reactivity. Ed. F. Hargreave, pp. 80-107, 1980.
10. Daniel, E.E., M. Kannan, C. Davis and V. Posey-Daniel. Ultrastructural studies on the neuromuscular control of human tracheal and bronchial muscle. Respiration Physiol. 63: 109-128, 1986.
11. Daniel, E.E. Gap junctions in smooth muscle. Chapter on Intercellular Communications. Ed. I. De Mello, Plenum Press, New York, Publisher. (In press).
12. Daniel, E.E., C. Davis and V. Sharma. Effects of endogenous and exogenous PGE_2 in neurotransmission in canine trachea. Can. J. Physiol. Pharmacol. (In press).
13. Daniel, E.E., F. Inoue, L.P. Jager, J. Jury and R. Serio. Excitatory junction potentials in canine trachealis smooth muscle cells mediated via an increased chloride conductance. Submitted to J. Physiol. (Lond.)
14. Danser, A.H.J., R. van den Ende, R.R. Lorenz, N.A. Flavahan and P.M. Vanhoutte. Prejunctional β_1-adrenoceptors inhibit cholinergic transmission in canine bronchi. J. Appl. Physiol. 62: 785-790, 1987.
15. Davis, C., M.S. Kannan, T.R. Jones and E.E. Daniel. The control of human airway smooth muscle (in vitro studies). J. Appl. Physiol. 53(5): 1080-1087, 1985.
16. Dewald, B., R. Rinder-Ludwig, U. Bretz and M. Boggiolini. Subcellular localization and heterogeneity of neutral proteases in neutrophilic polymorphonuclear leukocytes. J. Exp. Med. 141: 709-723, 1975.

17. Fabbri, L.M., H. Aizawa, S.E. Alpert, E.H. Walters, P.M. O'Byrne, B.D. Gold, J.A. Nadel and M.J. Holtzman. Airway hyperresponsiveness and changes in cell counts in bronchoalveolar lavage after ozone exposure in dogs. Am. Rev. Respir. Dis: 129: 288-291, 1984.
18. Foster, R.W., R.C. Small and A.H. Weston. Evidence that the spasmogenic action of tetraethylammonium in guinea pig trachealis is both direct and dependent in the cellular influx of calcium ion. Br. J. Pharmacol. 79: 255-263, 1983.
19a. Hirshman, C.A. and H. Downes. Airway responses to methacholine and histamine in basenji greyhounds and other purebred dogs. Respir. Physiol. 63: 339-346, 1986.
19b. Hirshman, C.A., D.R. Austin, W. Klein, J.M. Hanifin and W. Holber. Increased metachromatic cells and lymphocytes in broncheolar lavage fluid of dogs with airway hyper-reactivity. Am. Rev. Respir. Dis. 137: 482-487.
20. Holtzman, M.J., L.M. Fabbri, P.M. O'Byrne, B.D. Gold, H. Aizawa, E.H. Walters, S.E. Alpert and J.A. Nadel. Importance of inflammation for hyperresponsiveness induced by ozone. Am. Rev. Respir. Dis. 127: 686-690, 1983.
21. Honda, K. and T. Tomita. Electrical activity in isolated human tracheal muscle. Jap. J. Physiol. 37: 333-336, 1987.
22. Jones, T.R., M.S. Kannan and E.E. Daniel. Ultrastructural study of guinea pig tracheal smooth muscle and its innervation. Can. J. Physiol. Pharmacol. 58: 974-983, 1980.
23. Kannan, M.S. and E.E. Daniel. Structural and functional study of control of canine tracheal smooth muscle. Am. J. Physiol. 238: C27-C33, 1980.
24. Kannan, M.S., L.P. Jager, E.E. Daniel and R.E. Garfield. Effects of 4-aminopyridine and tetraethylammonium chloride on the electrical activity and cable properties of canine tracheal smooth muscle. J. Pharmacol. Exp. Ther. 227: 706-715, 1983.
25. Kirkpatrick, C.T. Excitation and contraction in bovine tracheal smooth muscle. J. Physiol (Lond.) 244: 263-281, 1975.
25c. Macklem, P.T. Bronchial hyporesponsiveness. Chest 87: 1585-1595, 1985.
26. Mansour, S. and E.E. Daniel. Responsiveness of isolated tracheal smooth muscle from normal and

sensitized guinea pigs. Can. J. Physiol. Pharmacol. (in press).
27. McCormack, G.S., R.H. Moreno, J.C. Hogg and P.D. Pare. Lung mechanics in papain-treated rabbits. J. Appl. Physiol. 60: 242-246, 1986.
28. Moreno, R.H., J.C. Hogg, and P.D. Pare. Mechanics of airway narrowing. Am. Rev. Respir. Dis. 133: 1171-1180, 1986.
29. O'Byrne, P.M., E.H. Walters, B.D. Gold, H.A. Aizawa, L.M.Fabbri, S.E. Alpert, J.A. Nadel and M.J. Holtzman. Neutrophil depletion inhibits airway hyperresponsiveness induced by ozone exposure. AM. Rev. Respir. Dis. 130: 214-219, 1984.
30. O'Byrne, P.M., E.H. Walters, B.D. Gold, H.A. Aizawa, L.M. Fabbri, M.J. Holtzman and J.A. Nadel. Indomethacin inhibits the airway hyperresponsiveness but not the neutrophil influx induced by ozone in dogs. Am. Rev. Respir. Dis. 130: 220-224, 1984.
31. Pack, R.J. and P.S. Richardson. The adrenergic innervation of the human bronchus: a light and electron microscopic study. J. Anat. 138: 493-502, 1984.
32. Small, R.C. Electrical slow waves and tone of guinea pig isolated trachealis muscle: effects of drugs and temperature change. Br. J. Pharmacol. 77: 45-54, 1982.
33. Sterk, P.J., E.E. Daniel, N. Zamel and F.E. Hargreave. Limited bronchoconstriction to methacholine using partial flow volume curves in non-asthmatic subjects. Am. Rev. Respir. Dis. 132. 272-277, 1985.
34. Sterk, P.J., E.E. Daniel, N. Zamel and F.E. Hargreave. Limited maximal airway narrowing in nonasthmatic subjects. Role of neural control and prostaglandin release. Am. Rev. Respir. Dis. 132: 865-870, 1985.
35. Sterk, P.J., M.C. Timmers and J.H. Dijkman. Maximal airway narrowing in humans in vitro: histamine compared with methacholine. Am. Rev. Respir. Dis. 134: 714-718, 1986.
36. Travia, J. and G.S. Salvesen. Human plasma proteinase inhibitors. Ann. Rev. Biochem. 52: 655-709, 1983.
37. Walters, E.H., P.M. O'Byrne, P.D. Graf, L.M. Fabbri and J.A. Nadel. The responsiveness of airway smooth muscle in vitro from dogs from airway hyperresponsive in vivo. Clinical Science 71: 605-611, 1986.
38. Woolcock, A.J., C.M. Salone and K. Yan. The shape of the dose-response curve to histamine in asthmatic and

normal subjects. Am. Rev. Respir. Dis. 130: 71-75, 1984.

39. Yip, P., B. Palombini and R.F. Coburn. Inhibitory innervation of the guinea pig trachealis muscle. J. Appl. Physiol. 50: 374-382, 1981.

DISCUSSION

Pare: You have said that there's more innervation in peripheral airways. How does that fit with what Peter Barnes has shown, that there are more dense cholinergic receptors in larger airways and what Ann Woolcock showed some years ago, that vagal stimulation produces more central, large airway stimulation?

Daniel: What's surprising is that the innervation was adrenergic nerves, as you look more peripherally.

Woolcock: These are still large airways.

Nadel: Let's call them 4-5 mm airways.

James: How soon can you see damage to the epithelium after ozone exposure?

Daniel: These were the dogs that we studied functionally, i.e. they had 2 acetylcholine dose response curves. So about 1 hour.

Nadel: Boatman et al. wrote a magnificent series of articles describing the electron microscopy of ozone if you want to pursue this.

Stephens: There is no doubt that there is good cell-to-cell coupling if you judge this by the magnitude of the space constant in tracheal smooth muscle. I have a problem trying to relate that to the numbers of gap junctions. Cardiac muscle people said ages ago that 5% of the total sarcolemna should be gap junction to allow adequate communication. Granted that the impedence properties of the two tissues may not be the same, do you have any estimate as to how much involvement of the sarcolemma in gap junctions must there be to provide adequate cell-to-cell communication?

Daniel: In a wide variety of smooth muscle the highest percentage ever observed by me, and I think anybody, is in the circular muscle of the gut where there's about 1-2% of the total sarcolemma which is occupied by gap junctions. The question we have not time to pursue is: is there an alternate route of cell-to-cell coupling not involving gap junctions?

Stephens: In our studies in dog trachea we don't see many cells penetrating to the very centre of a muscle bundle. How does stimulation of those cells occur?

Daniel: When we stimulate dog trachea to get an EJP we have to use a pulse train. Rarely can you get a response to a single pulse. However, when you get to second or third order bronchi, every pulse leads to an EJP. You have to build up the level of acetylcholine in the trachea in order to get a response.

Nadel: People have claimed that gap junctions may be responsible for presynaptic effects. Does that sound feasible to you?

Daniel: Not likely.

Thompson: You demonstrated evidence for a prejunctional β-adrenoceptor effect on EJP. Could you demonstrate that with contractile responses?

Daniel: We didn't study that. Vanhoutte and others have demonstrated the existence of a presynaptic control, but not a physiological role for it. I think there's general agreement that there is presynaptic modulation of release of acetylcholine by β receptors. This is the first demonstration that it's likely to be of physiological relevance.

Barnes: You say there are no gap junctions in human bronchi and that a possible defect in asthma may be an increase in gap junctions. Have you looked at this?

Daniel: I've looked at it quantitatively so far in the model of the Basenji-greyhound dogs of Carol Herschman. At every level there is a small significant increase in the density of gap junctions. Whether that is the explanation remains to be determined.

Mechanisms in Asthma: Pharmacology,
Physiology, and Management, pages 205–217

THE RELATIONSHIP BETWEEN ELECTROPHYSIOLOGICAL AND MECHANICAL EVENTS IN AIRWAYS SMOOTH MUSCLE

Roger C. Small, Robert W. Foster, John P. Boyle and Jane M. Davies.
Department of Physiological Sciences,
University of Manchester Medical School,
Manchester, M13 9PT, U.K.

ELECTRICAL PROPERTIES OF AIRWAYS SMOOTH MUSCLE: RESTING MEMBRANE POTENTIAL, SLOW WAVES AND RECTIFYING BEHAVIOUR.

For a variety of mammalian species, including humans, the resting membrane potential of trachealis cells usually lies within the range -45 to -65mV (Small and Foster, 1988). Smooth muscle from airways of smaller calibre has been little studied, but in the second generation bronchus (Souhrada et al., 1983) or bronchiole (Inoue and Ito, 1986) of the dog the resting membrane potential is close to, or may exceed, the upper limit of the range observed for trachealis cells.

Spontaneous electrical activity is relatively uncommon in airways smooth muscle but oscillations of membrane potential known as slow waves can be recorded from bovine and guinea-pig trachealis (Small and Foster, 1987). Slow waves of guinea-pig trachealis are resistant to antagonists at muscarinic cholinoceptors, antagonists at β-adrenoceptors, guanethidine, hexamethonium and tetrodotoxin (Honda et al., 1986; McCaig, 1986; Boyle et al., 1988). Slow waves are therefore unlikely to result from the activity of intramural cholinergic or noradrenergic neurones. Since the slow waves of guinea-pig trachealis persist in the presence of concentrations of flurbiprofen or indomethacin which suppress mechanical tone (McCaig and Rodger, 1986; Boyle et al., 1988), their discharge is unlikely to be caused by prostaglandin synthesis. Slow wave discharge may therefore represent an intrinsic property of the smooth muscle cell.

Slow waves are abolished in a Ca^{2+} - free medium (Foster et al., 1983a; McCaig, 1986) or by organic inhibitors of Ca^{2+} influx (Ahmed et al., 1985; Small and Foster, 1986). These findings suggest that the depolarizing phase of the slow wave may result from an increase in membrane Ca^{2+} conductance. Accordingly the slow waves may represent a vestigial or aborted form of the action potential. The observations that spontaneous slow waves are often associated with tension development (Kirkpatrick, 1981; Small 1982; Souhrada et al., 1983; Honda et al., 1986) and that increases in slow wave frequency accompany the spasmogenic effects of acetylcholine, histamine or leukotriene D_4 (McCaig and Souhrada, 1980; Ahmed et al., 1984; McCaig and Rodger, 1986) lend support to this hypothesis.

Curiously, in guinea-pig trachealis, the maintenance of spontaneous mechanical tone does not depend on slow wave discharge. Organic inhibitors of Ca^{2+} influx such as verapamil and nifedipine can abolish slow waves without lowering mechanical tone (Ahmed et al., 1985; Small and Foster, 1986). Since spontaneous mechanical tone in this tissue is believed to be the result of prostaglandin synthesis, it may be that prostaglandins act to maintain tone principally by releasing Ca^{2+} from intracellular sites of sequestration. Such a mechanism would permit tone to be maintained in the absence of slow wave activity.

The cell membrane of airways smooth muscle exhibits rectifying behaviour in that the depolarization evoked by a pulse of outward transmembrane current is smaller than the hyperpolarization evoked by an inward transmembrane current pulse of the same size. This rectifying behaviour may explain why spike-like action potentials do not arise spontaneously in airways smooth muscle and why, in most cases, spikes cannot be evoked by excitatory stimuli (Small and Foster, 1987).

The K^+-channel inhibitor tetraethylammonium (TEA) reduces rectification in airways smooth muscle and allows action potential discharge in response to pulses of outward transmembrane current (Kirkpatrick, 1975; Kroeger and Stephens, 1975; Suzuki et al., 1976; Kannan et al., 1983; Ito and Itoh, 1984). Accordingly, it seems likely that plasmalemmal K^+-channels are involved in the rectifying behaviour of airways smooth muscle.

As yet relatively few attempts have been made to characterize the K^+-channels present in the plasmalemma of airways smooth muscle cells. However, patch clamp recordings from canine trachealis have identified a voltage-dependent K^+-channel. The opening of this K^+-channel is dependent on the concentration of Ca^{2+} on the cytoplasmic side of the membrane and can be inhibited by TEA (McCann and Welsh, 1986). Furthermore, studies of the outward K^+ current induced by a depolarising voltage step in trachealis cells (Klockner and Isenburg, 1985) suggest that the K^+ current has two distinct components. The more rapidly activating of these two currents may be dependent on Ca^{2+} entering the cell from the extra-cellular fluid while the more slowly activating of the two currents may be dependent on Ca^{2+} released from intracellular sites of sequestration. It is possible that these two currents are carried by different Ca^{2+}-dependent K^+-channels in the plasmalemma. However, characterization of these two K^+-channels and assessment of their relative importance in determining the electrical behaviour of the trachealis cell have yet to be performed.

ACTIONS OF SPASMOGENS

Potassium chloride (KCl) and TEA may cause spasm of airways smooth muscle by similar mechanisms yet the membrane potential changes evoked by these agents are not identical. KCl acting on trachealis evokes spasm accompanied by graded depolarization but not by the discharge of regenerative action potentials (Suzuki et al., 1976; Coburn and Yamaguchi, 1977; Farley and Miles, 1977; Foster et al., 1983b). TEA also causes depolarization of airways smooth muscle but the K^+-channel blocking properties of this agent allow the discharge of spike-like regenerative action potentials (Kirkpatrick, 1975; Kroeger and Stephens, 1975; Small, 1982; Kannan et al., 1983).

Double sucrose-gap experiments (Coburn and Yamaguchi, 1977) have shown that KCl-induced spasm is dependent on the depolarization for current pulses which return the membrane potential towards the control value also suppress the KCl-induced spasm. Equivalent experiments with TEA have yet to be performed but it is likely that the TEA-induced spasm is also potential-dependent.

There is substantial evidence (Small and Foster, 1988) that KCl- or TEA-induced spasm of airways smooth muscle is initiated by the opening of voltage-operated Ca^{2+} channels (VOCs) in the cell membrane. The ability of organic inhibitors of Ca^{2+} influx (e.g. verapamil and nifedipine) to suppress the spasm and Ca^{2+} influx promoted by KCl or TEA and the ability of Bay K8644 to potentiate KCl and TEA forms a major part of this evidence. Although the organic Ca^{2+} influx inhibitors suppress the spasm evoked by KCl or TEA they have relatively little effect on the evoked depolar- ization (Coburn, 1979; Imaizumi and Watanabe, 1981; Kannan et al., 1983). This suggests that Ca^{2+} movement through VOCs contributes little to the depolarization induced by these two spasmogens.

Agonists at muscarinic cholinoceptors and histamine H_1 receptors evoke spasm of airways smooth muscle by a mechanism which differs from that utilised by KCl and TEA. Acetylcholine (ACh) and carbachol cause spasm of trachealis which is accompanied by depolarization. Slow wave discharge is sometimes stimulated but regenerative action potentials are not observed (Kirkpatrick, 1975; Suzuki et al., 1976; Farley and Miles, 1977; Kannan et al., 1983; Souhrada et al., 1983; Ahmed et al., 1984). Histamine has similar electrophysiological effects in airways smooth muscle (Kirkpatrick, 1975; Suzuki et al., 1976; Souhrada et al., 1983; Ahmed et al., 1984). In guinea-pig trachealis the depolarization induced by ACh or histamine is often accompanied by rapid hyperpolarising transients (Ahmed et al., 1984) which may represent the opening of plasmalemmal K^+-channels triggered by the release of Ca^{2+} from intracellular sites of sequestration (Benham and Bolton, 1986). This Ca^{2+}-triggered K^+-channel opening tends to offset the ACh- or histamine-induced depolarization, and may be prevented by K^+-channel inhibitors such as TEA and procaine (Boyle et al., 1988).

Double sucrose-gap experiments (Coburn, 1979) have

shown that ACh-induced spasm of trachealis is not potential-dependent. Equivalent experiments with histamine yet to be performed but there is substantial evidence (Small and Foster, 1988) that the actions of ACh and histamine in initiating tension development in airways smooth muscle are largely independent of the opening of VOCs. ACh and histamine may initiate tension development principally by releasing Ca^{2+} from intracellular sites of sequestration. However, there is evidence that Ca^{2+} influx may be required for maintaining the tension developed in response to the administration of ACh or histamine (Cheng and Townley, 1983; Ahmed et al., 1985).

ACTIONS OF RELAXANTS

Agonists at β-adrenoceptors (e.g. isoprenaline) have mechano-inhibitory effects in trachealis muscle which are associated with hyperpolarisation and, in those tissues exhibiting spontaneous electrical activity, inhibition of slow wave discharge (Suzuki et al., 1976; Kirkpatrick, 1981; Small, 1982; Allen et al. 1985; Honda et al. 1986; McCaig, 1987). The suppression of these electrophysiological changes by propranolol (Kirkpatrick, 1981; Ito and Tajima, 1982; Allen et al., 1985; Honda et al., 1986) but not by phentolamine (Honda et al., 1986) suggests that they are mediated by the activation of β-adrenoceptors.

Electrotonic potentials evoked during the hyperpolarization induced by agonists at β-adrenoceptors are reduced in amplitude (Cameron et al., 1983; Ito and Tajima, 1982) indicating that the hyperpolarization results from an increase in membrane conductance, presumably to K^+. In guinea-pig trachealis the K^+-channels activated by agonists at β-adrenoceptors do not seem to be apamin-sensitive (Allen et al., 1985) or permeable to $^{86}Rb^+$ (Allen et al., 1986c).

Methylxanthines such as aminophylline and theophylline cause relaxation of guinea-pig trachealis and, in the upper part of their effective concentration range, hyperpolarization and slow wave suppression are also observed (Honda et al., 1986; Allen et al., 1986b). It is possible that methylxanthine-induced hyperpolarization results from the opening of plasmalemmal K^+-

channels for aminophylline can raise the membrane potential of guinea-pig trachealis to a value approaching the calculated K^+-equilibrium potential and the hyperpolarization can be reduced by K^+-channel inhibitors such as procaine and TEA (Allen et al., 1986b).

Several observations suggest that the hyperpolarization evoked by methylxanthines or by agonists at β-adrenoceptors is not essential for their relaxant effects. Firstly, low concentrations of these agents evoke relaxation with little or no change in membrane potential. Secondly, K^+-channel inhibitors such as procaine can antagonise the hyperpolarization without antagonising the relaxation. Thirdly, the methylxanthines and the agonists at β-adrenoceptors retain relaxant activity in a K^+-rich (120mM) medium. In such a medium K^+-channel opening cannot cause hyperpolarization because the K^+-equilibrium potential and the resting membrane potential are virtually coincident (Allen et al., 1985; Allen et al., 1986b). The membrane potential changes evoked by methylxanthines and agonists at β-adrenoceptors may therefore represent a by-product rather than an essential link in the process by which relaxation is evoked by these agents.

The hyperpolarization and slow wave suppression induced by methylxanthines and agonists at β-adrenoceptors can be mimicked by dibutyryl-cAMP and by forskolin (Honda et al., 1986). Accordingly, these membrane potential changes may result from the intracellular accumulation of cAMP.

BRL 34915 is a novel smooth muscle relaxant which causes hyperpolarization of guinea-pig trachealis attributable to plasmalemmal K^+-channel opening. The evidence suggests that the relaxant action of this compound may more directly depend on the membrane potential changes (or K^+-channel opening) than does the relaxation evoked by agonists at β-adrenoceptors or by methylxanthines (Allen et al., 1986a).

NEUROEFFECTOR TRANSMISSION

Field stimulation of cholinergic neurones in the

trachealis muscle of several mammalian species yields a wave of depolarization and a tension increment. Such responses can be abolished either by atropine or by tetrodotoxin (Cameron and Kirkpatrick, 1977; Ito and Tajima, 1981; Ito and Takeda, 1982; Inoue and Ito, 1986) suggesting that the wave of depolarization represents a cholinergic excitatory post-juctional potential (EPJP). Similar EPJPs have been recorded from ferret and guinea-pig trachealis in response to stimulation of extrinsic parasympathetic neurones (Coburn, 1984; McCaig, 1986). Repetitive stimulation of cholinergic neurones supplying airways smooth muscle may initiate a series of membrane potential oscillations or a larger EPJP surmounted by a small action potential (Inoue and Ito, 1986; McCaig, 1986).

Endogenous substances may attenuate cholinergic EPJPs possibly by inhibiting ACh release. In canine trachealis the amplitude of successive EPJPs declines as a result of prostaglandin synthesis (Ito and Tajima, 1981; Inoue et al., 1984; Inoue and Ito, 1985). Noradrenaline released from sympathetic neurones of cat or guinea-pig trachealis may reduce the size of cholinergic EPJPs (Ito and Tajima, 1982; McCaig, 1987).

When airways smooth muscle is subjected to field stimulation in the presence of an antagonist at muscarinic cholinoceptors, single pulses do not evoke discrete inhibitory post-junctional potentials (IPJPs) (Ito and Takeda, 1982; Inoue and Ito, 1986; Boyle et al., 1987). However, repetitive field stimulation in the presence of muscarinic cholinoceptor blockade or repetitive stimulation of extrinsic sympathetic nerves suppresses slow wave activity of guinea-pig trachealis (McCaig, 1986; Boyle et al., 1987). At sufficiently high stimulus frequencies hyperpolarization of trachealis muscle is observed (Ito and Takeda, 1982; McCaig, 1986; Boyle et al., 1987). This hyperpolarization is suppressed by propranolol (Ito and Takeda, 1982; McCaig, 1986; Boyle et al., 1987) and therefore represents a compound noradrenergic IPJP. Since electrotonic potentials are reduced in amplitude when evoked during the IPJP (Ito and Takeda, 1982) the IPJP represents an increase in membrane conductance, presumably to K^+ ion.

The effects of activating non-adrenergic non-cholinergic inhibitory (NANCI) neurones supplying airways smooth muscle can be observed by applying field stimulation in the presence of both muscarinic cholinoceptor blockade and β-adrenoceptor blockade. In feline and guinea-pig trachealis the relaxation evoked by the transmitter of the NANCI neurones occurs without change in resting membrane potential or membrane resistance (Ito and Takeda, 1982; Boyle et al., 1987). In guinea-pig trachealis field stimulation of NANCI neurones did not suppress slow wave activity yet slow wave discharge was depressed when the NANCI neurones were activated using nicotine (Boyle et al., 1987). This may suggest that slow wave suppression can be a feature of the action of the NANCI neurotransmitter provided that the transmitter is released in adequate amount.

ACKNOWLEDGEMENTS

The authors work has been supported by the Asthma Research Council, the British Lung Foundation, the North Western Regional Health Authority and the Wellcome Trust.

REFERENCES

Ahmed F, Foster, RW, Small RC (1985). Some effects of nifedipine in guinea-pig isolated trachealis. Br J Pharmac 84: 861-869.

Ahmed F, Foster RW, Small RC, Weston AH (1984). Some features of the spasmogenic actions of acetylcholine and histamine in guinea-pig isolated trachealis. Br J Pharmac 83: 227-233.

Allen SL, Beech DJ, Foster RW, Morgan GP, Small RC (1985). Electrophysiological and other aspects of the relaxant action of isoprenaline in guinea-pig isolated trachealis. Br J Pharmac 86: 843-854.

Allen SL, Boyle JP, Cortijo J, Foster RW, Morgan GP, Small RC (1986a). Electrical and mechanical effects of BRL34915 in guinea-pig isolated trachealis. Br J Pharmac 89: 395-405.

Allen SL, Cortijo J, Foster RW, Morgan GP, Small RC, Weston AH (1986b). Mechanical and electrical aspects of the relaxant action of aminophylline in guinea-pig isolated trachealis. Br J Pharmac 88: 473-483.

Allen SL, Foster RW, Morgan GP, Small RC (1986c). The relaxant action of nicorandil in guinea-pig isolated trachealis. Br J Pharmac 87: 117-127.

Benham CD, Bolton TB (1986). Spontaneous transient outward currents in single visceral and vascular smooth muscle cells of the rabbit. J Physiol 381: 385-406.

Boyle JP, Davies JM, Foster RW, Good DM, Kennedy I, Small RC (1988). Spasmogen action in guinea-pig isolated trachealis: involvement of membrane K^+-channels and the consequences of K^+-channel blockade. Br J Pharmac In press.

Boyle JP, Davies JM, Foster RW, Morgan GP, Small RC (1987), Inhibitory responses to nicotine and transmural stimulation in hyoscine-treated guinea-pig isolated trachealis: an electrical and mechanical study. Br J Pharmac 90: 733-774.

Cameron AR, Johnston CF, Kirkpatrick CT, Kirkpatrick MCA (1983). The quest for the inhibitory neurotransmitter in bovine tracheal smooth muscle. J exp Physiol 68: 413-426.

Cameron, AR, Kirkpatrick, CT (1977). A study of excitatory neuromuscular transmission in the bovine trachea. J Physiol 270: 733-745.

Cheng JB, Townley RC (1983). Pharmacological characterization of effects of nifedipine on isolated guinea-pig and rat tracheal smooth muscle. Archs Int Pharmacodyn 263: 228-244.

Coburn RF (1979). Electromechanical coupling in canine trachealis muscle: acetylcholine contractions. Am J Physiol 236: C177-C184.

Coburn RF (1984). Neural co-ordination of excitation of ferret trachealis muscle. Am J Physiol 246: C459-C466.

Coburn, RF, Yamaguchi T (1977). Membrane potential-dependent and -independent tension in the canine tracheal muscle. J Pharmac exp Ther 201: 276-284.

Farley, JM, Miles PR (1977) Role of depolarization in acetylcholine-induced contractions of dog trachealis muscle. J Pharmac exp Ther 201: 199-205.

Foster RW, Small RC, Weston AH (1983a). Evidence that the spasmogenic action of tetraethylammonium in guinea-pig trachealis is both direct and dependent on the cellular influx of calcium ion. Br J Pharmac 79: 255-263.

Foster RW, Small RC, Weston AH (1983b). The spasmogenic action of potassium chloride in guinea-pig trachealis. Br J. Pharmac 80: 553-559.

Honda K, Satake T, Takagi K, Tomita T (1986). Effects of relaxants on electrical and mechanical activities in the guinea-pig tracheal muscle. Br J Pharmac 87: 665-671.

Imaizumi Y, Watanabe M (1981). The effect of tetraethylammonium chloride on the potassium permeability in the smooth muscle cell membrane of canine trachea. J. Physiol 316: 33-46.

Inoue T, Ito Y (1985). Pre- and post-junctional actions of prostaglandin I_2, carbocyclic thromboxane A_2 and leukotriene C_4 in dog tracheal muscle. Br J Pharmac 84: 289-298.

Inoue T, Ito Y (1986). Characteristics of neuroeffector transmission in the smooth muscle layer of dog bronchiole and modifications by autacoids. J Physiol 370: 551-565.

Inoue T, Ito Y, Takeda K (1984). Postaglandin-induced inhibition of acetylcholine release from neuronal elements of dog tracheal tissue. J Physiol 349: 553-570.

Ito Y, Itoh T (1984). The roles of stored calcium in contraction of cat tracheal smooth muscle produced by electrical stimulation, acetylcholine and high K^+. Br J Pharmac 83: 667-676.

Ito Y, Tajima K (1981) Actions of indomethacin and prostaglandins on neuroeffector transmission in the dog trachea. J. Physiol 319: 379-392.

Ito Y, Tajima K (1982) Dual effects of catecholamines on pre-and post-junctional membranes in the dog trachea. Br J Pharmac 75: 433-440.

Ito Y, Takeda K (1982). Non-adrenergic inhibitory nerves and putative transmitters in the smooth muscle of the cat trachea. J Physiol 330: 497-511.

Kannan MS, Jager LP, Daniel EE, Garfield RE (1983). Effects of 4-aminopyridine and tetraethylammonium chloride on the electrical activity and cable properties of canine tracheal smooth muscle. J Pharmac exp Ther 227: 707-715.

Kirkpatrick CT (1975) Excitation and contraction in bovine tracheal smooth muscle. J Physiol 244: 263-281.

Kirkpatrick CT (1981). Tracheobronchial smooth muscle. In Bulbring E, Brading AF, Jones AW, Tomita T (eds): "Smooth Muscle: an Assessment of Current Knowledge", London: Edward Arnold, p385.

Klockner U, Isenburg G (1985). Calcium activated potassium currents as an indicator for intracellular Ca^{2+} transients (single smooth muscle cells from trachea and urinary bladder). Pflugers Archiv 405:R61.

Kroeger EA, Stephens NL (1975). Effect of tetraethylammonium on tonic airway smooth muscle: initiation of phasic electrical activity. Am J Physiol 228: 633-636.

McCaig DJ (1986). Electrophysiology of neuroeffector transmission in the isolated, innervated trachea of the guinea-pig. Br J Pharmac 89: 793-801.

McCaig DJ (1987). Effects of sympathetic stimulation and applied catecholamines on mechanical and electrical responses to stimulation of the vagus nerve in guinea-pig isolated trachea. Br J Pharmac 91: 385-394.

McCaig DJ, Rodger IW (1986). Electrophysiological effects of leukotriene D_4 in guinea-pig trachealis airways smooth muscle. Br J Pharmac 88: 399P.

McCaig DJ, Souhrada JF (1980). Alteration of electrophysiological properties of airways smooth muscle from sensitized guinea-pigs. Resp Physiol 41: 49-60.

McCann JD, Welsh MJ (1986). Calcium-activated K^+-channels in canine airway smooth muscle. J Physiol 372: 113-127.

Small RC (1982). Electrical slow waves and tone of guinea-pig isolated trachealis muscle: effects of drugs and temperature changes. Br J Pharmac 77: 45-54.

Small RC, Foster RW (1986). Airways smooth muscle: an overview of morphology, electrophysiology and aspects of the pharmacology of contraction and relaxation. In Kay AB (ed): "Asthma: Clinical Pharmacology and Therapeutic Progress", London: Blackwell Scientific, p101.

Small RC, Foster RW (1987). Electrophysiological behaviour of normal and sensitized airways smooth muscle. Am Rev Resp Dis. In press.

Small RC, Foster RW (1988). Electrophysiology of the airways smooth muscle cell. In Barnes PJ, Rodger IW, Thompson NC (eds): "Asthma: Basic Mechanisms and Clinical Management", London: Academic Press, in press.
Souhrada M, Klein JJ, Berend N, Souhrada JF (1983). Topographical differences in the physiological responses of canine airway smooth muscle. Resp Physiol 52: 245-248.
Suzuki H, Morita K, Kuriyama H (1976). Innervation and properties of the smooth muscle of the dog trachea. Jap J Physiol 26: 303-320.

DISCUSSION

Marthan: Have you repeated the experiments with receptor activation in the presence of barium?

Small: We've not used barium to analyse the mechanism of the noise. Klockner & Isenberg have studied single isolated trachealis cells and monitored the outward K^+ currents. They used a Ca^{2+} free medium containing EGTA and acetylcholine evoked an outward K^+ current which represents the release of Ca^{2+} from internal stores activating that K^+ channel.

Marthan: Would you expect there to be differences in the rectifying properties of the membrane in different species? In human isolated airway cells we cannot abolish the rectification in the presence of TEA and 4AP and we got no action potential. We did get action potentials with patch clamping using cesium in the pipette.

Small: I've only looked at guinea-pig trachealis but the K^+ rectification is abolished by TEA in dog and bovine trachealis.

Nadel: What can shift acetylcholine from a pathway which is independent of external calcium to one associated with membrane depolarization? Similarly, histamine induced contraction, where both pathways are involved, how does it shift from one to another and is this important in changing the way the muscle responds?

Small: Acetylcholine and histamine in the guinea-pig trachealis cause release of calcium from the internal stores. At low concentrations where the membrane potential changes, both these agents stimulate slow wave activity. If we believe that the depolarization phase of each slow wave represents a "puff" of calcium moving across the membrane into the cell, then we must accept that some calcium goes into the trachealis cells under the action of acetylcholine and histamine. If you look at an established spasm evoked by either of those agents and then expose the preparation to verapamil or nifedipine, then these are more effective in suppressing an evoked spasm rather than preventing the development of tension initially. Thus although release from intracellular stores is of major importance influx assumes a greater importance once tension has reached a peak and is then maintained.

Mechanisms in Asthma: Pharmacology,
Physiology, and Management, pages 219–230

EFFECT OF ACTIVE SENSITIZATION ON CANINE AIRWAY SMOOTH MUSCLE RESPONSIVENESS TO ADRENERGIC AND CHOLINERGIC MECHANISMS IN VITRO

Edwin A. Kroeger, Jerry M. Bergen and
Richard W. Mitchell

Department of Physiology, Faculty of
Medicine, University of Manitoba,
Winnipeg, Canada R3E 0W3

INTRODUCTION

Neural control of canine airway smooth muscle is effected primarily by acetylcholine released from parasympathetic nerves (Russell, 1978) and, to a lesser extent, by norepinephrine released from sympathetic nerves (Vermeire and Vanhoutte, 1979).

The roles of adrenergic and cholinergic neural mechanisms in the development of allergic bronchospasm have been the object of considerable experimental interest. These investigations have led to proposals involving a decreased beta-adrenoceptor set (Szentivanyi, 1968), increased responsiveness to alpha-adrenoceptor activation (Adolphson et al., 1971; Beinfield and Seifter, 1980) and alterations in cholinergic neural function, including the activation by irritant receptors of a bronchoconstrictor (vagal) reflex (Nadel, 1965) and decreased prejunctional inhibition of acetylcholine release by prostaglandin E_2 (Walters et al., 1984).

The present studies derived from our previous observations that the functional expression of alpha-adrenoceptor activation in canine tracheal smooth muscle (CTSM) requires an active component within the basal tone of the equilibrated muscle in vitro (Bergen and Kroeger, 1986) and that a correlate of active sensitization is an increased basal tone of this preparation (Antonissen et al., 1979). Our objectives were to determine, in CTSM from immunologically sensitized animals, whether responsiveness to alpha-adrenoceptor activation is increased and the involvement of cholinergic mechanisms in the increased basal tone.

METHODS

Dogs were sensitized to ovalbumen (OA) or ragweed (RW) by a technique developed by Pinckard et al. (1972) involving immunization at birth to either an OA-dinitrophenol conjugate (10 mg) or ragweed pollen extract (0.5 mg) with $Al(OH)_3$ (30 mg) as adjuvant for both. Animals with serum IgE titers >256 (as determined by passive cutaneous anaphylaxis in non-sensitized dogs) and which developed large increases in specific airflow resistance when challenged with inhalation of the sensitizing antigen (Kepron et al., 1977) were used as the source of sensitized tissue in these studies. These muscles consistently showed a Schultz-Dale response when exposed to the sensitizing antigen in vitro (Antonissen et al., 1979).

Adult animals were anesthetized with sodium pentobarbital (30 mg/kg, i.v.), the trachea excised and the muscle dissected into parallel-fibred strips approximately 1 cm long, and 0.15 cm wide (as per Stephens et al., 1969). Muscles were mounted isometrically near optimal length in 10 ml baths and the myograms recorded using Statham UC-3 force transducers connected to a Gould-Brush 2400 recorder. Equilibration of muscles (~90 min) was in physiological salt solution (PSS, in mM: NaCl,115; KCl,2.5; $NaHCO_3$,24; NaH_2PO_4,1.4; $MgSO_4.7H_2O$,2.5; $CaCl_2$,1.9 and dextrose, 5.6) aerated with 95% O_2/5% CO_2 and maintained at 37°C. Contractions were normalized, for statistical purposes, by calculating tension in g/cm^2.

Drugs used in these experiments were obtained from the Sigma Chemical Co (St. Louis, MO) and their concentrations expressed in final bath concentrations.

RESULTS AND DISCUSSION

The possibility that alpha-adrenoceptor-related mechanisms are altered with sensitization was addressed first by examining the responses of muscles to tyramine, which releases NE from neural stores, as well as the responses to exogenous NE and adrenergic antagonists. The responses to tyramine (figure 1) show a dose-

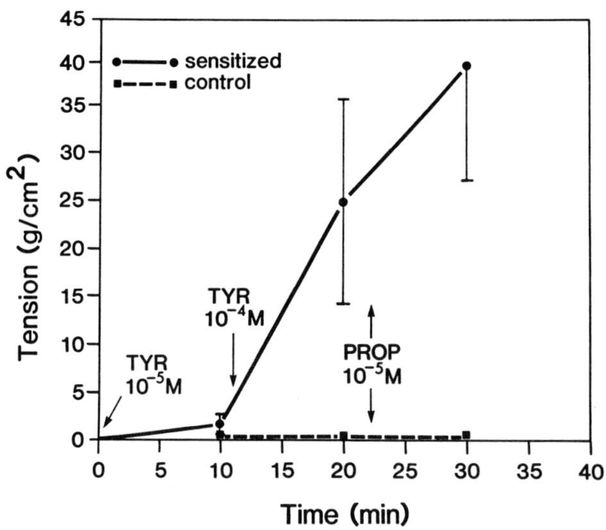

Figure 1. Effect of tyramine (TYR) and propranolol (PROP) on tone in CTSM from control (n=7) and OA-sensitized (n=10) dogs. Data points represent the mean ± SE of plateau responses.

related contractile response which was potentiated by propranolol, thus suggesting that NE released from sympathetic nerve terminals may modulate tone in CTSM and that its contractile effects are antagonized by beta-adrenoceptors. Control, non-sensitized muscles, however, did not respond to tyramine even in the presence of propranolol, thus indicating the specificity of the effect of tyramine and the qualitative change effected by sensitization. In order to determine the maximum responsiveness of these muscles to exogenous NE, propranolol-pretreated muscles were exposed to cumulatively increasing doses of NE and tyramine (figure 2). The strong maximal response was completely inhibited by phentolamine.

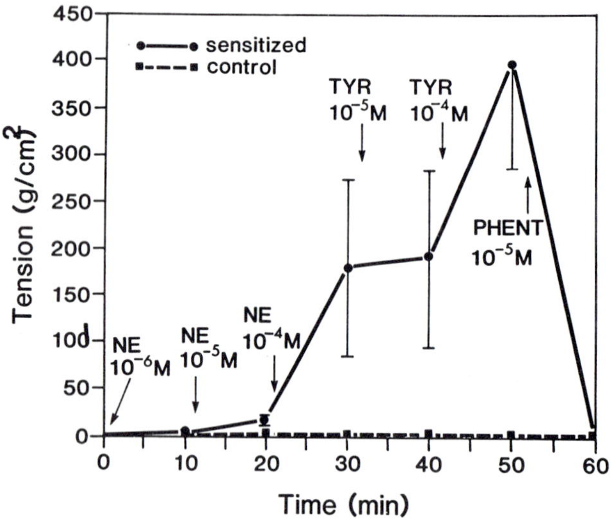

Figure 2. Effect of norepinephrine (NE), tyramine (TYR) and phentolamine (PHENT) on tone in propranolol-pretreated (10^{-5}M) CTSM from control (n=5) and OA-sensitized (n=9) dogs. Data points represent the mean $\pm$ SE of plateau responses.

Non-sensitized muscles, once again, did not respond to NE at any concentration even in the presence of tyramine though it should be noted that, when basal tone is elevated, as in the presence of elevated $[K]_o$, control CTSM also contracts in response to NE (Bergen and Kroeger, 1986) and the above-noted differences between control and sensitized muscles are abolished. Thus the response to alpha-adrenoceptor activation appears to be qualitatively changed in sensitized muscles, perhaps as a result of a change in basal tone although the possibility of increased alpha adrenoceptor-agonist binding, as occurs in lungs of allergic guinea pigs (Barnes et al., 1980) was not directly tested.

In order to evaluate the possibility of a cholinergic involvement in the altered alpha-adrenoceptor-mediated events, experiments were designed to examine the effect of sensitization on basal tone, responses to cholinergic nerve stimulation and exogenous acetylcholine. Figure 3 illustrates some of the mechanical characteristics of the sensitized- and littermate-control muscles. In their responses to electrical field

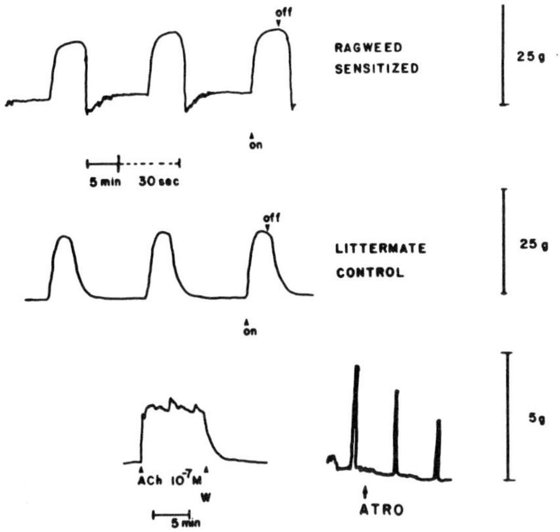

Figure 3. Representative mechanical responses of RW-sensitized and littermate control muscles to electrical field stimulation (60 Hz, "on/off"), acetylcholine (ACh) and atropine (ATR).

(nerve) stimulation, sensitized muscles produced a sustained plateau and their non-stimulated (basal) tension gave evidence of an active component with phasic spontaneous activity. The basal tension of control tissues, in contrast, shows no sign of an active component or spontaneous activity as is consistent with our previous observations that this muscle is incapable, due to its strong outward rectification (Kroeger and Stephens, 1975), of producing action potentials. The plateau of the response to electrical stimulation is also not maintained in control CTSM. Spontaneous phasic mechanical activity is, however, frequently seen in control muscles exposed to low concentrations of acetylcholine. Further evidence in support of a role for this neurotransmitter in the elevated basal tension of sensitized muscle is the observation that treatment with atropine caused a relaxation of basal tone in sensitized, but not control muscles.

Since field-stimulated contractions such as those seen in figure 3 are almost completely inhibited by atropine as well as by tetrodotoxin (Bergen and Kroeger, 1986), field stimulation provides a useful tool for evaluating cholinergic mechanisms in this muscle. The stimulus-response relationships in control and sensitized CTSM (figure 4) showed a significant leftward shift in

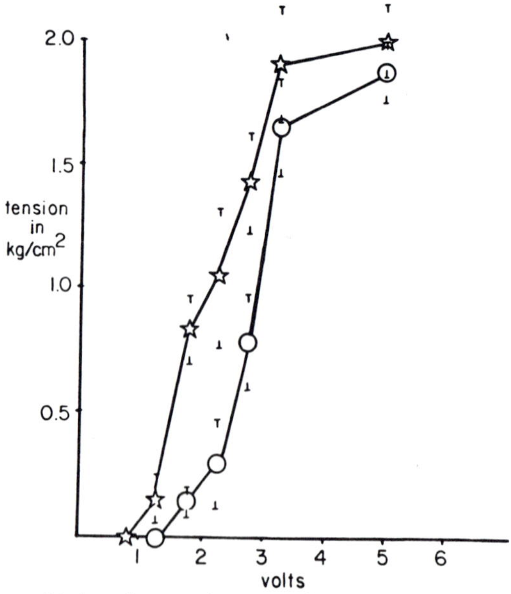

Figure 4. Stimulus (60 Hz)-response relations in control (circles, n=5) and RW-sensitized (stars, n=5) CTSM. Means ± SEM are shown.

the response of sensitized muscles to electrical stimulation and suggested the possibilities of increased neurotransmitter release, up-regulation of muscarinic receptors and/or decreased cholinesterase activity in sensitized muscle. Since these mechanical data were normalized in terms of cross-sectional area of muscle, smooth muscle hypertrophy/hyperplasia could be discounted as contributory factors.

In order to discriminate between the above possibilities, the dose-response relation to acetylcholine was investigated. The results (figure 5) showed a significantly increased response in sensitized CTSM over a broad range of

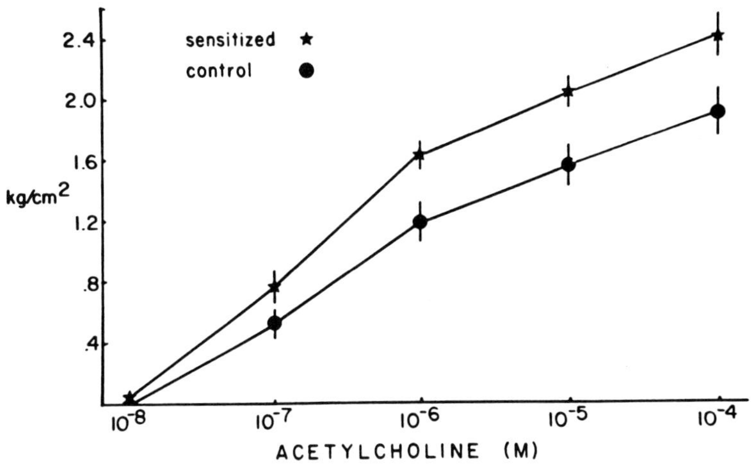

Figure 5. Dose-response relation of RW-sensitized- (stars, n=8) and littermate control (circles, n=5) CTSM. The ED_{50} values were 4.1 ± 1.0 X 10^{-7}M and 8.0 ± 1.4 X 10^{-7}M for sensitized and control muscles, respectively.

concentrations. While these results could be interpreted in terms of a non-specific increase in muscle responsiveness, it should be noted that the potentiation in response of sensitized muscles to increased $[K]_o$ is reversed by atropine

(Mitchell et al., in press), thus once again focussing attention on the cholinergic basis for the altered responsiveness. These results indicated that an increase in acetylcholine released from neural elements need not be postulated. In order to differentiate between altered receptor set and cholinesterase activity, dose-response relationships were studied in the presence of the cholinesterase inhibitor eserine. Since higher concentrations of this agent cause an increase in basal tone, a low dose (10^{-8}M) was used in these studies. The results (figure 6) show that eserine abolished the difference in the responses of

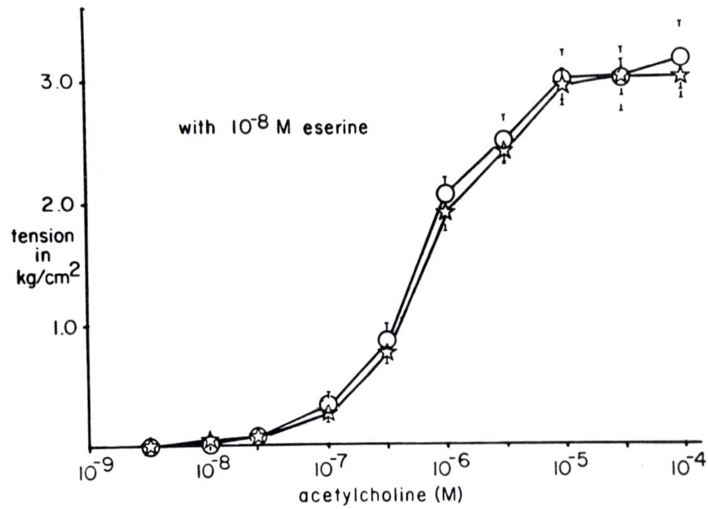

Figure 6. Dose-response relation of RW-sensitized (stars, n=5) and littermate control (circles, n=6) CTSM to ACh in the presence of eserine.

control and sensitized CTSM to acetylcholine. Since the dose-response relation of these respective muscles to carbachol, which is not hydrolysed by cholinesterase, was also not significantly different (Mitchell et al., in press) these findings were inconsistent with a primary effect of sensitization on the muscarinic receptor set and suggested the possibility of a decrease in cholinesterase activity in sensitized muscles. Measurement of cholinesterase activity in homogenates of the respective muscles (2-nitro-5-mercaptobenzoate method of Ellman et al., 1961) confirmed our expectation as sensitized muscles showed a significant decrease (~20%) in cholinesterase activity.

The model within which we interpret the effects of sensitization on basal tone, responses to field stimulation and alpha-adrenoceptor activation involves a primary decrease in cholinesterase activity. The resulting increase in acetylcholine concentration at muscarinic receptors could account for the increased basal tone and, thus, allow the expression of alpha-adrenoceptor activation as well as potentiate responses to nerve stimulation. Previous studies by ourselves (Bergen and Kroeger, 1986) and others (Kneussl and Richardson, 1978; Ohno et al., 1981; Leff et al., 1982) have shown airway tone to be a necessary prerequisite in that process.

Since our previous studies had shown an atropine-sensitive component in the mechanical response to increased $[K]_o$ (Bergen and Kroeger, 1986) it was important to determine whether the potentiation of mechanical responses to NE in sensitized muscles represented a specific interaction of cholinergic and adrenergic mechanisms or a non-specific concomitant of the increased tone. Our observations (unpublished) that atropine 1) did not alter the response to NE in muscles in which tone had been elevated in the presence of 23 mM K^+ but 2) abolished the response of resting ragweed-sensitized muscles to NE suggested a non-specific, tone-related mechanism as is consistent with the conclusion of Barnes et al. (1983) concerning a role for voltage-sensitive Ca channels.

In conclusion, the present observations suggesting a functional relationship between adrenergic and cholinergic mechanisms regulating tone in sensitized airways complement those of Suzuki et al. (1976) in defining the relevance of adrenergic mechanisms in allergic airways disease.

ACKNOWLEDGEMENTS

This work was supported by grants MA4765 and MA2604 from the Medical Research Council of Canada.

REFERENCES

Adolphson RS, Abern SB, Townley RG (1971). Human and guinea pig respiratory smooth muscle - Demonstration of alpha adrenergic receptors. J Allergy 47:110-111.

Antonissen LA, Mitchell RW, Kroeger EA, Kepron W, Tse KS, Stephens NL (1979). Mechanical alterations of airway smooth muscle in a canine asthmatic model. J Appl Physiol 46:681-687.

Barnes PJ, Dollery CT, MacDermot J (1980). Nature (Lond) 285:569-571.

Beinfield WH, Seifter J (1980). Contraction of dog trachealis in vivo: Role of alpha-adrenergic receptors. J Appl Physiol 48:329-336.

Bergen J, Kroeger EA (1986). Adrenoceptor-mediated responses of canine tracheal smooth muscle. J Pharmacol Exp Ther 238:679-684.

Ellman GL, Courtney KD, Andres V Jr, Featherstone VE (1961). A new and rapid colorimetric determination of cholinesterase activity. Biochem Pharmacol 7:88-95.

Kepron W, James JM, Kirk B, Sehon AH, Tse KS (1977).A canine model for reagenic hypersensitivity and allergic bronchoconstriction. J Allergy Clin Immunol 59:64-69.

Kneussl MP, Richardson JB (1978). Alpha-adrenergic receptors in human and canine tracheal and bronchial smooth muscle. J Appl Physiol 45:307-311.

Kroeger EA, Stephens NL (1975). Effect of tetraethylammonium on tonic airway smooth muscle: initiation of phasic electrical activity. Am J Physiol 228:633-636.

Leff AR, Munoz NM, Shoulberg N (1982). Alpha-adrenergic contractile properties of canine tracheal muscle in vitro. Fed Proc 41:1355.

Mitchell RW, Kroeger EA, Kepron W, Stephens NL (in press). Local parasympathetic mechanisms for ragweed sensitized canine trachealis hyperresponsiveness. J Pharmacol Exp Ther

Nadel JA (1965). Structure-function relationships in the airways: bronchoconstriction mediated via vagus nerves or bronchial arteries; peripheral lung constriction mediated by pulmonary arteries. Med Thorac 22:231.

Ohno Y, Watanabe M, Kasuya Y (1981). Manifestation of latent alpha-excitatory response in the canine tracheal smooth muscle preparation - relation to basal tone. Arch Int Pharmacodyn Ther 251:205-216.

Pinckard RN, Halonen M, Meng AL (1972). Preferential expression of anti-bovine serum albumin IgE homocytotropic antibody synthesis and anaphylactic sensitivity in the neonatal rabbit. J Allergy Clin Immunol 49:301.

Russell JA (1978). Responses of isolated canine airways to electric stimulation and acetylcholine. J Appl Physiol 45:690-698.

Stephens NL, Kroeger EA, Mehta JA (1969). Force-velocity characteristics of respiratory airway smooth muscle. J Appl Physiol 26:685-692.

Suzuki H, Morita K, Kuriyama H (1976). Innervation and properties of the smooth muscle of the dog trachea. Jpn J Physiol 26:303-320.

Szentivanyi A (1968). The beta adrenergic theory of atopic abnormality in bronchial asthma. J Allergy 42:203-232.

Vermeire PA, Vanhoutte PM (1979). Inhibitory effects of catecholamines in isolated canine bronchial smooth muscle. J Appl Physiol 46:787-791.

Walters EH, O'Byrne PM, Fabbri LM, Graf PD, Holtzman PJ, Nadel JA (1984). Control of neurotransmission by prostaglandins in canine trachealis smooth muscle. J Appl Physiol 57:129-134.

DISCUSSION

Seale: How do you measure the decrease in acetylcholinesterase activity, and what do you think the mechanism whereby sensitization decreases acetylcholinesterase activity might be?

Kroeger: We used the 5 mercapto benzoate method for measuring acetylcholine in ground-up tissues. As to mechanisms, it occurs in both actively and passively sensitized tissues but I have no idea as to how this occurs.

Benveniste: Do you believe that the changes that you see are related to the immunization of the animal or to the presence of the antibody on the cell - did you do passive transfer experiments to see if you can reproduce these results?

Kroeger: We did not do passive transfer, but these tissues were taken from animals which have not seen a challenge for some considerable time. They have also been in the organ bath for a while.

P. Barnes: It's possible that there could be some defect in a muscarinic autoreceptor in this preparation that gives you enhanced acetylcholine release. We have some preliminary clinical evidence for this in asthma. Have you looked for autoreceptors in this preparation?

Kroeger: No - I must point out that the change in acetylcholine release does not seem to be the major factor since the response with eserine showed we did not enhance responsiveness. So I would suggest that the cholinesterase is likely to be physiologically more important.

Mechanisms in Asthma: Pharmacology,
Physiology, and Management, pages 231–254

MECHANISMS OF INCREASED SHORTENING OF SENSITIZED AIRWAY SMOOTH MUSCLE

Newman L. Stephens, S.K. Kong and C.Y. Seow
Department of Physiology, Faculty of Medicine, University of Manitoba, Winnipeg, Manitoba, Canada R3E 0W3

INTRODUCTION

Were it not for the existence of asthma perhaps no great interest would have developed in research dealing with airway smooth muscle (ASM) function. This is partly due to the fact, as pointed out by Otis (1983) that, while speculations abound, there is no clear idea as to what actually is the function of smooth muscle in the airways. This uncertainty notwithstanding, the high incidence of asthma all over the world, especially among children, points out the need to study the physiology and patho- physiology of airway smooth muscle. In this context it is worth pointing out that suitable animal models will play an important role since, for obvious reasons, human airway smooth muscle is difficult to come by.

Study of airway smooth muscle is important for another reason that extends to beyond elucidation of the pathogenesis of asthma. This refers to the fact that insight obtained from airway smooth muscle research (especially that dealing with its biochemical properties) may help us understand how movement is initiated and regulated in a host of non-muscular contractile systems. These employ an acto-myosin system akin to that of mammalian smooth muscle and radically different from that of striated muscle. Examples of nonmuscular contractile systems are cilia of tracheo-bronchial epithelium and of the Fallopian tubes, spermatozoa, mitosis in cells, exocytosis of neurotransmitters from presynaptic neural membranes, macrophages, fibroblasts, platelets and slime moulds.

In this chapter we will deal with determining whether airway smooth muscle from sensitized animals demonstrates increased shortening in vitro. If so, it could provide a test tube model of allergic bronchoconstriction. We will also describe studies, based on new analytical techniques, that help us understand important factors determining the muscle's capacity to shorten. Briefly these consist of two processes. Firstly and importantly, study of what has been termed, by striated muscle investigators, the internal resistance to shortening. If a structure exists intracellularly that impedes shortening, then increased compliance of this hypothetical structure could permit development of the increased bronchoconstriction of asthma. The second is study of the maximum velocity of shortening. By itself it does not tell us whether increased velocity could necessarily result in increased shortening, but only whether whatever shortening is seen develops over a shorter time frame. It is not difficult to imagine a situation in which, though the muscle enjoyed increased ability to shorten it could not realize that ability if the velocity of shortening was critically low.

Structure

What follows is focused mainly on the relationship between airway smooth muscle mechanics and allergic bronchoconstriction. However to conduct reliable mechanical experiments certain structural requirements have to be satisfied. The most important are 1), that the major portion of the tissue to be mounted for study should consist of muscle. Smooth muscles vary considerably in their content of collagen and elastin. Fortunately more than 75% of content of canine tracheal tissue is muscle and thus results of both mechanical and biochemical experiments relate directly to properties of airway smooth muscle, and 2), that the muscle cells in the strip are arranged parallel to each other.

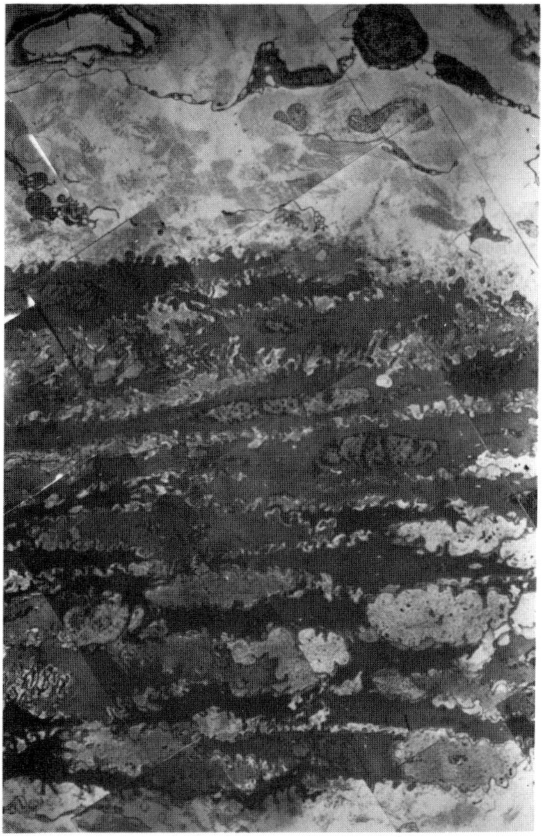

Figure 1. Montage made from low power electromicrographs of longitudinal sections of isometrically contracted canine tracheal smooth muscle (x 1,920)

Figure 1 shows a low power electron micrograph of a bundle of canine tracheal smooth muscles at their optimal length and stimulated supramaximally by electrical means. Fixation has been carried out at the peak of an isometric tetanic contraction. The sole purpose is to show that in contraction the muscle cells remain parallel to each other in the longitudinal axis. Hence all the force developed by the muscle can be measured by a suitably aligned force transducer.

It must be pointed out that demonstrating the cells are parallel to each other is not sufficient with respect to correct measurement of force. Models have been produced (Fay et al. 1984) that indicate the contractile filaments are oriented obliquely across the cell and hence force could not be optimally measured by a transducer aligned with the longitudinal cellular axis. Not all agree with the idea that the contractile filaments are obliquely arrayed. Gabella (1975) and Small (1985) being notable exceptions.

The best way to determine the optimal orientation is to determine it experimentally, according to Herlihy's method (1980). In this, helical strips are cut at a variety of angles and the maximum normalized forces developed by them compared. The optimal cut is that associated with the greatest maximal force. Using this method we found that the optimal cut is in the longitudinal axis of the muscle strip and it is this type of strip that is used for all our experiments.

Another consideration is that in situ the canine trachealis muscle is situated external to an epithelial membrane which if retained in in vitro preparations could present serious diffusion limitation problems. For this reason and to reduce inertial and frictional forces the membrane is always dissected away. To date we have not found any evidence, at least in the canine trachealis, to indicate that an epithelial derived relaxing factor is produced in this tissue. Its presence has been reported in the canine bronchus (Vanhoutte - personal communication).

The next point to clarify is to what extent is the canine trachealis a reasonable model for smooth muscle from those airways where allergic bronchoconstriction occurs. Our previous studies (unpublished) have shown that with respect to mechanical properties muscle from airways down to the sixth generation is qualitatively similar to that of trachealis. There are of course differences in neural control (Russel, 1978) and pharmacological responses.

The final point to deal with is to determine to what extent is canine trachealis a model for human central airways that are the locus for broncochonstriction in the early asthmatic response. From such studies as have been conducted on human tracheal and bronchial tissues (Daniel et al. 1986) qualitative similarities exist. However differences in neural control exist, an important one being that while the dog does not possess a nonadrenergic, noncholinergic inhibitory nervous system, the human does.

MECHANICAL PROPERTIES

Length-Tension Studies

Figure 2 depicts conventional length-tension curves obtained from canine tracheal smooth muscle. With respect to the pathogenesis of abnormal bronchoconstriction the point of interest is that at L_{max} (the optimal length) resting tension is very low. Furthermore as deduced, from the curves shown (Stephens and Van Niekerk, 1977), the trachealis can shorten to a theoretical minimum length of 0.10 L_{max}. When isotonic shortening is measured the minimum length attained is about 0.30 L_{max} (Stephens and Van Niekerk, 1977). This magnitude of so-called supercontraction could very easily shut down the airway. The question then is what prevents normal people from not developing severe bronchostriction. Macklem (personal

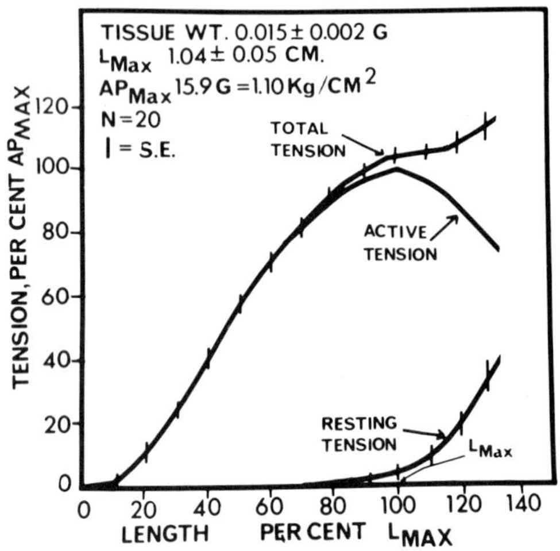

Figure 2. Length-tension curves for canine tracheal smooth muscle. (Reprinted with permission from: Stephens, N.L. et al., J. Appl. Physiol. 1969, 26:685)

communication) has suggested that, <u>in vivo</u>, activation of the nonadrenergic noncholinergic inhibitory nervous system (putative transmitter vasoactive intestinal polypeptide or VIP) inhibits contraction and thus prevents abnormal bronchoconstriction. The nerve fibres for this system are carried in the vagal nerve and the "braking action" of the VIP on cholinergic contraction of airway smooth muscle has been remarked on by other investigators.

Another explanation is that as these muscles shorten <u>in vivo</u>, their intensity of activation diminishes (Stephens, 1987) - a phenomenon, termed reduced activation at short length, shown to be present in both skeletal and cardiac muscle - and this puts a brake on further shortening. Any reduction in the operation of the brake could result in asthma. Figure 3 shows length-tension curves for tracheal smooth

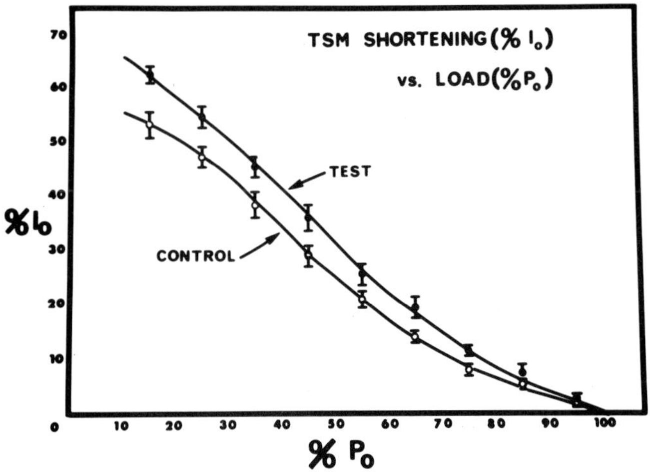

Figure 3. Plot of changes in length during isotonic shortening at different loads for control and sensitized canine trachealis. (Reprinted with permission from: Antonissen, L.A., et al. J. Appl. Physiol. 1974)

muscle obtained from sensitized dogs and litter mate controls relatively early in the course of the sensitization. The animals were about 2 months of age. No significant difference in maximum tetanic tension (P_o) is seen. Had purely isometric studies been conducted one would have concluded the sensitized muscle was normal. However a clear cut difference in maximum shortening is evident. This points out the importance of isotonic studies in detecting early disease. Furthermore isotonic shortening is the appropriate parameter to study, as it is the <u>in vitro</u> analogue to <u>in vivo</u> bronchoconstriction.

Studies to determine the mechanism for the increased shortening of sensitized airway smooth muscle. While many studies have been carried out in a variety of striated and smooth muscles to determine the cause for changes in maximum velocity of shortening, very few have been carried out to elucidate the mechanism responsible for increased shortening. This is even more true for smooth muscle.

One factor that could influence magnitude of shortening is an internal resistance to shortening. The evidence that such a phenomenon exists is straightforward. If one stretches a muscle to beyond L_{max} and then releases it, it returns to L_{max}. Furthermore, if one allows a stimulated muscle to shorten maximally and then removes the stimulus the muscle re-elongates to its original length. It is as if there was an elastic resistance to shortening and stretching. In the shortening mode this resistor undergoes compression and stores potential energy. When the stimulus is turned off the resistor re-expands and restores the muscle to its original length.

The hypothesis we tested is that increased compliance of the internal resistor would facilitate increased shortening of the muscle. To test this a method was developed to delineate the length-tension curve of the internal resistor. Figure 4 shows a depiction of the Voigt model for contraction. When a load is applied to an activated muscle it is transferred to the muscle's contractile element via the spring-like series elastic component (SEC). The maximal velocity attained by the contractile element would be an inverse function of the magnitude of the load. If however the external load was suddenly changed to zero by application of a so-called zero load clamp then the muscle would shorten at maximum velocity. It is evident however that as shortening develops the spring denoting the parallel elastic component (PEC) would relax from its slightly stretched

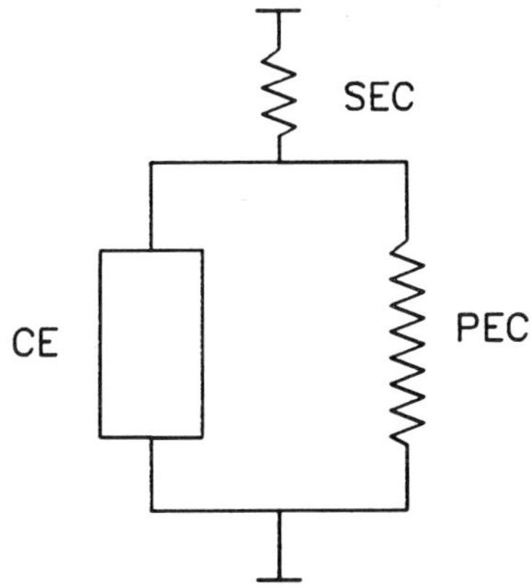

Figure 4. Schematic representation of Voigt Model

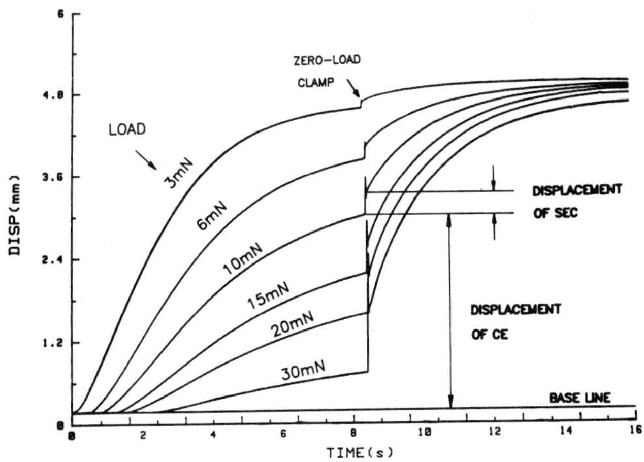

Figure 5. Experimental records of shortening versus time of a strip of canine tracheal smooth muscle set at optimal length initially. The contractile element length was obtained by subtracting the displacement of the contractile element and the series elastic component from the optimum muscle length (L_{max} or l_o). The maximum velocity (V_o) for each length was obtained by measuring the slope of the shortening curve 100 msec after the zero load clamp. The time chosen is arbitrary.

state at L_{max}. With further shortening of the contractile element the parallel component would be compressed further thus imposing an internal load on the contractile element whose velocity would be diminished proportionately.

The critical assumption we make at this point is that the force-velocity curve for the muscle's contractile element is the same regardless of whether the loading is internal via the compressed parallel elastic component or external via the series elastic component.

It is possible to measure maximum velocities of shortening at different contractile element lengths when the external load has been clamped to zero. Figure 5 shows a series of shortening records in which the maximally stimulated muscle was allowed to shorten isotonically. At any point in time the length of the contractile element was a function of the magnitude of the load. At the instant shown in the records zero load clamps were applied. A rapid transient due to the shortening of the unclamped series elastic component is seen in each trace, followed by a slower transient that represents shortening of the contractile element. The maximum velocity attained during this phase is plotted against the calculated contractile element length. Once a suitable range of contractile element lengths had been explored velocity-contractile element length curves were plotted and are shown in Fig. 6. The curvilinear relationship is well seen. A quadratic function best fitted the data. In terms of physiological significance it is evident that for the first 25% of shortening velocity is almost independent of length.

Conventional force-velocity curves were obtained. These were elicited by applying a range of loads after quick-release at the same time at which the studies of the internal resistor had been conducted.

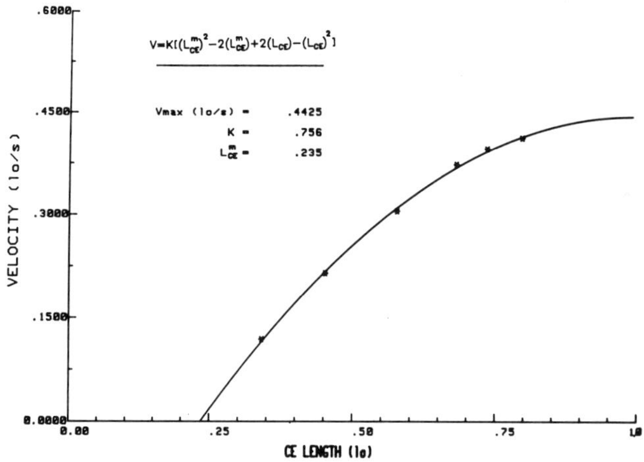

Figure 6. V_O versus contractile element length curve obtained from data in Fig. 5.

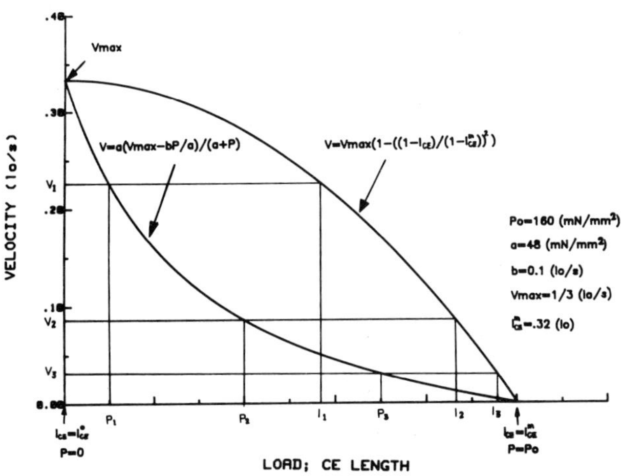

Figure 7. Curves of Fig. 6 superimposed on a force-velocity curve for the same muscle. Note the abscissa represents load for the force-velocity curve and CE length for the length-velocity phase plane.

Figure 7 shows the superimposition of the velocity at zero load versus contractile element curve and the force-velocity curve. From analysis of these curves tension-extension data for the internal resistor or the parallel elastic component can be obtained. For example at a selected velocity, say V_1 the corresponding load point P_1 can be read off the force-velocity point. This represents the load on the contractile element produced by extension of the series elastic component resulting from the external load. Reading the velocity-length (note that the abscissa depicts both length and load) curve for the PEC one determines the length (l_1) at which v_1 develops. The P_1 and l_1 values thus describe a point on the tension-extension curve of the internal resistor. Several points can be obtained and are plotted in Fig. 8 resulting in delineation of the

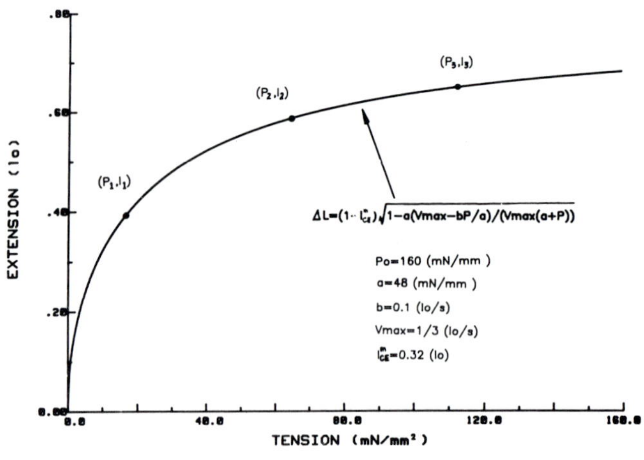

Figure 8. Tension-Compression curve for the PEC obtained from Fig. 7.

tension-extension curve. The figure also shows the empirical equation that best fits the data points.

A similar analysis was carried out for

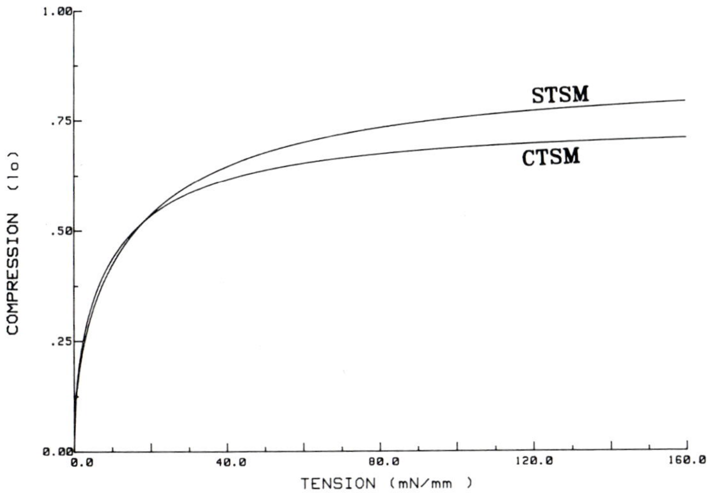

Figure 9. Tension-Compression curves for sensitized and control canine trachealis.

records obtained from sensitized canine trachealis. The two curves are shown in Fig. 9. They reveal that the internal resistor (or parallel elastic component) of the sensitized tracheal muscle is more compliant than that of the control. This could account for the increased bronchoconstriction of asthma or allergic bronchoconstriction.

What the mechanism is for the increased compliance of the internal resistor in the sensitized trachealis is unknown. While collagen and elastin and other structures in the extracellular and extra-fascicular spaces are strong contenders there are others that should be considered. At cellular level the cytoskeleton could play a very important role.

It is now recognized that the cytoskeleton is a very important component of any cell and especially of the smooth muscle cell. Furthermore it forms an exquisitely organized network around and through the sarcomeres of striated muscle (Wang and Ramirez-Mitchell, 1983). In skeletal muscle the major components of the system are nebulin, titin and desmin. Horowits et al. (1986) reported that changes induced in nebulin and titin by low doses of ionizing radiation of skinned skeletal muscle cells resulted in reduced ability of the cells to generate both passive tension in response to stretch and active tension in response to calcium. These experiments highlight the importance of the cytoskeleton in muscle contraction.

Titin and nebulin have not been found in smooth muscle. However this may be because appropriate polyacrylamide gels have not been utilized. The lowest concentration used is about 3.5% and the very large molecular weight proteins may have found it impossible to enter the gel. Studies using 2% polyacrylamide need to be carried out.

On the other hand there are a large number of small molecular weight cytoskeletal proteins present in smooth muscle (Rasmussen et al., 1987) such as filamin, α and β desmin, vimentin, vinculin, plectin, α-actinin and synemin. In addition 4 low molecular weight (18,000 to 30,000 dalton) cytosolic proteins and a separate 23,000 dalton protein have been reported by the same authors. While some or all of these could contribute to the structure of the internal resistor, it may be mentioned *en passant* that Rasmussen (1987) has shown that these proteins are phosphorylated late in the contraction. He has developed a theory that the sustained phase of contraction is not maintained by slowly cycling or latch crossbridges but by these proteins. Relaxation is brought about by a gelsolin induced solation.

Velocity of Shortening

The maximum velocity of shortening (V_o or V_{max}) is a mechanical parameter much studied in striated muscle mechanics. Its importance is clear since effective use of these muscles (cardiac and skeletal) either to effect movement rapidly or to pump adequate volumes of blood is an indirect function of the velocity of shortening, although, in the final analysis, the successful outcome depends upon shortening.

For example in the case of the heart, to maintain an adequate minute volume, regardless of what the V_o is, unless the stroke volume i.e. the magnitude of muscle shortening, is adequate the minute volume will be inadequate. Conversely, given that a certain amount of muscle shortening is necessary to maintain an adequate stroke output it is evident that unless the velocity is adequate also the desired amount of shortening will not be achieved.

Because of the above arguments it was deemed necessary to measure V_o in the sensitized canine trachealis where an increased capacity to shorten had already been demonstrated. It must be admitted that as smooth muscle is not generally called upon to make very rapid length adjustments in vivo, V_o is not as important a consideration as in striated muscle.

Calculations based on the data obtained from the curves in figure 10 revealed that while maximum isometric force production (P_o) in the sensitized tracheal did not differ from that in the control, V_o was significantly increased in the former.

In vascular smooth muscle shortening is effected by the recruitment of crossbridges that initially cycle at a normal rate, but very soon in the contraction slow down. This slowing either affects all bridges uniformly or is the result of the retarding effect of a few newly

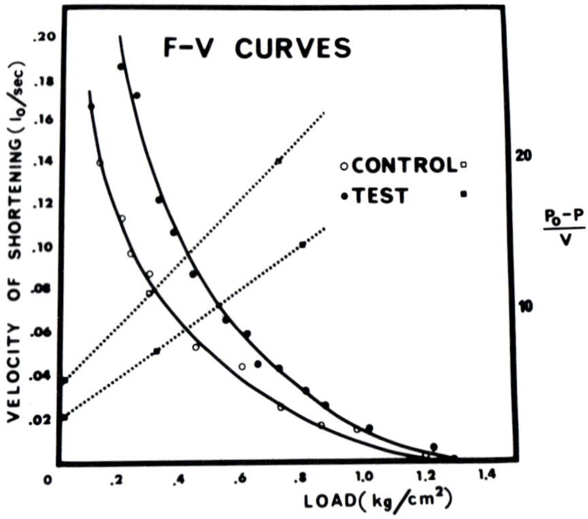

Figure 10. Force-velocity curves for control and sensitized canine tracheal smooth muscles. Linearized transforms are also shown - the right hand ordinate refers to them. (Reprinted with permission from Antonissen et al. J. Appl. Physiol. 1979)

developed latch bridges (Dillon et al. 1981; Stephens et al. 1986). It is therefore necessary to determine whether the increased V_o of the sensitized muscle shown in Fig. 10 reflects activity of the early bridges or of the late latch bridges if such bridges exist in the trachealis also.

Figure 11 shows length changes resulting from the application of zero load clamps at different points in time during the course of a lightly-loaded isotonic contraction. At each point a rapid transient is seen that represents the elastic recoil of the muscles series elastic component. This is followed by a slow transient, depicting the subsequent and slower shortening of the muscle's contractile element. The maximum slope of this transient represents

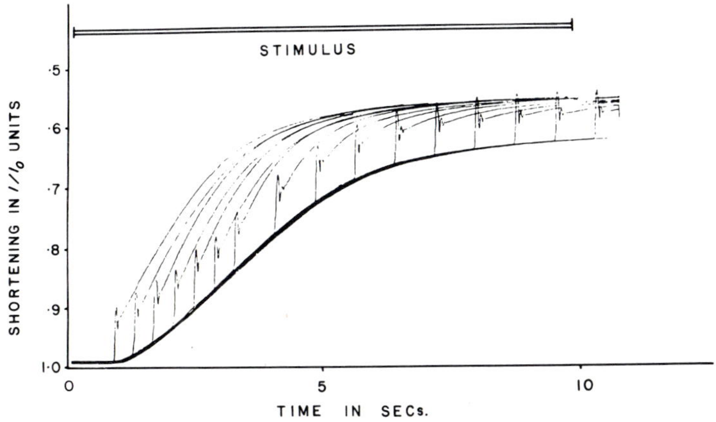

Figure 11. Records of zero load clamps applied at different moments during the course of a lightly loaded isotonic contraction (Reprinted with permission from Stephens et al. Am. J. Physiol. C435-C442, 1986)

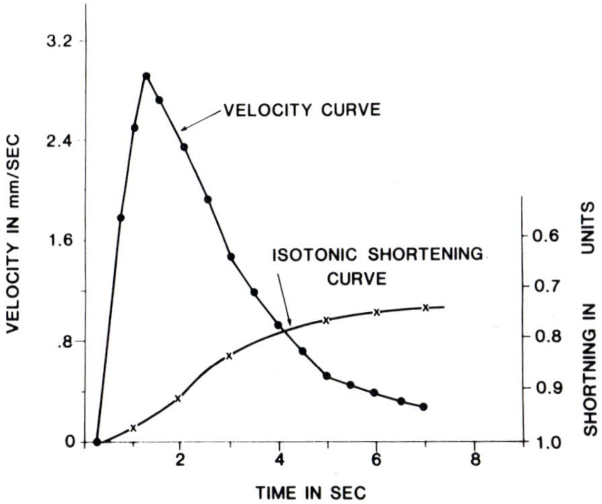

Figure 12. Plot of V_o (obtained from Fig. 11) versus time (Reprinted with permission from Am. J. Physiol. 251:C435-C442, 1986)

the V_o for that particular load.

Figure 12 shows a plot of the V_o's of figure 11 as a function of time. It is clear that maximum velocity of shortening varies markedly with time. Peak V_o is attained very early in the shortening (about 1.75 sec) and falls off rapidly, presumably as latch bridges become operative. This figure confirms that two types of crossbridges, or two varieties of activities in the same crossbridges exist in canine airway smooth muscle.

Table 1 shows an analysis of force-velocity parameters obtained from sensitized and control tracheal smooth muscles. The important finding

CANINE TRACHEAL SMOOTH MUSCLE

	sensitised	control
P_o (kg/cm^2)	1.482	1.50
$\Delta L max$ (l_o)	0.643	0.531
t_T (sec)	8.33	5.50
V_o-3sec (l_o/s)	0.401	0.296
V_o-8sec (l_o/s)	0.121	0.128

Table 1. Force-velocity constants for canine sensitized and control tracheal smooth muscles obtained at 3 sec. and 8 sec. during an isotonic contraction.

is that, only at 3 sec. is V_o greater in the sensitized muscle. At 8 sec. there is no difference in velocity. Maximum shortening (ΔL_{max}) is also greater in the sensitized muscle. Analysis and breakdown of the total shortening showed that 75% of the shortening was complete at the 3 second mark. Thus the major mechanical changes manifested by the sensitized muscle are almost complete within 3 sec. i.e. are produced by normally cycling bridges. The transition time (t_T) is significantly greater in sensitized muscle. We have defined this as the time, in the course of a lightly preloaded isotonic contraction, when normally cycling bridges become converted to slow. The table shows that not only are crossbridges of sensitized muscle cycling more rapidly but they remain in this mode for longer than those of control muscle. These two factors contribute to the increased shortening.

As myosin ATPase of smooth muscle differs radically from that of striated, inasmuch as calcium stimulates activity in the former while inhibiting it in the latter, any study to determine the cause of increased V_o must include studies of calcium metabolism. However we elected to commence our studies of the mechanism of increased V_o by measuring myofibrillar ATPase activity - a more directly related parameter.

Figure 13 shows that the myofibrillar ATPase activity of sensitized muscle is faster than that of control. This could account for the increased V_o of sensitized muscle.

The next series of experiments were carried out to elucidate the mechanism of the increased ATPase activity. The first possibility is that myosin ATPase activity is the resultant of the activities of two myosin heavy chain isozymes much as is seen in skeletal (Silberstein and Lowey, 1981) and cardiac muscle (Hoh et al.

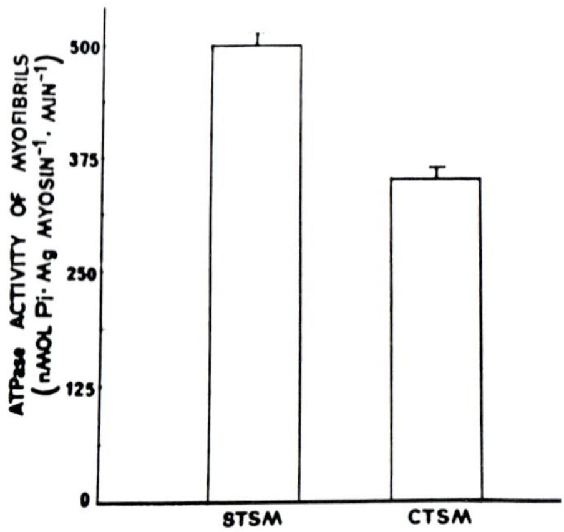

Figure 13. Histograms of mean (± SE) myofibrillar ATPase activity obtained from sensitized (STSM) and litter mate control (CTSM) tracheal smooth muscle.

1978, Schwartz et al. 1978). One of the isozymes could have a faster ATPase activity than the other. In conditions where V_o increased a transition could develop wherein the fast form could increase at the expense of the slow. Fig. 14 shows that two myosin isozymes do indeed exist in the canine trachealis. However no statistically significant difference in myosin band pattern is seen between protein obtained from the sensitized and control trachealis muscles. Thus difference in isozyme patterns cannot account for the increased V_o seen in sensitized muscles. The only remaining mechanism to explain the increased V_o is an increase in myosin light chain (20,000 dalton) phosphorylation. In normal smooth muscle regulation of contractile protein activity is not brought about by tropomin C, which, in fact, is totally missing from smooth muscle. It is effected by calcium-calmodulin dependent activation of a myosin light chain kinase that

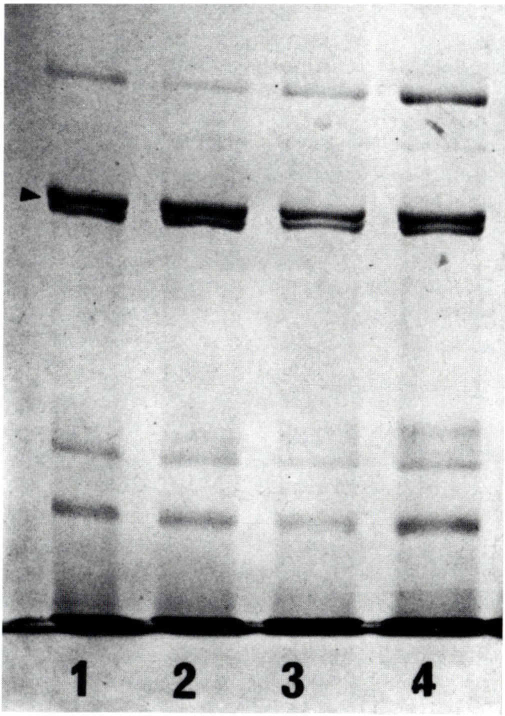

Figure 14. Polyacrylamide gel (4%) electrophoretograms of crude extracts of sensitized and control tracheal smooth muscles. The arrow head indicates the two isoforms of myosin heavy chains. Western blotting and the use of specific antibodies confirmed that neither of these bands originated from a non smooth muscle myosin. 1. Crude extract of litter mate control trachealis. Extraction was carried out employing pyrophosphate. 2. Crude pyrophosphate extract of sensitized trachealis. 3. Crude Guba-Straub medium extract of control trachealis. 4. Crude Guba-Straub medium extract of litter mate control trachealis.

phosphorylates the light chain. A linear relation between light chain phosphorylation and actomyosin ATPase activity has been demonstrated.

We have measured light chain phosphorylation in normal trachealis with the aid of 2-dimensional gel analysis and obtain similar results to those reported for other tissues (Sobieszek and Brenel 1975; Chacko 1981). Densitometric analysis enables the stoichiometry of light chain phosphorylation to be measured. Studies of phosphorylation in sensitized tracheal smooth muscle are shortly to be undertaken.

CONCLUSION

Studies of the mechanical and biochemical properties of airway smooth muscle have helped us understand some of the mechanisms that underlie the increased shortening of sensitized airway smooth muscle. Important findings are that most of the increased shortening is seen within the first three seconds of a contraction whose contraction time is 10 sec. The limit to shortening in normal airway smooth muscle appears to arise from a so-called internal resistance to shortening. This internal resistor is more compliant in sensitized muscle which accounts for the increased ability of the latter to shorten.

The increased shortening ability is associated with an increased velocity of shortening. This velocity increase only affects normally cycling crossbridges which are operative early in the contraction. This change is not due to any change in the distribution pattern of myosin heavy chain zones. By exclusion, it must be due to increased myosin light chain phosphorylation.

REFERENCES

Chacko S (1981). Effects of phosphorylation, calcium ion, and tropomyosin on actin-activated adenosine 5[1]=tri-phosphatase activity of mammalian smooth muscle myosin. Biochem. 20:702.

Daniel EE, Kannan M, Davis C, Posey-Daniel V (1986). Ultra-structural studies on the neuromuscular control of human tracheal and bronchial muscle. Resp Physiol 63:109.

Dillon PF, Aksoy MO, Driska SP and Murphy RA (1981). Myosin phosphorylation and the crossbridge cycle in arterial smooth muscle. Science 211:495.

Fay FS, Fogarty K, Fujwara K (1981). The organization of the contractile apparatus in sinble isolaged smooth muscle cells. In Stephens NL (ed): "Smooth Muscle Contraction." New York: Marcel Dekker, Inc. p. 75.

Gabella G (1975). Fine structure of smooth muscle. Philos Trans R Soc Lond (Biol) 265:7.

Herlihy JT (1980). Helically cut vascular strip preparation: geometrical considerations. Am J Physiol 238 (Heath Circ. Physiol. 7) 4107.

Hoh JH, McGrath PA, Hale PT (1978). Electrophoretic analysis of multiple forms of rat cardiac myosin: Effect of hypophysectomy and thyroxine replacement. J. Mol Cell Cardiol 10:1053.

Horwits R, Kempner ES, Bishor ME, Podolsky RJ (1986). A physiological role for titin and nebulin in skeletal muscle. Nature 323:160.

Otis, AB (1983). A perspective of respiratory mechanisms. J Appl Physiol 54:1183.

Rasmussen H, Takuwd Y, Park S (1987). Protein Kinase C in the regulation of smooth muscle contraction. The FASEB J 1(3):177.

Russel JA (1978). Responses of isolated canine airways to electric stimulation and acetylcholine. J Appl Physiol: Respirat Environ Exercise Physiol 45:690.

Schwartz K, Lecarpentier Y, Martin JL, Lompre AM, Mercadier JJ, Swynghedauw B (1981). Myosin isozymic distribution correlates with speed of myocardial contraction. J Mol Cell Cardiol 13:1071.

Small JV (1985). Geometry of actin-membrane attachments in the smooth muscle cell: the localisations of vinculin and -actinin. The Embo J 4(1):45.

Sobieszek A, Bremel R (1975). Preparation and properties of vertebrate smooth muscle myofibrils and actomyosin. Eur J Biochem 55:49.

Stephens NL, Kagan ML, Packer CS (1986). Time dependence of shortening velocity in tracheal smooth muscle. Am J Physiol 251 (Cell Physiol 20):C435.

Stephens NL, Van Niekerk W (1977). Isometric and isotonic contractions in airway smooth muscle. J Appl Physiol 26(6):685.

Wang, Ramirez-Mitchell R (1983). A network of transverse and longitudinal intermediate filaments is associated with sarcomeres of adult vertebrate skeletal muscle. The J of Cell Biol 96:562.

Mechanisms in Asthma: Pharmacology,
Physiology, and Management, pages 255–265

IS BRONCHIAL HYPERRESPONSIVENESS IN HUMANS A SMOOTH MUSCLE ABNORMALITY?

Johan C. de Jongste and Karel F. Kerrebijn

Department of Pediatric Pulmonology, University Hospital Rotterdam/Sophia Children's Hospital, Rotterdam, The Netherlands.

INTRODUCTION

Airway smooth muscle (ASM) is present from the trachea down to the membranous bronchioles, where it runs in helical strands around the airway circumference. Its physiological role is not entirely clear, but there is no doubt that, in asthma, the acute bronchoconstriction following exposure to nonspecific or allergic stimuli is due to exaggerated contraction of ASM. Many factors may be involved in the pathogenesis of this abnormal responsiveness of asthmatic ASM. One of these factors is an intrinsic abnormality of ASM itself. In order to examine this, several animal models have been developed that have features in common with human allergic bronchoconstriction. The research on human lung tissue, however, has been limited by the supply and by difficulties in obtaining stable and reproducible responses from human airway preparations _in vitro_. It seems nevertheless crucial to study human ASM from patients with bronchial hyperresponsiveness (BHR), because there are important species differences, and because there is no satisfactory animal model of spontaneous non-allergic asthma. This chapter will give a summary of our findings and those of others concerning the role of ASM in human bronchial responsiveness.

HYPERRESPONSIVENESS IN ASTHMA AND COPD

BHR is defined as an exaggerated bronchoconstrictor response to physical, pharmacological and chemical stimuli that do not have this effect in normals. BHR is a hallmark of asthma, where the degree of BHR is correlated with the severity of asthmatic symptoms (Neijens, 1983) and is regarded as a risk factor for the development of chronic airflow limitation (Weiss, 1986). Not only asthmatics, but also many patients with chronic obstructive pulmonary disease (COPD) respond to inhaled histamine or methacholine with a fall in FEV_1, although they generally lack the characteristic "twitchiness" of the airways and do not have the acute wheezing attacks of asthma. BHR in asthma and COPD has different characteristics. In many asthmatics with a normal baseline lung function, a severe bronchoconstriction can be provoked that causes respiratory distress, and makes it impossible to determine the maximal effect of the agonist, or response plateau. In most patients with COPD, however, the dose-response curve reaches a plateau at a relatively mild degree of airway narrowing (Sterk, 1985). The degree of BHR in COPD is correlated with baseline airway caliber (Ramsdale, 1984), whereas in asthma this relation is absent in patients who have a relatively normal baseline lung function. Furthermore, the bronchoconstriction in COPD, but not in asthma, seems to depend on which agonist is used (DuToit, 1986). These different characteristics of BHR in asthma and COPD suggest that the underlying mechanisms may be fundamentally different. Where geometric factors seem important in COPD (Moreno, 1986), the etiology of BHR in asthma is still poorly understood, which is reflected by a large number of hypotheses (Neijens, 1983; McFadden, 1984; Hargreave, 1986). The nonspecificity of asthmatic BHR suggests that the end-organ may be abnormal. Intrinsic defects of ASM may therefore play a role. Abnormalities of many factors that are involved in the contraction of ASM may produce hyperresponsiveness. Before examining putative mechanisms, the question needs to be answered first whether there is hyperresponsiveness of ASM in humans with BHR.

STUDIES ON ASTHMATIC HUMAN ASM

Since 1982, a few reports on asthmatic human ASM function in vitro have been published. In some of these studies, an increased maximal tension development after histamine, cholinergic agonists and leukotriene (LT)C_4 has been observed (De Jongste, 1987a; Schellenberg, 1984, 1985). Others found normal or low contractions (Paterson, 1982; Roberts, 1984; Goldie, 1986; Cerrina, 1986), sometimes with a variably reduced sensitivity and maximal response to beta agonists (Paterson, 1982; Goldie, 1986; Cerrina, 1986). We have observed a pronounced non-specific increase in maximal isometric tension development of asthmatic human ASM obtained during surgery (figure 1). We also found normal relaxation responses to forskolin, a diterpene

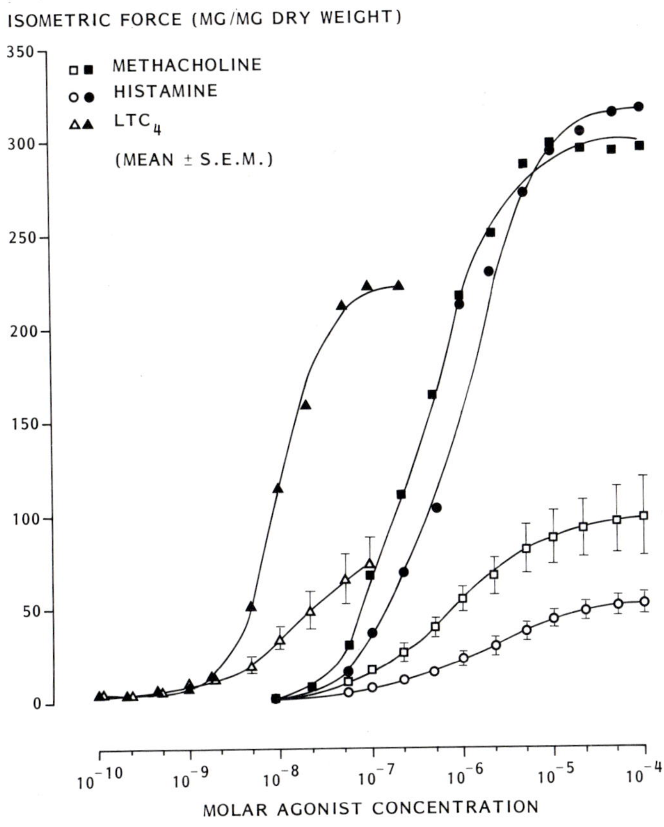

Figure 1. Isometric cumulative concentration-response curves of asthmatic (closed symbols) and non-asthmatic (open symbols) bronchiolar strips to histamine, methacholine and LTC_4. Asthmatic and non-asthmatic curves are from 1 and 10 subjects, respectively; asthmatic curves are the mean of triplicate measurements. The difference in maximal responses of asthmatic and non-asthmatic curves is significant for each agonist.

that stimulates cAMP production receptor-independently, and to l-isoproterenol (figure 2), whereas non-adrenergic inhibitory responses to electric field stimulation were low in bronchi from two asthmatics who were highly hyperresponsive in vivo ($PC_{20}FEV_1$: 1 mg/ml histamine) and had normal baseline lung function (De Jongste, 1987ab). Histologic examination of these asthmatic airways always showed marked ASM hypertrophy (figure 3). Although there seem to be important discrepancies in the results of the few in vitro studies on human asthmatic airways, these may be due to large differences in methodology and patient selection. It is remarkable, for instance, that increases in contractile force have been found in fresh tissue, and that impaired relaxation responses have been found in autopsy tissues from patients that died of asthma.

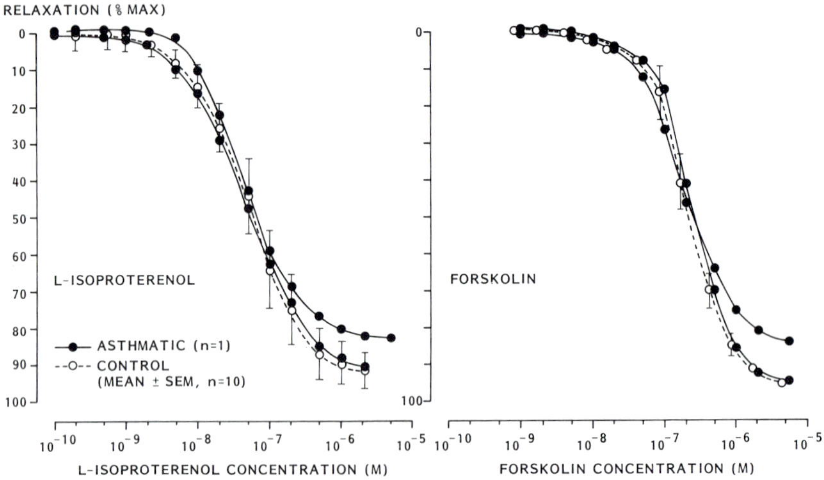

Figure 2. Isotonic cumulative concentration-response curves of human asthmatic (closed symbols) and non-asthmatic (open symbols) bronchiolar strips to l-isoproterenol and forskolin. Individual curves from 2 asthmatic subjects are shown; non-asthmatic curves are the mean of 10 separate experiments. Relaxations are expressed as a percentage of maximal relaxation in Ca-free buffer. Strips were precontracted with methacholine EC_{50}.

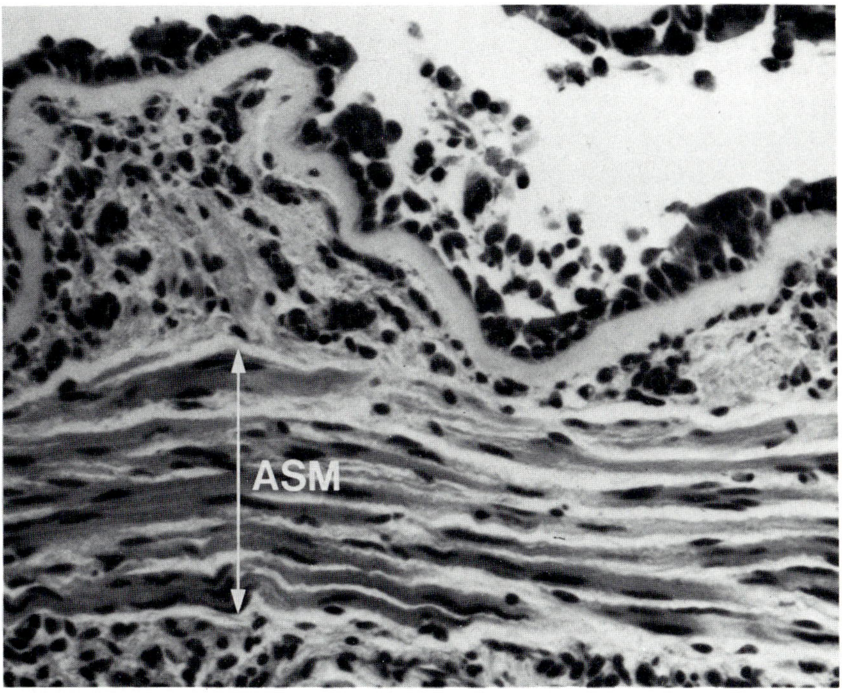

Figure 3. Histological section of a human asthmatic bronchus obtained during surgery from a stable non-smoking asthmatic patient who had a normal baseline lung function, but a highly increased bronchial responsiveness. Note the epithelial derangement, basal membrane thickening, infiltration of the submucosa with inflammatory cells with many eosinophils, and marked smooth muscle (ASM) hypertrophy (stain: hematoxilin/eosin, magnification 250x).

STUDIES ON NON-ASTHMATIC HUMAN ASM

More work has been done using ASM from well-defined populations of patients with and without COPD and BHR. There is now general agreement that, in COPD, the degree of BHR is not related to the sensitivity of ASM to contracting agonists (Vincenc, 1983; Armour, 1984ab; Roberts, 1984, 1985; Taylor, 1985; Cerrina, 1986; De Jongste, 1987c). Previous studies have mainly concentrated on the sensiti-

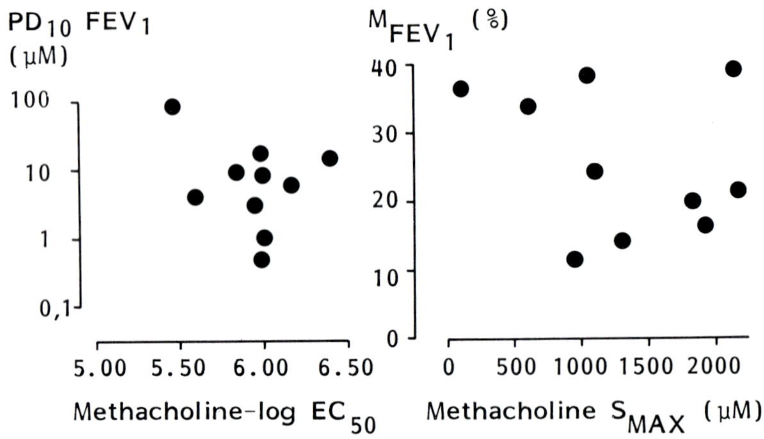

Figure 4. Comparison of in vivo and in vitro bronchial responses to methacholine in 10 non-asthmatic subjects. Left panel: relation between the $PD_{10}FEV_1$ in vivo and $-logEC_{50}$ to methacholine in vitro. Right panel: relation between mean % decline in FEV_1 at the response plateau in vivo (M_{FEV1}) and maximal shortening of ASM in vitro (S_{max}). No significant correlations were found.

vity of human ASM to constricting agents, expressed as the effective concentration that produces 50% of the maximal effect (EC_{50}); absolute responses and maximal effects showed a troublesome within-subject variability. By using carefully standardized techniques and a well-defined airway preparation, the bronchiolar strip, we reduced this variability sufficiently to detect differences in maximal responses between-subjects (De Jongste, 1985, 1986). We have compared the degree of in vivo BHR to methacholine with the methacholine responsiveness of ASM in vitro in 10 non-asthmatic subjects who underwent lung resection for malignancies, and found no relation between the maximal response plateau in vivo and the maximal isotonic contraction of ASM in vitro (De Jongste, 1987d) (figure 4). This suggested that, in non-asthmatic BHR, both the position and the maximal response plateau of the dose-response curve to inhaled methacholine are not determined by ASM function. Although

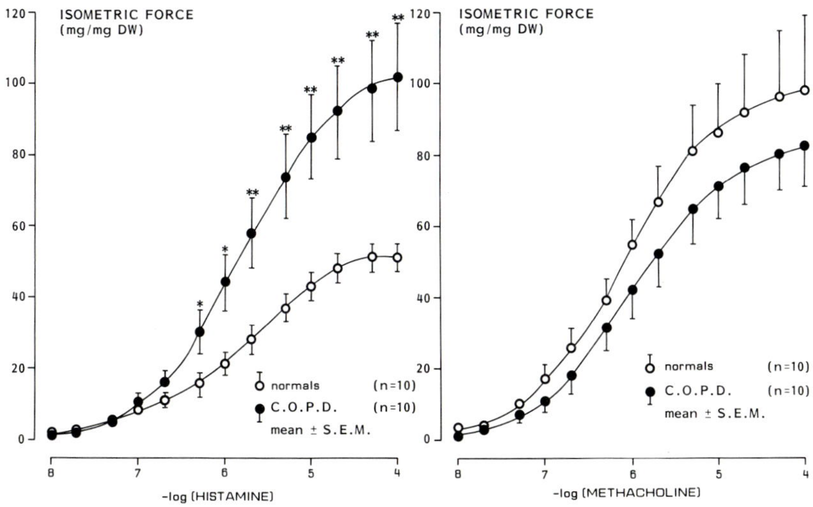

Figure 5. Isometric cumulative concentration-response curves to histamine (left panel) and methacholine (right panel) of bronchiolar strips from subjects with (closed symbols, n=10) and without (open symbols, n=10) COPD. The difference in maximal tension (T_{max}) after histamine is significant (Students t-test, $p < 0.05$).

these data and those in the literature indicate that, in COPD, BHR is not a smooth muscle abnormality, things may be different with respect to histamine. Histamine is more active in peripheral airways, and produces more airway narrowing than methacholine in COPD patients (DuToit, 1986). We have shown that the maximal response of bronchiolar ASM to histamine, but not to methacholine and LTC_4, is significantly higher in patients with COPD than in controls without COPD (De Jongste, 1987c) (figure 5). This suggests, that a histamine-specific hyperresponsiveness of ASM in small airways may be partly responsible for the exaggerated bronchoconstriction after inhaled histamine in COPD.

Unfortunately, no studies have been published on the effects of active or passive sensitization of human airways on ASM function. Several studies have suggested, however, that non-asthmatic allergic individuals may have a normal

ASM function (Vincenc, 1983; Armour, 1984a; Roberts, 1984, 1985).

Acute airway inflammation is probably important in the pathogenesis of BHR. We have examined human ASM function in relation to the degree of airway wall inflammation. In bronchioles from subjects with and without COPD a negative correlation was found between the severity of airway wall inflammation and the sensitivity of bronchiolar ASM to various contracting agonists, e.g. inflamed airways were less sensitive to methacholine than non-inflamed airways (De Jongste, 1987e). These results suggested that, in non-asthmatic subjects, chronic inflammation does not cause BHR via a direct effect on ASM.

Not only an increased contractility, but also a decreased relaxability of ASM could be important in BHR. This aspect has been examined in only few studies (Taylor, 1985; Cerrina, 1986), that showed no differences in mean relaxation responses of non-asthmatic ASM from subjects with and without BHR. We have also found similar mean relaxation responses to l-isoproterenol and forskolin of bronchiolar segments from patients with and without COPD. It seems, therefore, that, in non-asthmatic BHR, there is no intrinsic defect of ASM relaxation.

CONCLUSIONS

Comparative _in vivo_-_in vitro_ studies have shown that, in non-asthmatic humans with BHR, the increased responsiveness of the airways _in vivo_ is not caused by an abnormal sensitivity of ASM to contracting stimuli, and is not due to an impaired relaxability to e.g. beta receptor stimulation. An increased histamine efficacy in small airways may, however, contribute to the _in vivo_ bronchoconstriction after histamine inhalation.

Because of the different nature of BHR in asthma and COPD, the results obtained with non-asthmatic human ASM may not be relevant to asthmatic BHR. The few data on asthmatic human ASM seem inconsistent and contradictory, but can be interpreted in the following way: Dependent on the degree of smooth muscle hypertrophy, there is a non- specific increase in asthmatic ASM strength, as suggested by _in vitro_ studies on fresh airways from stable asthmatics. Hypertrophy and hyperplasia of ASM is a pathological characteristic of asthmatic airways (Hossain, 1973) that may lead to BHR because a stronger muscle will more easily overcome the elastic recoil forces that may normally prevent excessive airway narrowing. Studies on autopsy tissue from asthmatics who died during attacks suggest, that an impaired beta receptor function may occur during severe asthma attacks, which fits the clinical observation that beta agonists are excellent bronchodilators in asthmatic patients, but are usually not very effective during severe attacks.

The study of asthmatic human ASM is progressing slowly due to the limited supply. Furthermore, the techniques that have been used to study human ASM function have serious disadvantages. Bronchial strips are not muscle preparations, but contain many other components such as connective tissue, epithelium and inflammatory cells, that may influence muscle function. It seems unlikely, therefore, that the role of ASM in asthmatic BHR will be clarified without a change in research strategies. Now human ASM cells can be obtained safely from mild asthmatics and healthy volunteers by bronchoscopy, can be cultured with preservation of contractile function, and be used for biochemical, electrophysiological and functional studies, it is likely that the question whether, in asthma, BHR is a smooth muscle abnormality will definitely be answered in due time.

REFERENCES

Armour CL, Black JL, Berend N, Woolcock AJ (1984a). The relationship between bronchial hyperresponsiveness and airway smooth muscle structure and reactivity. Respir Physiol 58:223.

Armour CL, Lazar NM, Schellenberg RR, Taylor SM, Chan N, Hogg JC, Paré PD (1984b). A comparison of in vivo and in vitro human airway reactivity to histamine. Am Rev Respir Dis 129:907.

Cerrina J, Le Roy Ladurie M, Labat C, Raffestin B, Bayol A, Brink C (1986). Comparison of human bronchial muscle responses to histamine in vivo with histamine and isoproterenol agonists in vitro. Am Rev Respir Dis 134:57.

De Jongste JC, Van Strik R, Bonta IL, Kerrebijn KF (1985). Measurement of human small airway smooth muscle function in vitro with the bronchiolar strip preparation. J

Pharmacol Methods 14:111.
De Jongste JC, Mons H, Van Strik R, Bonta IL, Kerrebijn KF (1986). Human small airway smooth muscle responses in vitro: actions and interactions of methacholine, histamine and leukotriene C_4. Eur J Pharmacol 125:9.
De Jongste JC, Mons H, Bonta IL, Kerrebijn KF (1987a). In vitro responses of airways from an asthmatic patient. Eur J Respir Dis 71:23.
De Jongste JC, Mons H, Bonta IL, Kerrebijn KF (1987b). Cholinergic and non-adrenergic inhibitory nerve-mediated responses of isolated human airways in COPD and asthma. Am Rev Respir Dis 135:A 181.
De Jongste JC, Mons H, Block R, Bonta IL, Frederiksz AP, Kerrebijn KF (1987c). Increased in vitro histamine responses in human small airway smooth muscle from patients with chronic obstructive pulmonary disease. Am Rev Respir Dis 135:549.
De Jongste JC, Sterk PJ, Mons H, Timmers M, Kerrebijn KF (1987d). Comparison of maximal airway narrowing in vivo and small airway smooth muscle contractility in vitro in non-asthmatic humans. Bull Europ Physiopathol Respir 23:317s.
De Jongste JC, Mons H, Van Strik R, Bonta IL, Kerrebijn KF (1987e). Comparison of human bronchiolar smooth muscle responsiveness in vitro with histological signs of inflammation. Thorax, in press.
DuToit JI, Woolcock AJ, Salome CM, Sundrum R, Black JL (1986). Characteristics of bronchial hyperresponsiveness in smokers with chronic airflow limitation. Am Rev Respir Dis 134:498.
Goldie RG, Spina D, Henry PJ, Lulich KM, Paterson JW (1986). In vitro responsiveness of human asthmatic bronchus to carbachol, histamine, β adrenoceptor agonists and theophylline. Br J Clin Pharmacol 22:669.
Hargreave FE, Dolovich J, O'Byrne PM, Ramsdale EH, Daniel EE (1986). The origin of airway hyperresponsiveness. J Allergy Clin Immunol 78:825.
Hossain S (1973). Quantitative measurement of bronchial muscle in men with asthma. Am Rev Respir Dis 107:99.
McFadden ER (1984). Pathogenesis of asthma. J Allergy Clin Immunol 73:413.
Moreno RH, Hogg JC, Paré PD (1986). Mechanisms of airway narrowing. Am Rev Respir Dis 133:1171.
Neijens HJ, Duiverman EJ, Kerrebijn KF (1983). Bronchial responsiveness in children. Pediatr Clin North Am 30:829.
Paterson JW, Lulich KM, Goldie RG (1982). The role of

β adrenoceptors in bronchial hyperreactivity. In: Morley J, ed. Bronchial hyperreactivity. London: Academic Press, p 19.

Ramsdale EM, Morris MM, Roberts RS, Hargreave FE (1984). Bronchial responsiveness to methacholine in chronic bronchitis: Relationship to airflow obstruction and cold air responsiveness. Thorax 39:912.

Roberts JA, Raeburn D, Rodger IW, Thomson NC (1984). Comparison of in vivo airway responsiveness and in vitro smooth muscle sensitivity to methacholine in man. Thorax 39:837.

Roberts JA, Rodger IW, Thomson NC (1985). Airway responsiveness to histamine in man: Effect of atropine on in vivo and in vitro comparison. Thorax 40:261.

Schellenberg RR, Foster A (1984). In vitro responses of human asthmatic airway and pulmonary vascular smooth muscle. Int Archs Allergy Appl Immunol 75:237.

Schellenberg RR, Duff MJ, Foster A, Paré PD (1985). Asthmatic bronchial reactivity in vitro. Proc Can Soc Clin Invest A 202.

Sterk PJ, Daniel EE, Zamel N, Hargreave FE (1985). Limited bronchoconstriction to methacholine using partial flow-volume curves in non-asthmatic subjects. Am Rev Respir Dis 132:272.

Taylor SM, Paré PD, Armour CL, Hogg JC, Schellenberg RR (1985). Airway reactivity in chronic obstructive pulmonary disease. Failure of in vivo methacholine responsiveness to correlate with cholinergic, adrenergic or non-adrenergic responses in vitro. Am Rev Respir Dis 132:30.

Vincenc KS, Black JL, Yan K, Armour CL, Donnelly PD, Woolcock AJ (1983). Comparison of in vivo and in vitro responses to histamine in human airways. Am Rev Respir Dis 128:875.

Weiss ST, Speizer FE (1984). Increased levels of airways responsiveness as a risk factor for development of chronic obstructive lung disease. Chest 86:3.

Yan K, Salome CM, Woolcock AJ (1985). Prevalence and nature of bronchial hyperresponsiveness in subjects with chronic obstructive pulmonary disease. Am Rev Respir Dis 132:25.

Mechanisms in Asthma: Pharmacology,
Physiology, and Management, pages 267–280

IS AIRWAY HYPERRESPONSIVENESS A SMOOTH MUSCLE ABNORMALITY?

Judith Black, Roger Marthan, Carol Armour and Peter Johnson.
Department of Pharmacology, University of Sydney
N.S.W. 2006, Australia.

INTRODUCTION

If the airway hyperresponsiveness which is the hallmark of asthma is a smooth muscle abnormality, then airway smooth muscle from individuals who are hyperresponsive to inhaled agonists in vivo should exhibit hyperresponsiveness in vitro. In pharmacological terms, the increase in responsiveness in vitro could be seen as a shift to the left in the response curve to contractile agonists, an increase in the maximal contractile response or a combination of these (Figure 1).

Alternatively hyperresponsiveness could be represented by a shift to the right in the response curve to relaxant agonists, a decrease in the maximal relaxant response, or a combination of these (Figure 1).

We have studied the in vitro response to histamine of bronchial smooth muscle resected from subjects whose responsiveness to inhaled histamine was tested prior to surgery. These subjects were not asthmatic but smokers, some of whom exhibited airway hyperresponsiveness (Vincenc et al., 1983). We found no positive correlation between the degree of in vivo hyperresponsiveness and in vitro response to histamine and this result was subsequently confirmed by others using a variety of contractile agonists (Armour et al., 1984a, 1984b; Roberts et al., 1984, 1985; Cerrina et al., 1986).

There are three possible explanations for these findings. Firstly, aspects of the experimental protocol such as the method of recording in vitro changes in muscle tone and

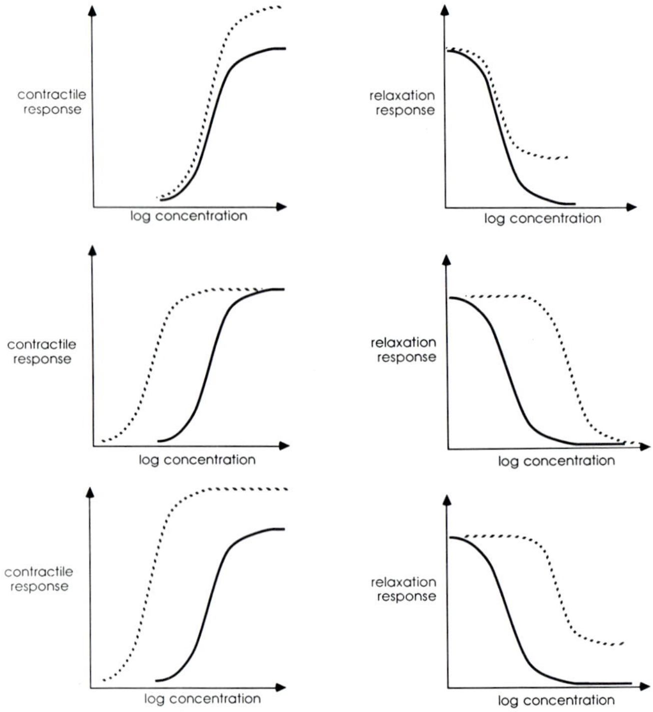

Figure 1. Theoretical response curves representing airway hyperresponsiveness as an abnormality in the in vitro response of airway smooth muscle to contractile (left panel) or relaxant (right panel) agonists.

type of muscle preparation studied could have accounted for the lack of correlation between in vivo and in vitro responses. Subsequent studies (de Jongste et al., 1987b) have suggested however, that whether changes in tone are recorded isotonically or isometrically has little influence on results. We have shown that whether bronchial preparations are spirally cut or studied as intact tubes has minimal effect on contractile response (unpublished observation). Secondly, it may be that in order to demonstrate hyperresponsiveness in vitro, the continuous production of an inflammatory mediator with a short half-life is necessary (see Armour et al., this volume). Thirdly, it is possible that the airway hyperresponsiveness observed in the smokers we studied differs markedly from that which is characteristic of asthma. Airway tissue from asthmatic subjects is rarely available for in vitro investigation, and thus only a limited number of studies has been performed. The results of these are summarised in Table 1 and it is apparent that no consistent pattern of either increase in contractile response or decrease in relaxant response has emerged so far.

Table 1. Studies of responses to contractile and relaxant agonists on airway tissue from asthmatic subjects.

Study	n	Hist.	Chol.	Leuk.	Iso.	Theo.	Forsk.
a	2	-		-			
b	1	↑	-	-			
c	1		-				
d	1	-					
e	5	-			↓		
f	7	-	↓		↓	-	
g	1	↑	↑	↑	-		-

a: Dahlen (1983); b: Schellenberg (1984); c: Roberts (1984); d: Roberts (1985); e: Cerrina (1986); f: Goldie (1986); g: De Jongste (1987a). n indicates number of asthmatic subjects. Arrows denote an increase (↑) or decrease (↓) and - no change compared with tissue from non-asthmatic subjects, in response to histamine, cholinergic stimuli, leukotrienes, isoprenaline, theophylline and forskolin.

It would seem to be beneficial to consider under what circumstances, in our laboratory, shifts in in vitro response curves as described above can be demonstrated in human bronchial tissue and to attempt to formulate a hypothesis relating to in vitro hyperresponsiveness.

1. DECREASE IN TEMPERATURE

We have observed a shift in response curves to carbachol when the temperature of the physiological solution bathing the tissue is reduced from 37°C to 20°C (Black et al., 1984).

Two successive cumulative concentration response curves (CCRC) were obtained in each bronchial tissue. In test tissues, the second CCRC was carried out at 20°C while in control tissues the temperature was maintained at 37°C. When second CCRC were compared mean maximal responses to carbachol were potentiated, and this is shown in Figure 2. No potentiation of contractile responses to histamine or KCl were observed with a decrease in temperature.

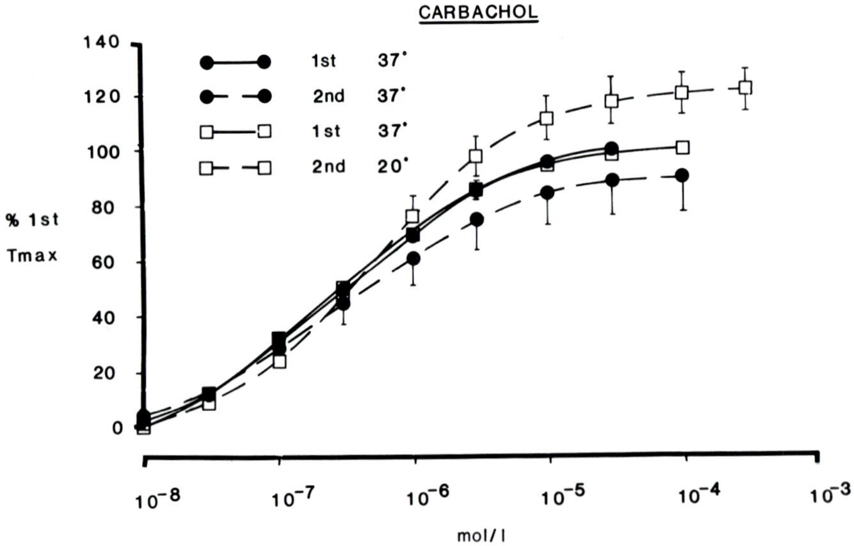

Figure 2. Mean cumulative concentration response curves (CCRC) for carbachol from 7 experiments. In all tissues, the first curves were carried out at 37°C. In half the tissues, second CCRC were carried out at 20°C while the rest were studied at 37°C. Vertical bars indicate SEM.

2. THE CALCIUM VOLTAGE DEPENDENT CHANNEL (VDC) AGONIST BAYK8644.

The second set of experimental conditions under which in

vitro response curves are shifted occurs in the presence of the calcium VDC agonist BAYK8644 (Marthan et al., 1987). This compound is thought to alter the "gating behaviour" of the VDC by inducing an increase in the probability of opening the channel and/or by increasing the duration of the channel opening (Hess et al., 1984; Callewaert and Droogmans, 1985). Two successive CCRC to histamine, KCl or carbachol were obtained in each bronchial tissue. In test tissues, the second CCRC was carried out in the presence of BAYK8644, 10^{-6} M. When test and control tissues were compared, BAYK8644 produced significant shifts to the left in the response curves to histamine and KCl (Figure 3) while responses to carbachol were unaffected.

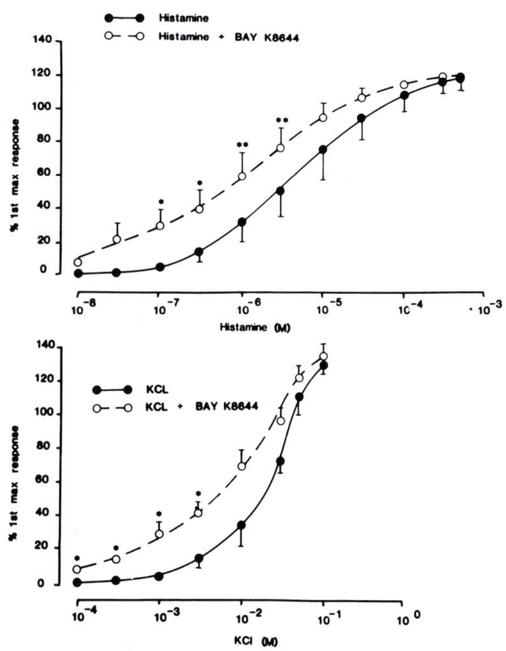

Figure 3. Mean second cumulative concentration response curves (CCRC) for KCl (n=5) and histamine (n=6) in the absence and presence of BAYK8644. Vertical bars indicate SEM; * ($P \leq 0.05$) and ** ($P < 0.01$) indicate a response in BAYK8644-treated tissues that was significantly different from the corresponding response in control tissues.

3. PASSIVE SENSITIZATION OF HUMAN BRONCHUS AND THE EFFECT OF BAYK8644 ON CONTRACTILE RESPONSES.

In this series of experiments human bronchial spiral strips were passively sensitized by incubation in serum with a high RAST titre to the house dust mite antigen Dermatophagoides (D.) farinae. Sensitization was confirmed by the presence of a contractile response to the addition of D. farinae. Control strips were incubated in serum with a total IgE of less than 10 units per litre, and these did not contract in response to D. farinae. Contractile responses

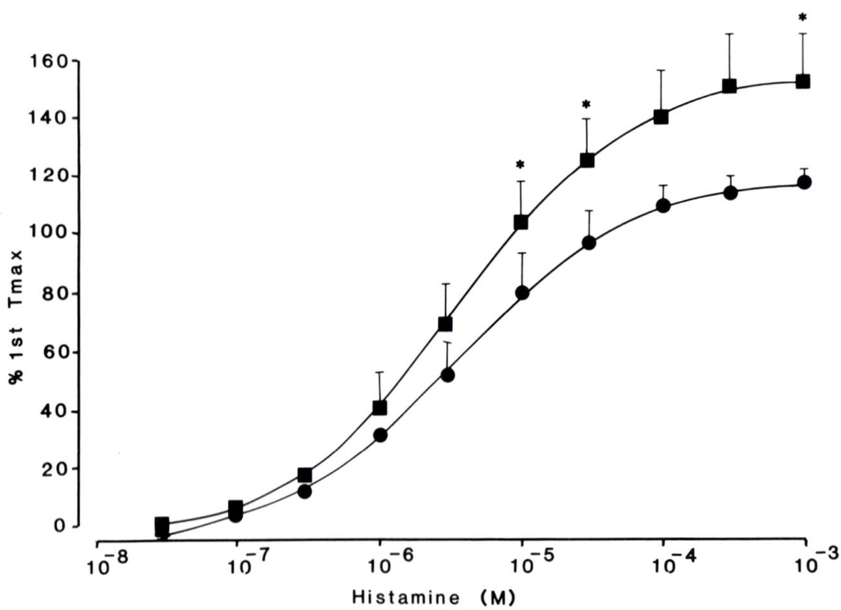

Figure 4. Mean second cumulative concentration response curves (CCRC) for histamine in non-sensitized ●—● and sensitized ■—■ tissues. Points are the mean values from 7 experiments and vertical bars indicate SEM. * denotes a significant difference ($P<0.05$) from the corresponding value in control tissues.

to histamine in sensitized strips were potentiated compared with those in control, non-sensitized strips (Figure 4). Sensitization did not potentiate responses to KCl or carbachol.

When sensitized strips were treated with BAYK8644, response curves to KCl lay to the left of non-sensitized, BAYK8644-treated strips and there was also an increase in the maximal response. The combination of sensitization and BAYK8644 did not potentiate carbachol responses.

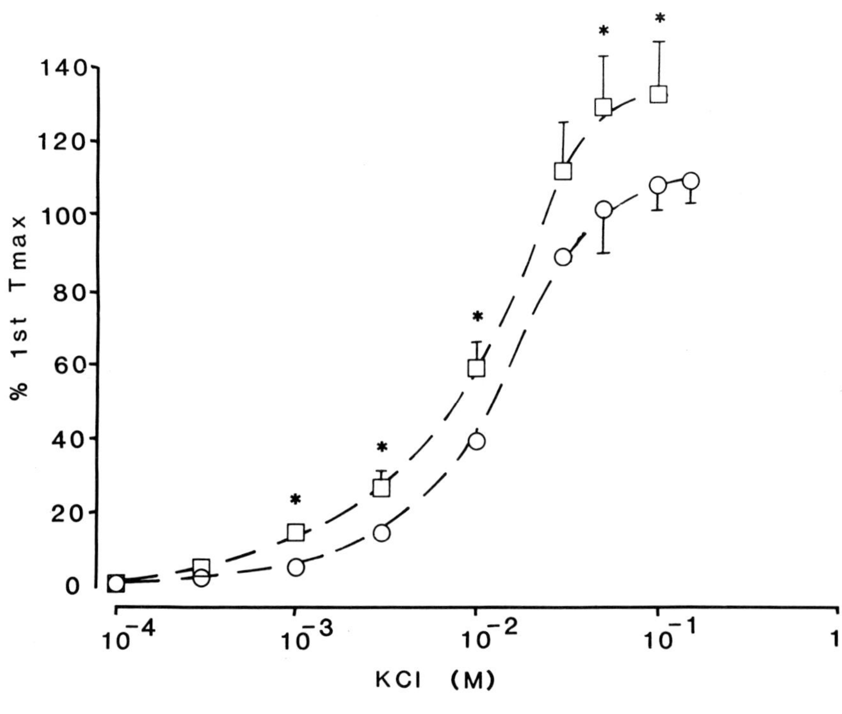

Figure 5. Mean second cumulative concentration response curves (CCRC) for KCl in the presence of BAYK8644 (10^{-6} M) in non-sensitized O—O and sensitized □--□ tissues. Points are the mean of 7 experiments and vertical bars indicate SEM. * denotes a significant difference (P<0.05) from the corresponding value in control tissues.

DISCUSSION

The results of these three studies have shown that hyperresponsiveness is demonstrable in vitro in human isolated bronchial tissue. A decrease in temperature potentiates carbachol responses. BAYK8644 produces shifts in response curves to KCl and histamine without affecting carbachol responses. Passive sensitization shifts response curves to histamine and KCl in the absence and presence of BAYK8644 respectively. We postulate that the differences observed between these agonists reflect differences in the way they mobilise calcium, the cytosolic concentration of which ultimately determines excitation-contraction coupling. A rise in cytosolic calcium concentration can occur if calcium enters the cell via the VDC, receptor operated channels or the leak pathway, or via release of calcium from intracellular stores. We have previously shown (Black et al., 1986; Marthan et al., 1987) that the contractile response to histamine and KCl involves activation of the VDC. Since sensitization alters histamine responses and sensitization with BAYK8644 affects KCl responses, activation of the VDC would explain the effects of these stimuli. By contrast, our findings (Black et al., 1986) that the action of carbachol appears to be independent of the VDC would explain why carbachol responses are not affected by sensitization or BAYK8644. There is evidence to suggest (Marthan et al., 1986) that in human airways the contractile response to cholinergic stimulation results from release of calcium from intracellular stores. Studies in animal airway tissue (Grandordy et al., 1986) indicate that this is mediated via inositol triphosphate formation. It is possible that the potentiation of contractile responses to carbachol observed with temperature reduction is mediated via an action on this mechanism of excitation-contraction coupling.

CONCLUSION

Airway hyperresponsiveness may be a smooth muscle abnormality. Hyperresponsiveness can be demonstrated in vitro under certain conditions. These would seem to be associated with various patterns of calcium mobilisation, some of which are dependent on the VDC and others which are independent of this channel.

ACKNOWLEDGEMENT

This study was supported by the National Health and Medical Research Council of Australia. Roger Marthan was a recipient of an Australian-European Award from the Commonwealth Department of Education in Australia.

REFERENCES

Armour CL, Black JL, Berend N, Woolcock AJ (1984a). The relationship between bronchial hyperresponsiveness to methacholine and airway smooth muscle structure and reactivity. Respir Physiol 58:223-233.

Armour CL, Lazar NM, Schellenberg RR, Taylor SM, Chan N, Hogg JC, Pare PD (1984b). A comparison of in vivo and in vitro human airway reactivity to histamine. Am Rev Respir Dis 129:907-910.

Black JL, Armour CL, Shaw J (1984). The effect of alteration in temperature on contractile responses in human airways in vitro. Respir Physiol 57:269-277.

Callewaert G, Droogmans G (1985). Transient inward current through Ca channels in isolated smooth muscle cells of the guinea-pig ileum. Effect of the dihydropyridine agonist BAYK8644. Arch Int Pharmacodyn Ther 278:169.

Cerrina J, Le Roy Ladurie M, Labat C, Raffestin B, Bayol A, Brink C (1986). Comparison of human bronchial muscle response to histamine in vivo with histamine and isoproterenol agonists in vitro. Am Rev Respir Dis 134:57-61.

Dahlen SE, Hansson G, Hedquist P, Bjorek T, Granstrom E, Dahlen B (1983). Allergen challenge of lung tissue from asthmatics elicits bronchial contraction that correlates with the release of leukotrienes C_4, D_4, E_4. Proc Natl Acad Sci USA 80:1712-1716.

Goldie RG, Spina D, Henry PJ, Lulich KM, Paterson JW (1986). In vitro responsiveness of human asthmatic bronchus to carbachol, histamine, β-adrenoceptor agonists and theophylline. Br J Clin Pharmac 22:669-676.

Grandordy BM, Cuss FM, Sampson AS, Palmer JB, Barnes PJ (1986). Phosphatidylinositol response to cholinergic agonists in airway smooth muscle: relationship to contraction and muscarinic receptor occupancy. J Pharmac Exp Ther 238:273-279.

Hess P, Lansman JB, Tsien RW (1984). Different mode of Ca channel gating behaviour favoured by dihydropyridine Ca agonists and antagonists. Nature 311:538-44.

de Jongste JC, Mons H, Bonta IL, Kerrebijn KF (1987a). Human asthmatic airway responses in vitro - a case report. Eur J Respir Dis 70:1-7.

de Jongste JC, Mons H, Van Strik R, Bonta IL, Kerrebijn KF (1987b). Comparison of isometric and isotonic responses of human small airway smooth muscle in vitro. J Pharmacol Methods, in press.

Marthan R, Armour CL, Johnson PRA, Black JL (1987). The calcium channel agonist BAYK8644 enhances the responsiveness of human airway muscle to KCl and histamine but not to carbachol. Am Rev Respir Dis 135:185-189.

Marthan R, Savineau JP, Mironneau J (1986). Acetylcholine-induced contraction in human isolated bronchial smooth muscle: Role of an intracellular calcium store. Respir Physiol 67:127-135.

Roberts JA, Raeburn D, Rodger IW, Thomson NC (1984). Comparison of in vivo airway responsiveness and in vitro smooth muscle sensitivity to methacholine in man. Thorax 39:837-843.

Roberts JA, Rodger IW, Thompson NC (1985). Airway responsiveness to histamine in man: effect of atropine on in vivo and in vitro comparison. Thorax 40:261-67.

Schellenberg RR, Foster A (1984). In vitro responses of human asthmatic airway and pulmonary vascular smooth muscle. Int Archs Allergy Appl Immunol 75:237-241.

Vincenc KS, Black JL, Yan K, Armour CL, Donnelly P, Woolcock AJ (1983). Comparison of in vivo and in vitro responses to histamine in human airways. Am Rev Respir Dis 128:875-879.

DISCUSSION

Mitchell: An alternative way to look at the relationship between in vivo and in vitro responsiveness would be to take a situation in which you know there is an vitro difference, i.e. species or a preparation, in which there is a difference between two drugs in vitro and then do the appropriate experiment in vivo. I am not aware of any such studies.

Daniel: A comment on the limitations of the dose-effect curve as a measure of hyperresponsiveness. It cannot take into account any changes in cell-to-cell coupling, secondly it won't reflect changes in membrane properties such as loss of rectification and the ability of the cells to produce action potentials. Thus we should not assume from studies of dose effect curves that we know fully how to evaluate hyperresponsiveness.

Nadel: How can this be solved?

Daniel: If we can obtain asthmatic tissues or if we have a satisfactory model of hyperresponsiveness by examining cell-to-cell coupling directly, there are ways to do that and also by looking at the membrane properties of fresh asthmatic tissue.

Pare: Dr de Jongste, did you correct your g tension for the amount of muscle?

de Jongste: It was corrected for the weight of the preparation and that's not the muscle.

Landau: Peter Macklem has suggested that normal individuals have a controlled shortening, whereas the asthmatic has the shortening one would expect from their length-tension relationships that Neuman Stephens showed. Our data in infants suggests that this hypothesis could be true - that there is in all infants an increased responsiveness and a control is gradually acquired during the first two years of life. On that basis of normals having a control mechanism which is not present in asthmatics, would it be possible for that control mechanism to be still within the smooth muscle, or do we have to start looking outside the smooth muscle?

Black: I think it's a very good point. I don't know if

it's in the smooth muscle.

de Jongste: It may be in the innervation - we don't know.

Goldie: We have published data concerning beta receptor responsiveness in asthmatic lung and in normal lung and our data run absolutely contrary to yours. I wouldn't be at all surprised to see normal beta-adrenergic function or adenylate cyclase function in the asthmatics you've looked at, given that baseline lung function was completely normal. What is absolutely necessary is the demonstration of a fully-blown inflammatory response and severe asthma before reduced beta-adrenergic function is involved. Could you comment on the work of Cerrina et al. who have correlated reduced beta receptor function with increased disease severity? Tony Bai also has data indicating reduced beta-adrenergic funtion. The responsiveness to spasmogens in your results is again explanable in terms of patient selection.

de Jongste: The paper by the group from Paris may be a bit confusing. The subjects called asthmatic in that study also had a COPD component in their disease and had a severe baseline airway obstruction. It may thus be confusing to regard these subjects as asthmatic.

Stephens: In terms of looking at relaxation - what happens in vivo is first isometric force development of the muscle, and isotonic shortening. Relaxation is the reverse - first the relaxation of length change and then the isometric force. Unless you are looking at that you might miss what relaxation is really doing. So I would suggest doing a quasi-isotonic experiment.

de Jongste: That is a more difficult kind of experiment to do, but you are right.

Whicker: I have studied isoprenaline-induced relaxation responses in surgically resected bronchus. We have studied seven asthmatics, and when we compare them to non-asthmatics there is no difference in the isoprenaline responses.

Goldie: The patients in our study died in status asthmaticus. Asthma is a dynamic disease which varies in severity and I think we're all comparing different states of the disease.

Mapp: Were the patients taking β_2 agonists regularly? What do you mean when you say that chronic inflammation is not relevant to explain bronchial hyperresponsiveness?

de Jongste: The patients did not use beta agonists for a few weeks before surgery - they used beclomethasone. The inflammation was chronic because it was from subjects with chronic obstructive lung disease. They didn't have signs of acute inflammation and we didn't find signs of hyper-responsiveness in their muscle.

Benveniste: A technical point - the studies by Cerrina and Brink are done at my lab. They keep their resected lung samples in the fridge overnight and do the experiments the next day. The problem is, does this change the responsiveness, i.e. should the experiments be done immediately?

Black: Johan de Jongste has done extensive studies on this.

de Jongste: We looked at the responses of fresh tissue directly from the theatre and then stored it for a night, then two nights. The pharmacological responsiveness remains stable for at least two days after surgery and that's not true for field stimulation responses.

Bai: We've looked at six asthmatics who have died - four in status asthmaticus and one who died from a coronary and one in a car accident. Five of our six definitely showed decreased beta-adrenergic responsiveness post mortem. Histamine and cholinergic responses were not different. In status asthmaticus as we know clinically beta responsiveness is decreased.

Thompson: Another methodological consideration - people who work with isolated tissue describe curves in terms of EC_{50} and maximal response. But what part of the in vitro dose response curve is relevant to the in vivo situation?

Daniel: In vivo, you are dealing with mediators which are inhaled or arriving through the bloodstream. They do not arrive simultaneously, or at all, in every place and so I don't know how you can compare that with the in vitro situation where you are ultimately perfusing every cell.

Walters: Some of that could be answered by Neuman Stephens and colleagues. Their dogs are hyperresponsive in vivo - are there any correlations between their in vivo hyperresponsiveness and the various phenomena they've shown in vitro?

Stephens: We haven't done a systematic comparison. The dogs are hyperresponsive to allergen and the methacholine responses seem to parallel what we see in vitro. The other point I wanted to make was that force velocity and length tension are not affected by storage for one, two or three days.

Pare: In normal subjects you can do a complete dose response curve in vivo. You can give doses of inhaled agonist which result in maximal airway smooth muscle shortening because you get a plateau on the dose response curve. Ann Woolcock's group have shown that, and so have we.

Daniel: How is that relevant to what I said?

Pare: Well, you were saying that in vitro may have nothing to do with in vivo because you cannot get complete dose response curves.

Daniel: That is not what I said. I said when you apply a mediator or an agonist through the epithelium by inhalation or through the bloodstream, it will not reach equilibrium. It will arrive at some cells and not other cells and therefore cell-to-cell coupling plays a role. In vitro the agonist arrives ultimately at every cell and so other factors such as cell-to-cell coupling or membrane properties will not be manifest.

Pare: I think if you double the dose of inhaled drug and get no more response it must mean that you've reached a state of equilibrium.

Daniel: I'm sorry, that's just dead wrong.

Stephens: What are the experiments which need to be done to determine what is the basic cause of asthma?

Benveniste: The dogma may be wrong. Maybe we need another dogma. We have to identify the mechanisms, identify agonists and antagonists and as soon as the antagonists are proven non-toxic, give them to man.

Physical Factors

Mechanisms in Asthma: Pharmacology,
Physiology, and Management, pages 283–299

HEAT AND WATER LOSS FROM THE AIRWAYS AS A PROVOKING STIMULUS FOR ASTHMA

Sandra D Anderson and Christine M Smith

Department of Thoracic Medicine
Royal Prince Alfred Hospital
Camperdown, NSW, AUSTRALIA 2050

When air is inspired it needs to be heated and humidified in the airways before it reaches the alveoli. The numbers of airways involved in this process will depend on the heat and water content of the air inspired and the rate of ventilation. During exercise the rate of ventilation may increase to 30 times the value at rest. Thus large volumes of air are required to be humidified and heated in a relatively short time (McFadden, 1983). Under temperate conditions, 80% of the heat loss is due to vaporisation of water to humidify the air, the remaining heat being lost in bringing the air to body temperature. The number of generations of airways required to humidify the air is not known but will depend upon the water available and the rate at which it is returned to those airways.

The source of water available to humidify the air is the periciliary fluid lining the airway mucosa. This fluid, which is composed of more than 90% water, contains chloride, sodium, potassium, and calcium ions (Boat and Matthews, 1973). The amount of water available from this fluid at any one time can be calculated by knowing the surface area of the mucosa and the depth of the fluid. Using the morphometric measurements of Weibel (1963) and an exaggerated depth of 10 microns for the periciliary fluid (more likely to be 5-7 microns) we have calculated that the first 10 generations of airways has only 1 ml of fluid and even up to 16 generations only 6-7 mls are available (Anderson, 1987b).

The rate of water loss from the airways when dry air of between minus 20°C to plus 42°C is breathed varies between

27-33 mg per L (Anderson et al., 1985; Eschenbacher and Sheppard, 1985). This means that under resting conditions there is a loss of between 0.15-0.35 ml per min. During exercise, rates can increase up to 3.5 ml per min and even light exercise will use 1 ml or more per minute. To accommodate an increase in water loss of this magnitude, it is necessary for some physiological adaptation to occur and this has been observed in response to breathing warm dry air but only after 15 minutes (Tabka et al., 1987). In the short term the rate of return of water to the airway lumen would not appear to meet the requirements of evaporative loss. This has been demonstrated by a reduction in water content of the expired air from 31 to 27 mg per L (Tabka et al., 1987). Thus with time it is likely that more and more airways will be required to humidify the air so that 14 or so of the 23 generations of airways are involved in the process of conditioning dry air at high flow rates. Beyond the 14th generation the surface area of the airway mucosa increases enormously and the amount of fluid available to humidify the air is sufficient to permit full saturation at body temperature before the alveoli are reached.

There are two consequences of evaporative water loss from the airways. The first is that the airways will be cooled below body temperature. The process of cooling of the airway mucosa is a natural defense mechanism to conserve both heat and water. As conditioned air from the alveoli passes back over the airways which were cooled during inspiration, some heat and water is returned to the mucosa. Even so, whenever the inspired air is drier or cooler than the body, the nett effect will be a loss of heat and water from the airway mucosa.

The second consequence of evaporative water loss will be an increase in the concentration of ions in the periciliary fluid of the airways and thus a transient increase in osmolarity of this fluid. The loss and return of water by evaporation and condensation with each respiratory cycle means that the perciliary fluid is under dynamic change in terms of its ion concentration. A nett loss of water of 0.15-0.35 ml per min, which is normal with resting ventilation, is probably necessary to maintain normal airway temperature and osmolarity. With exercise however, this loss is exceeded and changes are predicted to occur in the osmolarity of the periciliary fluid (Anderson, 1984).

It is the loss of heat and water from the respiratory mucosa which is thought to be the stimulus for the acute development of airway narrowing, 5 to 10 minutes after exercise or isocapnic hyperventilation, in 80% of patients with asthma. Clinically, this airway response to exercise is known as exercise-induced asthma (EIA). In most asthmatic patients EIA resolves spontaneously within an hour but it can be reversed within minutes by giving a beta-sympathomimetic by aerosol. Fifty percent of patients who recover spontaneously are refractory to the effects of heat and water loss for at least 1 hour. EIA can be abolished by preventing the loss of heat and water from the airways and this can be achieved by breathing fully saturated air at temperatures between 32 and 37°C (Anderson, 1987a; Lockhart et al., 1985).

The nature of the airway narrowing induced by cooling and a change in osmolarity is not known. It is thought that smooth muscle contraction, vagal reflexes, mucosal oedema and a reactive hyperemia all contribute to the increase in airway resistance after exercise. Studies using pharmacological agents have given some insight into the mechanism by which changes in temperature and osmolarity induced by hyperpnea can lead to narrowing of the airways. Thus EIA can be prevented by taking sodium cromoglycate or a beta-sympathomimetic immediately before exercise, although the actual loss of heat and water remains unchanged. EIA may also be partially inhibited by anti-histamines taken either by aerosol or orally in high doses. In a small proportion of patients EIA is prevented by anticholinergic agents, alpha-adrenoceptor agonists, and calcium channel blockers and they are more efficacious when administered as aerosols. The amount of therapy required to prevent severe EIA may be modified after 4 to 6 weeks treatment with aerosol corticosteroids (Anderson, 1987b).

There has been some controversy as to whether cooling or hyperosmolarity of the airway mucosa is the primary stimulus by which exercise and hyperventilation induce airway narrowing in patients with asthma (Anderson, 1985). Direct measurements of airway temperature during hyperpnea have been made in both asthmatic and normal subjects and have clearly demonstrated that there is a reduction in airway temperature in response to breathing cold dry air at high rates of ventilation. Most of the reduction in temperature occurs in the first 4 minutes of hyperpnea when a steady state is reached (McFadden and Pichurko, 1986). Unfortunately there have been no direct measurements made of airway temperature in human subjects breathing hot dry air although studies reporting changes in retrotracheal temperature imply that some reduction in temperature does occur under these inspired air conditions. The fact that the severity of the airway responses in asthmatics are similar while breathing hot or cold dry air (Eschenbacher and Sheppard, 1985; Hahn et al., 1984) does however suggest that similar numbers of airways are involved in the humidifying process.

There is no direct evidence that evaporative water loss during exercise in patients with EIA creates a hyperosmolar environment. It is known however that evaporative water loss does lead to an increase in osmolarity of the respiratory tract fluid, both in animals and in man. The osmolarity of the respiratory tract fluid has been measured in patients with laryngectomies and shown to be 359 milliosmoles (Boat and Matthews, 1973; Potter, 1967). Similar quantitative findings have been made in dogs merely by changing from nose to mouth breathing at resting ventilation for 10 minutes (Man, 1979).

Although there are no direct measurements of osmolarity of the periciliary fluid before and after exercise, it is known that patients with asthma can have an attack provoked by increasing the osmolarity of their respiratory tract by inhaling hyperosmolar aerosols of saline or dextrose (Eschenbacher, 1984; Schoeffel et al., 1981). Under these conditions airway temperature should remain relatively unchanged compared with exercise. In fact, the change in lung function recorded in response to an osmotic load produced by inhaling an aerosol of hyperosmolar saline is similar to the change in lung function produced by the osmotic load of evaporative water loss. This is evidence in support of osmolarity being an important stimulus to EIA (Smith and Anderson, 1986; 1987).

The precise mechanism whereby an increase in osmolarity or a reduction in temperature of the bronchial mucosa leads to airway narrowing in patients with asthma is unknown. However there are a number of tissues and cells in the airways which could be affected by a change in physical environment (see Figure reproduced from Anderson, 1985, with permission). For example an increase in osmolarity, or a decrease in temperature could have a direct effect on epithelial cells, mast cells, submucosal cells, nerves, blood vessels, or smooth muscle.

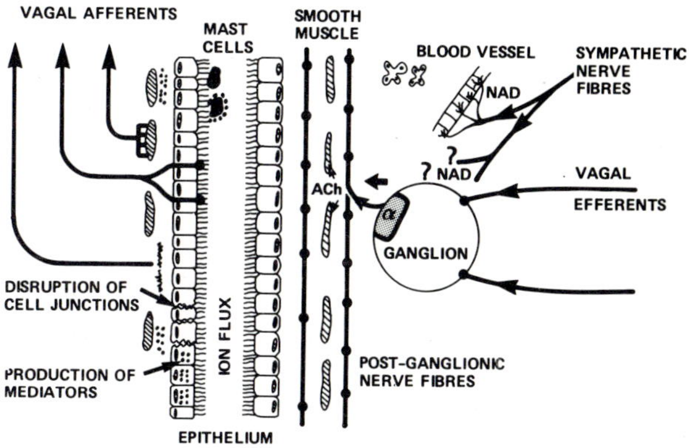

Schematic diagram of the human airways illustrating the various pathways and events that may occur in response to respiratory water and heat loss. α = α -adrenoceptor.

Epithelial cells act as a barrier between the airway lumen and the sub-mucosa. A breakdown in the integrity of this barrier is one of the well-known pathological changes associated with severe asthma. One of the important functions of the epithelial cells is the production of substances which have potential to modulate the bronchoconstrictor response to a variety of known stimuli (Butler et al., 1987; Farmer, 1987; Goldie et al., 1986; Hunter et al., 1985; Laitenan et al., 1985). Because a reduction in airway temperature and an increase in osmolarity are normal responses to evaporative water loss, it is possible that epithelial cells respond to these stimuli by producing substances which normally inhibit or prevent the cascade of events which results in airway narrowing. When the integrity of the epithelium is damaged, not only is the natural barrier to the physical environment destroyed but the role of these cells in regulating other events, such as water return to the lumen, may also be compromised.

Prostaglandin E_2 is just one example of a substance

likely to play a regulatory role by inhibiting bronchial smooth muscle contraction (Butler et al., 1987; Flavahan et al., 1985). Prostaglandin E_2 is produced by gut epithelial cells in response to a hyperosmolar stimulus (Assouline et al., 1977) and it may also be produced by airway epithelium which is embryologically similar in origin. PGE_2 levels increase in the peripheral blood in response to exercise (Satake et al., 1981) and they are thought to play a role both in the bronchodilating effects which are observed during the exercise and the refractory period which follows EIA (Anderson, 1987a; O'Byrne et al., 1986).

Another substance, epithelial-derived relaxant factor (EDRF), as yet unidentified is thought to play an important role in protecting the airways. Airways denuded of their epithelium have enhanced responses to both histamine and carbachol, and fail to produce prostaglandins in response to arachidonic acid (Butler et al., 1987; Flavahan et al., 1985; Goldie et al., 1986). These findings suggest that the epithelium plays an important role in modifying responses to naturally occurring substances which may explain its importance in modulating smooth muscle responsiveness.

Epithelial cells are also thought to be important in maintaining the depth of periciliary fluid which is normally about 5-7 microns. To increase the volume of periciliary fluid, water moves from the epithelial cells to the airway lumen in association with the active transport of chloride ions. However under normal circumstances the airways, at least the peripheral ones, act as an absorptive rather than secretory surface for water (Kilburn, 1968). The volume of water moving up the mucociliary escalator is thought to be absorbed along with sodium ions and chloride ions so that the nett flow of water is normally from the airway lumen to the sub-mucosa. The increase in the concentration of these ions in the periciliary fluid, as a result of evaporative water loss, could conceivably change the direction of water flux across the airways. It may be that active transport of chloride ions is not necessary before water will cross the respiratory epithelium and the osmotic gradient caused by evaporative water loss may be sufficient to enhance the movement of water towards the airway lumen. It may be predicted however that any process which inhibits the return of water to the airways, either by the mucociliary escalator or across the epithelial cells e.g. bacterial infection, will enhance the airway responses to mucosal water loss and those interventions which promote the return of water to the airways e.g. beta-sympathomimetics, will inhibit the airway responses to water loss.

One aspect of an increase in osmolarity of the fluid lining the epithelial cells which is not well understood is the potential to alter the permeability of the cells or their junctions. Disruption of tight junctions in response to hyperosmolarity has been described in toad bladders (Wade and Karnovsky, 1974). Presumably any change in permeability would allow for more rapid movement of water and other substances across paracellular pathways. It is now recognised that nerves are present between epithelial cells and that they are well positioned to be affected by a change in the physical or chemical environment of the airways. Cooling of these nerve endings as a result of heat loss may inhibit the normal release of neuropeptides so that excess is released on rewarming of the airways after cooling. Axon reflexes, which are also thought to play a role in modulating airway calibre in asthmatics, may be themselves modified by changes in airway osmolarity and temperature.

The network of blood vessels which forms the bronchial circulation which surrounds the airways can be found just beneath the epithelial cells in the sub-mucosa (Deffebach, 1987). This circulation which carries less than 1% of the cardiac output is thought to be important in conditioning the inspired air, and for the delivery and clearance of substances to and from the airway mucosa (Holroyde, 1986). It has recently been suggested that a change in the permeability of the post-capillary venules of this circulation permits exudation of plasma products which results in mucosal oedema (Persson, 1986). As mucosal oedema is another characteristic feature of the pathology of asthma, the control of these blood vessels is important in patients with asthma. It is thought that the bronchial circulation is the origin of the water supplied to the airway lumen. Factors which modify this circulation might also affect the dynamics of heat and water exchange in the airways. By absorbing and clearing the mediators produced by cells in the airway lumen or sub-mucosa, it is also likely that this circulation acts as an important barrier to the bronchial smooth muscle. There is also a potential for this circulation to modify the action of topically administered drugs.

Bronchial circulation increases in response to a number of agents known to cause bronchial smooth muscle contraction, e.g. histamine, methacholine, prostaglandin F_2 alpha (Lakshminarayanan et al., 1985; Parsons et al., 1985). Changes in bronchial circulation in response to heat loss have also been investigated. Most studies which have used dry air, either hot or cold, have shown an increase in bronchial artery blood flow (Baile et al., 1985). Changes in the bronchial circulation in response to a hyperosmolar stimulus, in the absence of a change in temperature, has not yet been reported. One of the consequences of a reduction in airway temperature due to conditioning the inspired air is thought to be a reactive hyperemia of the blood vessels of the bronchial circulation. Indeed it is this hyperemia which is considered to be important in the airway narrowing which follows exercise and hyperventilation (McFadden, 1986) but this has not been proven. Hyperemia may also occur in response to the release of mediators of the inflammatory response.

The activation of leucocytes is an important event which follows challenge with the stimulus of heat and water loss (Lee et al., 1983, 1984; Moqbel et al., 1986). A change in permeability of blood vessels, together with the release of chemotactic substances and subsequent attraction of white cells to the mucosa may be important events which follow an abnormally high loss of heat and water from the airways.

There have been a number of studies to determine if smooth muscle is directly affected by a reduction in temperature or an increase in osmolarity. Studies of human lung tissue _in vitro_ have shown that a reduction in temperature to $20^{o}C$ enhances contractile responses to carbachol but not histamine or potassium chloride (Black et al., 1984). By contrast, there is a reduction in contractile effects of carbachol and histamine when osmolarity was increased to 440 mOsm (Finney et al., 1987).

The precise mechanism by which heat and water loss from the respiratory mucosa can provoke an attack of asthma is unknown. It is likely however, that the events which result in acute airflow limitation involve the release of mediators from osmotically sensitive cells in the airway lumen (Tomioka et al., 1984). These mediators could act either directly to cause airway narrowing by oedema or smooth muscle contraction, or indirectly to produce other substances which cause the airway to narrow.

It would appear from pharmacological studies that histamine is an important mediator of the airway responses to heat and water loss (O'Byrne et al., 1983; Patel, 1984). As the source of histamine is the mast cell it is likely that this cell plays a relevant role in the events following heat and water loss. Recently human lung mast cells (HLMC) have been shown to be very sensitive to changes in osmolarity and temperature <u>in vitro</u>. Thus the release of histamine from HLMC is optimal between 640 and 770 milliosmoles at 32°C and can occur after exposure to the hyperosmolar stimulus for 60 sec or less (Eggleston et al., 1987). The release of histamine from HLMC is calcium dependent and is enhanced in the presence of anti-IgE (Eggleston, 1985). These ideal conditions for histamine release are very likely to occur after 3 to 4 minutes of exercise in atopic asthmatic subjects. Evaporative water loss would not only serve to cool the airways to 32°C but also increase the ion concentration to change the required concentration of calcium. The fact that HLMC release histamine rapidly, that is within 2 minutes, is in keeping with the time course of bronchoconstriction observed in asthmatics following challenge with both exercise and hyperosmolar aerosols. The efficacy of sodium cromoglycate in preventing the responses to changes in airway osmolarity is also supported by observations <u>in vitro</u>. Flint et al. (1985) have shown that HLMC, obtained by bronchoalveolar lavage, release histamine in response to hyperosmolar solutions and this release is significantly reduced by sodium cromoglycate.

The loss of heat and water from the respiratory mucosa is a potent stimulus to narrowing of the airways in patients with asthma. A reduction in mucosal temperature and an increase in the osmolarity of the periciliary fluid occur as a result of heat and water loss from the airways. These physical changes in the airways provide an ideal environment for the release of histamine and possibly other mediators from human lung mast cells. It is likely that these mediators act in a number of ways to cause the airways to narrow acutely in response to the heat and water loss induced by exercise.

REFERENCES

Anderson SD (1984). Is there a unifying hypothesis for exercise-induced asthma? J Allergy Clin Immunol 73:660-665.

Anderson SD (1985). Issues in exercise-induced asthma. J Allergy Clin Immunol 76:763-772.

Anderson SD (1987a). Exercise-induced asthma. In Middleton E, Reed C, Ellis Adkinson NF, Yunginger JW (eds): "Allergy: Principles & Practice (3rd Edition)", St. Louis: CV Mosby Company.

Anderson SD (1987b). Exercise-induced asthma: Stimulus, mechanism, and management. In Barnes PJ, Rodger I, Thomson NC (eds): "Asthma: Basic Mechanisms and Clinical Management," London: Academic Press.

Anderson SD, Schoeffel RE, Black JL, Daviskas E (1985). Airway cooling as the stimulus to exercise-induced asthma - a re-evaluation. Eur J Respir Dis 67:20-30.

Assouline G, Leibson V, Danon A (1977). Stimulation of prostaglandin output from rat stomach by hypertonic solutions. Eur J Pharmacol 44:271-273.

Baile EM, Dahlby RW, Wiggs BR, Pare PD (1985). Role of tracheal and bronchial circulation in respiratory heat exchange. J Appl Physiol 58:217-222.

Black JL, Armour CL, Shaw J (1984). The effect of alteration in temperature on contractile responses in human airways in vitro. Respirat Physiol 57:269-277.

Boat TF, Matthews L-RW (1973). Chemical composition of human tracheo-bronchial secretions. In Dulfano MJ (ed): "The Fundamentals and Clinical Pathology of Sputum," Springfield, Illinois: Thomas, p 243-273.

Butler GB, Adler KB, Evans JN, Morgan DW, Szarek JL (1987). Modulation of rabbit airway smooth muscle responsiveness by respiratory epithelium. Am Rev Respir Dis 135:1099-1104.

Deffebach ME, Charan NB, Lakshminarayan S, Butler J (1987). The bronchial circulation: Small, but a vital attribute of the lung. Am Rev Respir Dis 135:463-481.

Eggleston PA (1984). Interaction between hyperosmolar and IgE-mediated histamine release from basophils and mast cells. Am Rev Respir Dis 130:89-91.

Eggleston PA, Kagey-Sobotka A, Lichtenstein LM (1987). A comparison of the osmotic activation of basophils and human lung mast cells. Am Rev Respir Dis 135:1043-1048.

Eschenbacher WL, Sheppard D (1985). Respiratory heat loss is not the sole stimulus for bronchoconstriction induced by isocapnic hyperpnea with dry air. Am Rev Respir Dis 131:894-901.

Eschenbacher WL, Boushey HA, Sheppard D (1984). Alteration of osmolarity of inhaled aerosols cause bronchoconstriction and cough, but absence of permeant anion causes cough alone. Am Rev Respir Dis 129:211-215.

Farmer SG (1987). Airway smooth muscle responsiveness: modulation by the epithelium. TIPS 8:8-10.

Finney MJB, Anderson SD, Black JL (1987). The effect of non-isotonic solutions on human isolated airway smooth muscle. Respir Physiol 69:277-286.

Flavahan NA, Aarhus LL, Rimele TJ, Vanhoutte PM (1985). Respiratory epithelium inhibits bronchial smooth muscle tone. J Appl Physiol 58:834-838.

Flint KC, Hudspith BN, Leung KBP, Pearce FL, Brostoff J, Johnson NMcI (1985). The hyperosmolar release of histamine from bronchoalveolar mast cells and its inhibition by sodium cromoglycate. Thorax 40:A717.

Goldie RG, Papadimitriou JM, Paterson JW, Rigby PJ, Self HM, Spina D (1986). Influence of the epithelium on responsiveness of guinea-pig isolated trachea to contractile and relaxant agonists. Br J Pharmac 87:5-14.

Hahn A, Anderson SD, Morton AR, Black JL, Fitch KD (1984). A re-interpretation of the effect of temperature and water content of the inspired air in exercise-induced asthma. Am Rev Respir Dis 130:575-579.

Holroyde MC (1986). The influence of epithelium on the responsiveness of guinea-pig isolated trachea. Br J Pharmacol 87:501-507.

Hunter JA, Finkbeiner WE, Nadel JA, Goetzl EJ, Holtzman MJ (1985). Predominant generation of 15-lipoxygenase metabolites of arachidonic acid by epithelial cells from human trachea. Proc Natl Acad Sci 82:4633-4637.

Kilburn KH (1968). A hypothesis for pulmonary clearance and its implications. Am Rev Respir Dis 98:449-463.

Lakshminarayanan S, Jindal SK, Kirk W, Butler J (1985). Increases in bronchial blood flow following bronchoconstriction with methacholine and prostaglandin F_2 alpha in dogs. Chest 87:183S-184S.

Laitinen LA, Heino M, Laitinen A, Kava T, Haahtela T (1985). Damage of the airway epithelium and bronchial reactivity in patients with asthma. Am Rev Respir Dis 131:599-606.

Lee TH, Assoufi BK, Kay AB (1983). The link between exercise, respiratory heat exchange, and the mast cell in bronchial asthma. The Lancet March 5, p 520.

Lee TH, Nagakura T, Papageorgiou N, Cromwell O, Iikura Y, Kay AB (1984). Mediators in exercise-induced asthma. J Allergy Clin Immunol 73:634-639.

Lockhart A, Regnard J, Dessanges JF, Florentin D, Lurie A (1985). Asthme post-exercice et post-hyperventilation. Bull Eur Physiopathol Respir 21:399-409.

Man SFP, Adams GK, Proctor DF (1979). Effects of temperature, relative humidity, and mode of breathing on canine airway secretions. J Appl Physiol:Respirat Environ Exercise Physiol 46:205-210.

McFadden ER (1983). Respiratory heat and water exchange: Physiological and clinical implications. J Appl Physiol:Respirat Environ Exercise Physiol 54:331-336.

McFadden ER, Pichurko BM (1985). Intraairway thermal profiles during exercise and hyperventilation in normal man. J Clin Invest 76:1007-1010.

Moqbel R, Durham SR, Shaw RJ, Walsh GM, MacDonald AJ, Mackay JA, Carroll MP, Kay AB (1986). Enhancement of leukocyte cytotoxicity after exercise-induced asthma. Am Rev Respir Dis 133:609-613.

O'Byrne PM, Jones GL (1986). The effect of indomethacin on exercise-induced bronchoconstriction and refractoriness after exercise. Am Rev Respir Dis 134:69-72.

O'Byrne PM, Thomson NC, Morris M, Roberts RS, Daniel EE, Hargreave FE (1983). The protective effect of inhaled chlorpheniramine and atropine on bronchoconstriction stimulated by airway cooling. Am Rev Respir Dis 128:611-617.

Parsons GH, Kramer GC, Link DP, Lantz BMT, Gunther RA, Green JF, Cross CE (1986). Studies of reactivity and distribution of bronchial blood flow in sheep. Chest 87:180S-182S.

Patel KR (1984). Terfenadine in exercise induced asthma. Brit Med J 285:1496-1497.

Persson CGA (1986). Role of plasma exudation in asthmatic airways. The Lancet November 15, p 1126-1128.

Potter JL, Le Roy WM, Spector S, Lemm J (1967). Studies on pulmonary secretions. II. Osmolality and the ionic environment of pulmonary secretions from patients with cystic fibrosis, bronchiectasis, and laryngectomy. Am Rev Respir Dis 96:83-87.

Satake T, Kato M, Takagi K, Ozawa T (1981). Role of prostaglandins in exercise-induced asthma. Adv Physiol Sci 10:369-377.

Schoeffel RE, Anderson SD, Altounyan RE (1981). Bronchial hyperreactivity in response to inhalation of ultrasonically nebulised solutions of distilled water and saline. Brit Med J 283:1285-1287.

Smith CM, Anderson SD (1986). Hyperosmolarity as the stimulus to asthma induced by hyperventilation? J Allergy Clin Immunol 77:729-736.

Smith CM, Anderson SD (1987). An investigation of the hyperosmolar stimulus to exercise-induced asthma. Aust NZ J Med 17(4):513.

Tabka Z, Ben Jebria A, Guenard H (1987). Effect of breathing dry warm air on respiratory water loss at rest and during exercise. Respirat Physiol 67:115-125.

Tomioka M, Ida S, Shindoh Y, Ishihara T, Takishima T (1984). Mast cells in bronchoalveolar lumen of patients with bronchial asthma. Am Rev Respir Dis 129:1000-1005.

Wade JB, Karnovsky MJ (1974). Fracture faces of osmotically disrupted zonulae occludents. J Cell Biol 62:344-350.

Weibel ER (1964). Morphometrics of the lung. In Fenn WO, Rahn H (eds): "Handbook of physiology, respiration section 3," Washington, DC: American Physiological Society Vol 1, p 285-307.

Discussion on Paper of S.D. Anderson

Pare: You calculate your dose-response curves with the rate of water loss, do you think it is the rate of water loss that is important or the absolute water loss?

Anderson: I think it has to be both. I think that a critical rate and critical amount of water loss has to occur to get the maximal response. This concept is supported by our knowledge of exercise-induced asthma. Both the intensity and duration of exercise are important determinants of the severity of the airway response. Unfortunately the scientific community has not accepted reporting amount of water loss only, and there is a requirement to give the time over which this water is lost. I think both the rate and total amount of water loss should be reported in studies using exercise and isocapnic hyperventilation.

Kerrebijn: From a clinical point of view, it has been found that asthma and exercise-induced asthma is less in a dry cool environment, such as in the alpine climate, compared with the severity in the lowlands. We have had the same experience in our country. We find in winter time when its freezing, most children with asthma are far better and have less symptoms than when it is warmer and more humid.

Anderson: I know from living in Sydney that I would probably attribute that to the presence of allergens and in particular the house dust mite. The house dust mite does not live above 3 or 4 thousand feet. There is a recent study from Simon Godfrey's group that shows that exposure to allergen does definitely enhance the response to exercise in patients with asthma.

Lee: Sandy, as you know I am one of those converted to the osmolarity hypothesis but one of the problems that I have, and I always get asked about and I'm sure that you do too, is that your calculations do have a number of assumptions attached to them. It would be much more elegant if we were able to measure osmolarity directly. Now you say you can't do it during exercise. Why is that?

Anderson: Well it is not that we can't do it but if we do it may be difficult to interpret the answers. Jay Nadel has pointed out to me many times, that once you start putting something down the airway you will immediately change the water fluxes across the epithelium. Remember the calculation shows that something less than 1 ml is available in the first 10 generations. Collecting enough fluid to make meaningful measurements will be difficult. There is however an abstract from the Boucher group (Am Rev Respir Dis 1984; 129:A315) studying normals at rest and presumably they will study the effects of exercise as well.

James: I am interested in the increased muscle sensitivity with cooling that Judith Black referred to this morning. How cool does the muscle have to get to show a change in sensitivity, and when does that effect start to occur? Also how far does the cooling that occurs on the airway surface extend. Does it extend to the smooth muscle?

Anderson: In Judy Black's study (Black et al 1984; Respirat Physiol 57:269-277) the temperature was 20°C which is lower than we would get even with subfreezing air. I don't know the answer to the second question but Peter Pare may as he has made temperature measurements in dogs.

Pare: We measured mucosal temperature by putting a thermistor into the airway lumen and pulled it back until we got a dampening of the temperature fluctuations with breathing and measured mucosal temperature. We didn't pull it back enough to measure what muscle temperatures might do.

Anderson: The smooth muscle temperature is likely to fall because the retrotracheal temperature falls in response to breathing cold or even warm air at high flow rates (Eschenbacher et al 1985; Am Rev Respir Dis 131:894-901). I think that the observation by Eggleston et al (Am Rev Respir Dis 1987; 135:1043-1048) showing that 32°C is the optimal temperature for human lung mast cell release of histamine is interesting. If the airways are below this temperature during exercise the airway response may be delayed or inhibited until the temperature increases to 32°C during recovery after exercise.

Landau: In reference to Professor Kerrebijn's comment, I think we have to be careful about interpreting observations from people moving from one geographical area to another. There are many variables that are altered under these conditions and when control trials are carried out the hypotheses fall down. With regard to exercise-induced asthma, and tachyphylaxis, do you still think it is mediator depletion or could it be a change in the effect of osmolality on mediator release.

Anderson: That could be the case, I now wonder if the hyperosmolar environment created by the initial test leads to an improved water return to the airways so that on the second test the stimulus just isn't there. However we record refractoriness in only 50% of our patients. Work from Tak Lee's group has suggested that it is not mediator depletion although they did not measure all the mediators (Belcher et al 1988; J Allergy Clin Immunol in press).

Nadel: Could refractoriness be due to reactive hyperaemia?

Anderson: I considered that a long-time ago but I don't think it is the case as studies on heat and water loss have not shown any difference with repeated challenge (Anderson et al 1982; Eur J Respir Dis 63:472-480).

Nadel: How much increase in blood flow can you actually get?

Anderson: I don't know if the blood flow in the bronchial circulation increases in response to exercise. The flow rate is estimated to be between 35 and 50 ml per min at rest in humans. For this reason it is unlikely to be as important as the pulmonary circulation in returning heat to the airways. However the bronchial circulation is presumably the source of the water to be returned to the airways and in this respect it is vital.

Woolcock: The bronchial circulation may be greater in asthmatics.

Anderson: Yes I think that hypertrophy of the vessels was appreciated by the pathologists some years ago (Dunhill MS 1960; J Clin Pathol 13:27-33).

O'Byrne: We have been interested in the tachyphylaxis or refractoriness after exercise-induced asthma and showed that it is prevented by pre-treatment with indomethacin (Am Rev Respir Dis 1986; 134:69-72). This is also true of histamine tachyphylaxis in asthmatics. Prostaglandins are probably released in response to the constrictor stimulus and these then protect the airway from a subsequent stimulus.

Anderson: I know that hyperosmolarity will produce PGE_2 (Assouline et al 1977; Eur J Pharmacol 44:271-273). I wonder if that is a possibility with exercise?

O'Byrne: That is possibly the case but muscle contraction almost certainly releases PGE_2 as well. Perturbation of the airway mucosa also releases PGE_2, so there are a number of sites of production for prostaglandins.

Mechanisms in Asthma: Pharmacology,
Physiology, and Management, pages 301–315

NON-PHARMACOLOGICAL MODULATORS OF AIRWAY RESPONSIVENESS

Peter D. Paré and Alan L. James

St. Paul's Hospital Pulmonary Research Laboratory, University of British Columbia, Vancouver and Department of Pulmonary Physiology, Sir Charles Gairdner Hospital, Perth.

Although exaggerated airway narrowing in response to inhaled pharmacological agonists is considered a characteristic feature of asthma its mechanism remains elusive. The rapid onset and reversibility of the bronchoconstriction suggests that smooth muscle contraction and shortening is the cause of the induced "asthma". Although hyperresponsive smooth muscle is an attractive explanation for the phenomenon studies which have examined smooth muscle function _in vitro_ from patients with airway hyperresponsiveness _in vivo_ have not supported this hypothesis (2, 11). These studies suggest that it is a property of the in situ airway which forms the basis of non-specific bronchial hyperresponsiveness (NSBH).

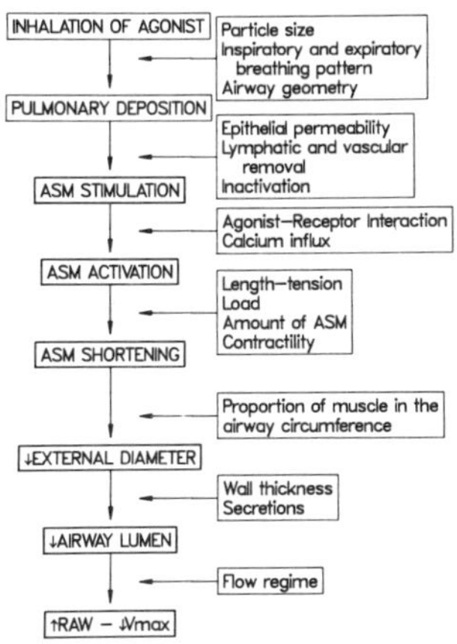

Fig. 1 Factors affecting the airway response to inhaled bronchoconstricting agonists

Figure 1 shows the steps which link inhalation of a bronchoconstricting stimulus and the ultimate airway narrowing which results; measured as an increase in airway resistance (↑R_{AW}) or a decrease in maximal expiratory flow (↓$\dot{V}_{MAX}$). The effect of an inhaled agonist is dependent on the extent and distribution of the intra pulmonary deposition of the drug. Factors which will increase total deposition or encourage localized deposition will increase the degree of obstruction for a given inhaled dose. The aerosol particle size, inspiratory and expiratory pattern and airway geometry will all affect this distribution. In narrowed airways air stream velocity will increase resulting in turbulent flow which may cause localized airway deposition and an apparent increase in airway responsiveness. Pharmacological agonists narrow airways by stimulating airway epithelial irritant receptors and initiating reflex bronchoconstriction, by causing direct smooth muscle activation, and by producing airway mucosal edema and mucous hypersecretion. To accomplish these effects the drugs must penetrate the airway epithelium, a relatively impermeable layer of epithelial cells joined by tight junction. Increased epithelial permeability could potentially produce "apparent" hyperresponsiveness by increasing the amount of mediator which reaches these end organs. Agonists that penetrate the epithelium may be removed or metabolized prior to having an effect. Increased or decreased bronchial vascular or lymphatic drainage of the airway interstitium may influence the local concentration of inhaled agonists at end organ receptor sites. Changes in the rate of inactivation of the drugs could similarly influence the ultimate response for a given concentration of nebulized and inhaled drug. Agonist that reaches receptors on smooth muscle, mucous producing cells and nerve endings will cause activation at these sites but the magnitude of the activation is dependent on the receptor number and kinetics and the availability of free calcium ions.

Airway smooth muscle activation causes smooth muscle shortening which ultimately narrows the airway. The amount of smooth muscle fibre shortening produced for a given activation is dependent on the length-tension characteristics of the muscle as well as the amount and contractile state of that muscle in relation to the load that the muscle must overcome to shorten. Smooth muscle contraction *in vivo* is not isotonic since shortening results in a progressive elastic load caused by distortion of airway connective tissue components such as cartilage and by the elastic recoil of the lung parenchyma. The balance between smooth muscle strength and these loads is an important determinant of the airway narrowing which follows smooth muscle activation. The airway narrowing produced by a given amount of smooth muscle shortening in an individual airway is also dependent on the proportion of that airway circumference occupied by muscle and on the thickness of the airway wall. Smooth muscle shortening will produce greater airway narrowing in an airway in which smooth muscle completely surrounds the lumen and in which the airway wall is thickened or the lumen narrowed with secretions. Finally the characteristic of the flow regime in narrowed airways could influence the relationship between decrease in airway lumen size and increase in R_{AW} or decrease in $\dot{V}MAX$.

Abnormalities at any one or combination of these steps could cause NSBH. Rather than discuss all the potential causes we will concentrate on the first two steps and describe three experiments which illustrate that these initial steps (prior to the inhaled agonist reaching the smooth muscle) may influence the measurement of NSBH.

In most studies of airway responsiveness it is the nebulized concentration or dose of agonist which is plotted as the dependent variable. In fact it is the dose of aerosol which reaches receptor sites in which we are most interested. Only a fraction of the nebulized "dose" reaches the lower respiratory tract. Much of the drug deposits in the apparatus, the nose, mouth and upper airway. The particle size and breathing pattern have important influences on the amount of nebulized drug that reaches the lower airway. In general large particles and more rapid flow rates result in greater impaction of particles in the upper airway. Rapid inspiratory flow results in exaggerated central deposition of large particles since impaction is encouraged by turbulence. For the same reason already narrowed airways will alter aerosol deposition by increasing the linear velocity of inspired air and encouraging central deposition. Ruffin et al (9) showed that the PC20 could be substantially decreased by inspiring rapidly during aerosol inhalation. The central deposition presumably has this effect by concentrating larger amounts of agonist at a localized site and because the large central airways are an important contributor to total airway resistance. Recently Smaldone et al (10) have shown that forced expiration during aerosol exposure leads to a preferential deposition of aerosol at flow limiting sites in central airways. We performed 2 inhalation dose response curves to nebulized methacholine in 13 subjects, 4 mild asthmatics and 9 normal subjects. During one challenge the subjects breathed with a fixed tidal volume but a spontaneous inspiratory and expiratory flow rate. During the second challenge the same tidal volume and inspiratory flow were used but forced expiration resulting in flow limitation was employed with each breath. Pulmonary resistance and FEV_1 were measured as estimates of airway narrowing. Aerosol deposition studies showed more central but not greater deposition with forced expiration.

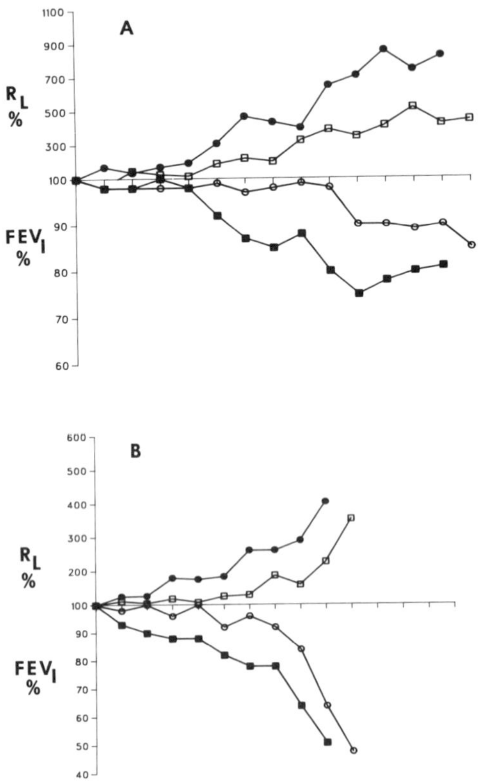

Fig. 2
a) Dose response curves in a normal subject. Changes in FEV_1 (lower panel) and pulmonary resistance (upper panel) in response to increasing concentrations of methacholine with quiet tidal breathing (open symbols) and with a forced expiratory pattern (closed symbols).
b) Dose response curve in an asthmatic subject.

The dose response curves from one normal subject is shown in Figure 2a. With forced expiration there is a shift to the left; lower concentrations of inhaled methacholine produce greater increases of RL and decreases of FEV_1. Although the position of the curves was shifted left the maximal response was not altered suggesting that different factors influence the position of the curve as opposed to the maximal response. A similar left ward shift is seen in a mildly asthmatic subject (Figure 2b) but in this instance no plateau or maximal response is apparent. A left ward shift was present in all subjects and in those in whom a PC20 FEV_1 could be calculated it decreased from 9.7 ± 6.7 mg/ml to 2.2 ± 7.2 mg/ml (geometric mean ± SD) during the force expiration challenge ($p < .001$). Similarly the inhaled concentration causing a 200% increase in RL decreased from 3.9 ± 5.7 mg/ml to 1.7 ± 5.5 mg/ml ($p < .001$). The results of this study suggest that the localized deposition of inhaled drug caused an apparent increase in "sensitivity" while not influencing the maximal response which is determined by the ability of the smooth muscle to shorten.

Once inhaled drug is deposited on the respiratory epithelium it must penetrate the epithelium to come in contact with irritant receptors, mucous glands and smooth muscle. Changes in permeability of the epithelium could influence what proportion of a pharmacological agonist reaches these receptors and therefore could influence the apparent airway responsiveness.

Cigarette smoke causes transient airway hyperresponsiveness in guinea pigs (4). To determine if increased mucosal permeability might be a factor in this change we measured airway responses to intravenous and inhaled acetylcholine in control and smoke-exposed guinea pigs (5). Conscious guinea pigs were exposed to the smoke from 6 cigarettes in a specially designed chamber. Immediately following air or smoke exposure they were anesthetized and studied in a body plethysmograph with a fluid filled eosophageal cannula to measure pleural pressure. Transpulmonary pressure, volume and flow signals were used to calculate pulmonary resistance before and after inhalation or intravenous injection of doubling doses of acetylcholine.

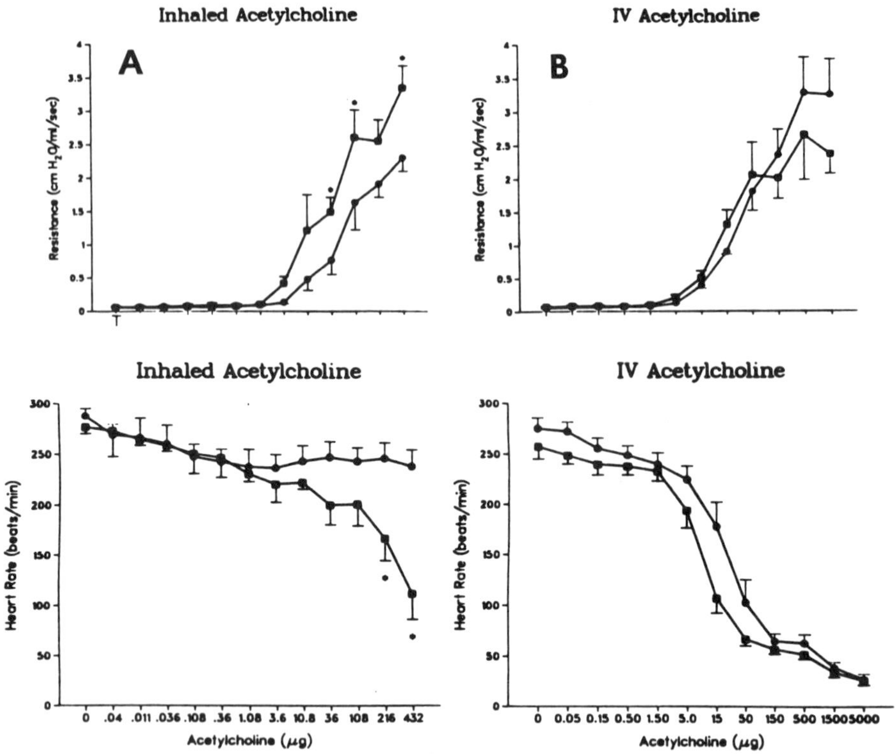

Fig. 3 Changes in pulmonary resistance (upper panels) and heart rate (lower panels) in response to increasing doses of inhaled (left) and intravenous (right) acetylcholine.

With inhaled acetylcholine there was a significant leftward shift of the dose response curve (see Figure 3a) but with intravenous acetylcholine the curves were not different (Figure 3b). This result could be due to altered deposition of aerosol or increased permeability. However the heart rate response to the two challenges suggested that changes in permeability explained the results. With intravenous drug the heart rate showed a dose dependent decrease in both exposure groups as one would expect from cholinergic stimulation. With inhaled drug the decrease was less but there was significantly more bradycardia with inhaled acetylcholine after smoke exposure. This suggests that more acetylcholine was reaching the systemic circulation because of increased epithelial permeability.

Although increased mucosal permeability has been demonstrated in animal models of airway hyperresponsiveness it is unclear whether it plays a role in the hyperresponsiveness of human asthma. A number of years ago we measured airway responsiveness and airway epithelial permeability in a group of normal and asthmatic subjects (3). We used nebulized technetium 99M labelled DTPA as our marker of epithelial permeability and delivered the aerosol preferentially to central airways by using a large particle size and rapid inspiratory flow rates. The disappearance of the radiolabel from the lung was measured with a gamma camera and its appearance in the blood was determined by counting samples of blood with a gamma counter. We found that the asthmatic subjects, despite marked increases in airway hyperresponsiveness, were not more permeable than normal subjects and in fact there was a non-significant tendency for their indices of permeability to be less than normal. These findings have been confirmed by O'Byrne et al (8) and suggest that increased permeability cannot explain the hyperresponsiveness seen in subjects with stable asthma. However epithelial permeability can be acutely increased by inhaled histamine (3) and distilled water aerosol (1). A similar change in epithelial permeability could explain the acute increase in responsiveness which accompanies viral infection, antigen exposure and inhalation of pollutants. Once inhaled pharmacologic agonists penetrate the airway epithelium they must diffuse through the interstitial space to reach the airway smooth muscle. The airway wall is highly vascular. The bronchial circulation forms 2 extensive plexuses of vessels, one lying external to the smooth muscle layer and one between the smooth muscle and the epithelium. There is a large blood flow to this subepithelial plexus of vessels and this blood flow can be modulated by a variety of mediators. Inhaled substances which penetrate the respiratory epithelium may be removed by the circulation prior to interaction with smooth muscle receptors. The potential importance of the bronchial circulation in modulating airway responses to inhaled pharmacologic agents has been demonstrated in a recent series of elegant experiments. Kelly et al (6) examined the importance of the pulmonary and bronchial circulations to the time course of peripheral airway narrowing caused by histamine aerosol. Peripheral lung resistance was measured by wedging a bronchoscope in small airways. A constant flow through the wedged bronchoscope exited the lung via collateral channels. By measuring the pressure at the bronchoscope tip a pressure flow curve of the peripheral lung units was obtained. Nebulization of histamine down the bronchoscope caused an increase in the pressure necessary to maintain the constant flow. When the nebulized histamine was stopped, the pressure returned toward the control value and it is the time constant of decay of this pressure which was used as an estimate of the recovery from bronchoconstriction. When the pulmonary or bronchial circulation was occluded there was a prolongation of the time course of recovery from histamine.

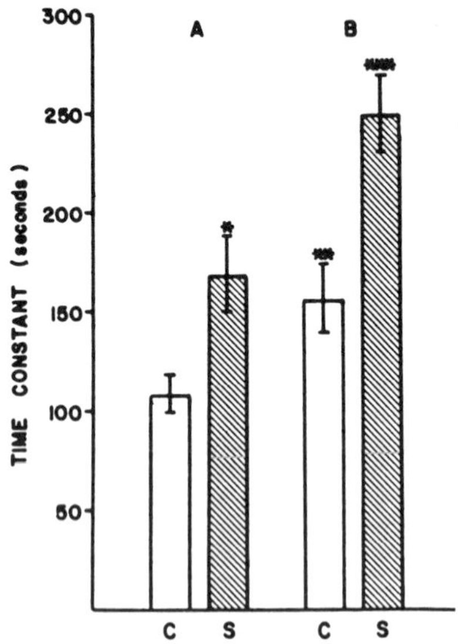

Fig. 4 The time constants for recovery from histamine with both circulations intact (open bar at left), occluded pulmonary circulation (hatched bar at left), occluded bronchial circulation (open bar at right) and with both occluded (hatched bar at right).
From Kelly et al (6), with permission from author and publisher.

The open bars on the left represent the time constant for recovery from bronchoconstriction with both the pulmonary circulation and the bronchial circulation intact. There is a significant prolongation of the time constant when the pulmonary circulation is obstructed indicating that in the periphery of the lung the pulmonary circulation is partially responsible for removal of mediator. When the bronchial circulation was occluded as shown by the second open bar the time constant was also prolonged. Finally when the pulmonary and bronchial circulation were both occluded the time constant for recovery was further prolonged.

Besides the actual physical removal of drug by blood flow and lymphatics, enzymatic inactivation could also be important in determining how much of an inhaled dose of agonist is available to interact with smooth muscle receptors. Kelly et al (7) found that the time course of the response to acetylcholine, unlike histamine, was not prolonged with vascular obstruction. Presumably the rate limiting step for acetylcholine was enzymatic degradation by cholinesterase. When they administered an anti-cholinesterase the action of acetylcholine was prolonged and was now affected by interruption of the blood supply.

In summary the changes in airway caliber (FEV_1 and RAW) induced by inhaled pharmacological agonists is a complex process far removed from the in vitro organ bath. The in vivo phenomenon known as bronchial hyperresponsiveness depends not only on the kinetics of agonist-receptor interaction, or the contractile response of the smooth muscle but is also influenced by the supply and removal of the nebulized drug in addition to the geometric factors which translate smooth muscle contraction into airway narrowing.

REFERENCES

1. Borland C, Chamberlain A, Minty B, Royston D, Higenbottam T (1983). Lung permeability changes after breathing a fine mist of distilled water but not after breathing cold air. Thorax 38:221.
2. Cerrina J, Ladurie ML, Labat C, Raffestin B, Bayol A, Brink C (1986). Comparison of human bronchial muscle responses to histamine in vivo with histamine and isoproterenol agonists in vitro. Am Rev Respir Dis 134: 57-61.
3. Elwood RK, Kennedy S, Belzberg A, Hogg JC, Paré PD (1983). Respiratory mucosal permeability in asthma. Am Rev Respir Dis 128:523-527.

4. Hulbert WC, Walker DC, Jackson A, Hogg JC (1981). Airway permeability to horseradish peroxidose in guinea pigs: the repair phase after injury by cigarette smoke. Am Rev Respir Dis 123:320-326.
5. James AL, Dirks P, Ohtaka H, Schellenberg RR, Hogg JC (1987). Airway responsiveness to intravenous and inhaled acetylcholine in the guinea pig after cigarette smoke exposure. Am Rev Respir Dis (in press).
6. Kelly L, Kolbe J, Mitzner W, Spannhake EW, Bromberger-Barnea B, Menkes H (1986). Bronchial blood flow affects recovery from constriction in dog lung periphery. J Appl Physiol 60:1954-1959.
7. Kelly LJ, Mitzner W, Spannhake EW, Bromberger-Barnea B, Menkes HA (1986). Pulmonary blood flow affects recovery from constriction in dog lung periphery. J Appl Physiol 60: 1554-1560.
8. O'Byrne PM, Dolovich M, Dirks R, Roberts RS, Newhouse MT (1984). Lung epithelial permeability: relation to non specific airway responsiveness. J Appl Physiol 57: 77-84.
9. Ruffin RE, Dolovich MB, Wolff RK, Newhouse MT (1978). The effects of preferential deposition of histamine in the human airway. Am Rev Respir Dis 117:485-492.
10. Smaldone GG, Messina MS (1985). Enhancement of particle deposition by flow-limiting segments in humans. J Appl Physiol 59:509-514.
11. Vincenc KS, Black JL, Yan K, Armour CL, Donnelly PO, Woolcock AJ (1983). Comparison of in vivo and in vitro responses to histamine in human airways. Am Rev Respir Dis 128:875-879.

Discussion on Paper by Peter Pare

N. Barnes: You suggested that your changes in responsiveness to methacholine are due to differences in deposition. I wonder if they could also be due to taking a forced inspiration or expiration. A change in the lung function from these manoeuvres in your subjects would be suggested by the fact that early on in your dose-response curve to methacholine you are already getting an effect. This effect is seen well before you're getting to doses of methacholine which will actually cause bronchoconstriction.

Pare: We studies normal subjects and repeated forced expirations don't usually cause bronchoconstriction in normal subjects. We didn't record any bronchoconstriction when we used phosphate-buffered saline as the control, either in the normals or the mild asthmatics we studied so I think the manoeuvres are unlikely to account for the change. What we didn't do was to repeat the forced exhalation manoeuvre without giving the doses of control or methacholine.

N. Barnes: We have found a small decrease in lung function after giving lots and lots of puffs from an aerosol. We found that it wasn't an effect of the inhaler, but rather it was caused by repeated inhalation. We also found this in normal subjects as well.

Pare: Very interesting.

N. Barnes: From your work on bronchial circulation in dogs you implied that the time course of histamine recovery should be different in normals and asthmatics.

Pare: No I'm not saying that at all, I'm just saying that one thing that could influence the airway responsiveness is the bronchial artery blood flow. I'm not saying that the bronchial artery blood flow <u>is</u> necessarily less in asthmatics, it is just <u>one</u> factor that has to be taken into account, <u>one</u> of the many.

N. Barnes: We have looked at the rate of recovery from histamine, LTC_4 and LTD_4-induced constriction and found that there is no difference between normals and asthmatics.

Pare: The rate of recovery from these stimuli may be important. Conceivably clearance could have affected the maximum response, if you have increased blood flow you may have less that reaches the muscle and have a sub-maximal response.

Fuller: I often wonder whether some of the small effects seen with vasodilating agents, such as the calcium antagonists and the alpha-blocker, prazosin, in exercise-induced and histamine-induced asthma, might be due to changes in the bronchial circulation. Do you know if anybody in the dog model has looked to see whether increasing the flow using these pharmacological agents has the opposite effect to what you show with inhibiting flow?

Pare: No I don't know of anybody who has studied that. Judy Black and I studied a couple of subjects who inhaled an alpha-agonist prior to inhaling histamine. We reasoned that alpha-agonists would constrict the bronchial vasculature and prolong, or make more acute, the effects of subsequently inhaled histamine. We only studied a couple of normal subjects and we didn't have any striking changes so we didn't carry on.

Anderson: Peter could you tell us what agent has been shown to constrict the bronchial vessels. I haven't seen any reference to a measurement of a reduction in bronchial artery blood flow. Everything seems to increase it rather than decrease it.

Pare: Alpha-agonists constrict bronchial arteries and that is about all.

Anderson: Do the bronchial arteries constrict in response to heat or water loss?

Pare: Nobody has measured that in humans although we have shown an increase in flow in the dog in response to heat and water loss.

P. Barnes: Well just to follow from that, we find that adrenaline is extremely effective in stopping leakage in the airways induced by a lot of different mediators, and we presume that it acts on the arteriolar side. It decreases the perfusion pressure in leaky vessels and that is the only thing we have found that does that. Also to follow up the point that Rick Fuller made, when we studied inhaled vasoactive intestinal peptide (VIP) in asthmatics, we found it had no effect on baseline lung function, but it did protect against histamine bronchospasm. VIP is extremely potent as a bronchial vasodilator and the possible explanation is that it is just increasing the removal of histamine from the sites of deposition.

Pare: In people who are bronchoconstricted VIP didn't relax?

P. Barnes: No.

Woolcock: Peter,when people make diagrams of asthma, they often include a picture of a leaky epithelium, implying that this is one of the factors in hyperresponsiveness. Do you know of any evidence in humans that the epithelial permeability is altered by any substance and affects bronchial dose-response curves to any mediator?

Pare: Well there are many things that affect bronchial mucosal permeability.

Woolcock: But have subsequent increases in response to either histamine or methacholine been shown in humans? It is easy to show in the guinea pig but it doesn't seem easy to show in humans.

Pare: In the human, cigarette smokers have increased airway responsiveness and cigarette smoke causes increased permeability but to say that those two are related is far fetched.

Anderson: We found a small increase in responsivenes to methacholine and histamine after water inhalation and we wondered if that was due to changes in permeability (Black et al 1985; Thorax 40:427-432).

Pare: We know that water does cause an increase in permeability (Borland et al 1983; Chest 83:934-935). However there is no study which has included the measurement of permeability and the measurement of responsiveness to methacholine or histamine after water inhalation.

Lockhart: If I may follow up on the effects of vasodilators and vasoconstrictors in humans. We have studied cardiac patients with very poor left ventricular function and compared their airway response to methacholine with that of cardiac patients with normal left ventricular function. When patients with a poor left ventricular function (which probably means they have a very high outflow pressure to the intrapulmonary bronchial circulation) inhaled methacholine they developed a remarkable hyperresponsiveness which was as severe as we measure in symptomatic asthmatics. This hyperresponsiveness to methacholine was entirely prevented when they were pre-treated with methoxamine given by aerosol. The preventative effect of the methoxamine was entirely offset by pre-treatment with the alpha antagonist indoramin. I think that these data show rather nicely that vasodilation of the bronchial circulation in the presence of a high output pressure causes leakage to take place in the wall of the vessel causing it to thicken. This thickening can be entirely offset by the use of an alpha agonist. If the alpha agonist were acting directly on the bronchial wall you would expect it to constrict the muscle and increase the secretion and therefore aggravate the effect of acetylcholine. However the alpha agonist did not aggravate the effect of acetycholine, rather it offset the response.

Pare: It is important to separate the influences on bronchial blood flow and bronchial vascular volume. If you can get a decrease in blood flow and increase in volume then the volume itself could narrow airways.

O'Byrne: I would like to reply to Ann Woolcock's question about changes in permeability and responsiveness. We had 3 subjects who inhaled allergen and we measured the permeability the day after their challenge when they were hyperresponsive. We couldn't show any difference in permeability compared with the measurement made the day before they had the allergen. Although the numbers were small and the study remains incomplete, we don't think that a permeability change can account for the increase in responsiveness following allergen challenge.

Nadel: In an animal, if you change the epithelial permeability and you increase the response of muscle, it does not demonstrate anything about the relationship between epithelial permeability and the access of a drug to the muscle. The point I want to make is that there are a number of the things that allow a drug to go across a membrane. For example, how hydrophilic it is, the molecular weight, whether it is transported - a whole series of things. I think that there have only been one or two experiments in the world on the actual movement of drugs and these have been with antibiotics. The number of studies that actually rigorously look at the flux of mediators or drugs across membranes are trivial. I don't accept that _in vivo_ or even an _in vitro_ study that shows an association, as a cause. I think it is tricky and it needs to be studied but I don't think that is has been shown.

Mechanisms in Asthma: Pharmacology,
Physiology, and Management, pages 317–329

EPITHELIAL DYSFUNCTION AND AIRWAY HYPERREACTIVITY IN ASTHMA

Roy G. Goldie, Lynette B. Fernandes, Paul J. Rigby and James W. Paterson.

Department of Pharmacology, University of Western Australia, Perth, Nedlands, 6009.

INTRODUCTION

The causes of the non-specific bronchial hyperreactivity associated with asthma (Boushey et al., 1980), are not established. Bronchoconstriction may be induced in asthmatics by many chemically dissimilar agents including methacholine, histamine and various occupational pollutants, at concentrations well below threshold for most non-asthmatic subjects. Inflammation-induced damage to the airway epithelium is commonly associated with asthma and may be causally linked to bronchial hyperreactivity (Laitinen et al., 1985). Bronchial hyperreactivity can also be induced in non-asthmatic subjects by inhalation of the inflammatory mediator, platelet activating factor (PAF) (Cuss et al., 1986) and by respiratory tract viral infections (Empey et al., 1976; Aquilina et al., 1980). Furthermore, respiratory viruses can provoke asthma attacks (Minor et al., 1976). Both PAF (Page et al., 1983) and respiratory viruses induce mucosal inflammation and epithelial damage (Hers, 1966).

EPITHELIUM-DERIVED RELAXANT FACTOR (EpDRF)

The airway epithelium limits the passage of large polar solutes to underlying airway wall structures. Inflammatory events disrupt epithelial cell tight junctions, increasing solute penetration of the airway mucosa (Ranga et al., 1983). Damage to epithelial structure may primarily result from the cytotoxic effects of eosinophil major basic protein (Gleich et al., 1983).

Airway hyperreactivity may be partly a consequence of epithelial damage and the compromise of this tissue as a barrier to the access of inhaled stimulants to airway smooth muscle, submucosal mast cells, irritant receptors and C fibre afferent nerves involved in mucosal axon reflexes (McFadden, 1984; Barnes, 1986; Hargreaves et al., 1986). However, recent evidence suggests that the epithelium also plays a more active role in protecting the airways from potentially obstructive stimuli.

Drug-induced bronchoconstriction in non-asthmatics is limited, whereas asthmatics continue to bronchoconstrict in a dose-related manner as if lacking some protective inhibitory mechanism (Woolcock et al., 1984). We have previously hypothesized that the airway epithelium releases a relaxant factor which modulates the responsiveness of the underlying smooth muscle to spasmogens (Goldie et al., 1986a). An airway epithelium-derived relaxant factor (EpDRF) generated in response to spasmogenic stimuli may provide such a protective "braking" mechanism in healthy lung. Epithelium-based protective mechanisms might be expected to be impaired or absent in asthma, since the bronchial epithelium has been shown to be damaged and may be shed from the airway luminal surface during asthma attacks (Cutz et al., 1978). It is well established that blood vessels produce an endothelium-derived relaxant factor (EDRF) in response to some vascular smooth muscle constrictor agents (Furchgott & Zawadzki, 1980).

We have examined the influence of gently removing the epithelium on responsiveness of guinea-pig tracheal ring preparations to contractile and relaxant agonists. We showed that the potency of histamine was about 4 fold greater in guinea-pig tracheal preparations denuded of epithelium than in intact preparations, while responsiveness to carbachol was not significantly altered (Goldie et al., 1986b). Maximal relaxant responses to isoprenaline, forskolin and theophylline were significantly reduced by epithelium stripping. However, responsiveness to the cyclic-GMP generator nitroglycerin was not significantly altered. We have subsequently shown that the potencies of 5-hydroxytryptamine, methacholine and the histamine H_1-agonist 2-pyridyl ethylamine, were also approximately 2, 3 and 4 fold greater respectively, in stripped than in intact tracheal rings, while the maximal relaxant response to nitroprusside was not significantly altered. These selective effects of epithelium stripping on drug action, indicate that loss of a diffusion barrier is not the mechanism of altered airway reactivity. Removal of the epithelium from human bronchial preparations also increased histamine and 5-hydroxytryptamine potencies by 2-4 fold. Similar results were obtained in guinea-pig trachea by Raeburn et al., (1986) and by Hay et al., (1986) and in airway tissue from several other species, including the dog (Flavahan et al., 1985). We have also shown an age-related attenuation of the influence of epithelium stripping (Fernandes et al., 1987), consistent with a decrease in the production of a relaxant factor, as has been described for vascular endothelium (Shimizu & Toda, 1986).

The airway epithelium may also behave as a site of loss for some agonists active at airway smooth muscle. Epithelial uptake of the relaxant beta-adrenoceptor agonist isoprenaline was suggested as the cause of its lesser potency in intact than in stripped guinea-pig trachea (Farmer et al., 1986). Another possibility is that some drug receptors in airway smooth muscle exist in a "cryptic", non-functional state in the presence of an intact epithelium and are only functionally revealed when the epithelium is damaged or lost. Such a mechanism has been postulated with respect to endothelium-dependent alpha-adrenoceptor function in bovine thoracic aorta (Carmen-Krzan, 1985). In reviewing the available evidence, Farmer (1987) concluded that EpDRF did exist in healthy lung and that the loss of EpDRF in asthma, may partially explain the bronchial hyperreactivity.

To confirm the existence of airway EpDRF, its production by donor epithelium and transfer to a recipient assay tissue had to be demonstrated. Tschirhart and Landry (1986) showed that the sensitivity of epithelium-denuded guinea-pig tracheal preparations to the contractile agonist substance P was 42 fold greater than that in intact preparations. This difference was markedly reduced in "sandwich preparations" in which an intact and an epithelium-denuded tracheal strip were closely juxtaposed, presumably as the result of the transfer of EpDRF. We have also demonstrated the transfer of EpDRF from intact guinea-pig tracheal tubes to both endothelium-denuded rat thoracic aorta preparations and epithelium-denuded rat tracheal preparations using a co-axial bioassay system. In addition, we have demonstrated relaxation of guinea-pig isolated trachea in response to a factor produced by cultured human airway epithelial cells challenged with histamine or acetylcholine. The relaxant factor appearing in superfusate from the epithelial cell culture in response to these spasmogens, was assayed by cascade onto an airway preparation denuded of epithelium.

The Nature of EpDRF

While the generation of an inhibitory chemical signal by the vascular endothelium has not been confirmed for all cases of endothelium-modulated drug responses, bioassay techniques have established the existence of such a substance in many instances. Cascade superfusion experiments have been instrumental in defining many of the characteristics of vascular EDRF.

Vascular EDRF behaves like a nitrodilator, increasing intracellular cyclic-GMP. It is neither a cyclooxygenase nor a lipoxygenase metabolite of arachidonic acid, but may be an unstable oxidation product of arachidonic acid (Peach et al., 1985). There is a continuous basal production and release of EDRF which can be increased by drugs including acetylcholine, histamine and bradykinin. Responses to EDRF are inhibited by some antioxidants including dithiothreitol and by the guanylate cyclase antagonist methylene blue. The chemical identity of EDRF has not been definitively established, primarily because of its highly labile nature. However, the most recent evidence suggests that EDRF and nitric oxide (NO) are identical (Palmer et al., 1987).

In rabbit airways, prostaglandin E2, a cyclooxygenase product of arachidonic acid metabolism, is produced by the epithelium and may be EpDRF or at least a component of EpDRF (Butler et al., 1987). Similarly, in guinea-pig trachea, arachidonic acid is converted to a relaxant prostanoid by the epithelium (Farmer et al., 1987). However, the sensitivity of epithelium-denuded or intact guinea-pig tracheal preparations to histamine was not altered in the presence of indomethacin, although the maximum response (Emax) was increased in intact preparations (Hay et al., 1986). We also observed no difference in either guinea-pig tracheal sensitivity or Emax to histamine in stripped or intact preparations. Furthermore, in both co-axial bioassay and superfusion cascade systems, human EpDRF was detected in the presence of indomethacin (5 μM), an inhibitor of cyclooxygenase. Relaxation responses were poorly sustained and only partially inhibited by the guanylate cyclase inhibitor methylene blue (10 μM). Thus, while vascular EDRF and human airway EpDRF have some characteristics in common, these factors are apparently not identical. It is probable that the chemical nature of EpDRF is different between species and in some, may be a heterogeneous mixture of smooth muscle relaxant compounds.

RESPIRATORY VIRUSES, BETA-ADRENOCEPTORS AND AIRWAY HYPERREACTIVITY

Bronchial obstruction is precipitated in asthma sufferers following the administration of beta-adrenoceptor antagonists such as propranolol. This is primarily caused by dominant parasympathetic, cholinergic nerve activity producing bronchial smooth muscle constriction, which reduces airway calibre and airflow. In the absence of such beta-antagonists, cholinergic activity is functionally opposed by inhibitory sympathetic activity mediated via beta-adrenoceptors. We have recently demonstrated significant beta-adrenoceptor hypofunction in bronchial preparations from severely asthmatic lung (Goldie et al., 1986b). We have also suggested that down-regulation of bronchial $beta_2$-adrenoceptors may be associated with hyper-reactivity to airway spasmogens in asthma (Paterson et al., 1982).

Rhinovirus-16 is one of the most common viral precipitants of bronchial asthma symptoms (e.g. wheeze). Parainfluenza and influenza-A viruses also trigger wheeze in children and adults (Hudgel et al., 1979; Tarlo et al., 1979). It is well established that upper respiratory tract viral infections induce airway inflammation and epithelial damage (Hers, 1966) and that hyperreactivity is associated with these events (Empey et al., 1976). However, virally precipitated asthma and hyperreactivity may also involve reduced airway beta-adrenoceptor function.

Several studies provide evidence for the attenuation of beta-adrenoceptor function by respiratory viruses. The inhibitory effect of isoprenaline on lysozymal enzyme release from human granulocytes was impaired in the presence of viral particles including influenza and rhinovirus-16, which can cause respiratory tract infections (Bush et al.,

1978; Busse et al., 1980). Similarly, influenza viral particles decreased the beta-adrenoceptor-mediated release β-glucuronidase from polymorphonuclear leukocytes (PMN) as well as PMN rosette formation with erythrocytes, induced by isoprenaline (Lee, 1980). In addition, infection with parainfluenza-3 virus reduced the ability of the beta-agonist sulfonterol to inhibit ovalbumin-induced contractions of tracheal preparations from sensitized guinea-pigs (Buckner et al., 1981). It is possible that respiratory viral infections initially induce bronchial beta-adrenoceptor hypofunction, which then results in bronchial obstruction.

The epithelium, as well as the smooth muscle of guinea-pig trachea, contains an abundance of beta-adrenoceptors (Goldie et al., 1986a). Furthermore, EpDRF is apparently produced in response to the spasmogen histamine and to the beta-adrenoceptor agonist isoprenaline. Thus, virally-induced bronchospasm may be initiated by attenuation of beta-adrenoceptor function in airway smooth muscle, as well as in epithelial cells (reducing EpDRF production).

Viral particles from different classes utilize different mechanisms to attach to the surface of target cells prior to internalization. It has recently been shown that reovirus-3 particles contain a surface binding site with many of the properties of mammalian beta-adrenoceptors (Co et al., 1985). In addition, the tissues known to bind reovirus-3, such as heart, brain and skeletal muscle, also contain beta-adrenoceptors. Reovirus-3 may also possess a site which recognizes beta-adrenoceptors on cell membranes (Co et al., 1985). Attachment of the virus to cell surface beta-adrenoceptors may be a prerequisite to their internalization.

It is possible that previously documented viral attenuation of beta-adrenoceptor function in PMN's and in guinea-pig trachea occurred as a result of the binding of viral particles to these receptors. Similarly, binding of these virus types to human airway beta-adrenoceptors would be expected to reduce function. In severe asthmatics with pre-existing bronchial beta-adrenoceptor hypofunction, a further reduction in function may follow the binding of viral particles such as rhinovirus-16, parainfluenza and influenza. This would cause an additional shift in the balance towards bronchoconstrictor cholinergic dominance of the autonomic control of airway calibre and thus promote bronchial hyperresponsiveness to spasmogens.

SUMMARY

It is clear that the central airway epithelium plays an important role in restricting access of inhaled solutes to sub-epithelial airway wall structures. Non-specific airway hyperreactivity to spasmogens in asthma may result partly as a consequence of the compromise of the epithelium as a barrier to solute diffusion. However, impaired epithelial production and release of smooth muscle relaxant factor(s) may also contribute to airway hyperresponsiveness. Virally precipitated asthma also involves inflammation-induced epithelial damage. Beta-adrenoceptor hypofunction induced by respiratory viruses may also contribute to bronchial obstruction.

REFERENCES

Aquilina A, Hall W, Douglas R, Utell M (1980). Airway reactivity in subjects with viral upper respiratory infections: the effects of exercise and cold air. Am Rev Resp Dis 122: 3-10.

Barnes PJ (1986). Asthma as an axon reflex. Lancet 1: 242-245.

Boushey HA, Holtzman MJ, Sheller JR, Nadel JAY (1980). Bronchial hyperreactivity. Am Rev Resp Dis 121: 389-413.

Buckner CK, Clayton DE, Ain-Shoka AA, Busse WW, Dick EC, Shult P (1981). Parainfluenza 3 infection blocks the ability of a beta-adrenergic receptor agonist to inhibit antigen-induced contraction of guinea-pig isolated airway smooth muscle. J clin Invest 67: 376-384.

Bush R, Busse WW, Flaherty D, Washauer D, Dick E, Reed C (1978). Effects of experimental rhinovirus 16 infection on airways and leucocyte function in normal subjects. J Allergy clin Immunol 61: 80-87.

Busse WW, Anderson CL, Dick EC, Warshauer D (1980). Reduced granulocyte response to isoproterenol, histamine, and prostaglandin E1 after in vitro incubation with rhinovirus 16. Am Rev Resp Dis 122: 641-646.

Butler GB, Adler KB, Evans JN, Morgan DW, Szarek JL (1987). Modulation of rabbit airway smooth muscle responsiveness by respiratory epithelium. Am Rev Resp Dis 135: 1099-1104.

Carmen-Krzan M (1985). Role of endothelium in the binding of [^{3}H]-prazosin to the aortic α_1-adrenergic receptors. Eur J Pharmac 111: 137-138.

Co MA, Gaulton GN, Tominaga A, Homcy CJ, Fields BN, Green MI (1985). Structural similarities between the mammalian beta-adrenergic and reovirus type 3 receptors. Proc Nat'l Acad Sci USA 82: 5315-5318.

Cuss FM, Dixon CMS, Barnes PJ (1986). Effects of inhaled platelet activating factor on pulmonary function and bronchial responsiveness in man. Lancet 2: 189-192.

Cutz E, Levison H Cooper DM (1978). Ultrastructure of airways in children with asthma. Histopath 2: 407-421.

Empey DW, Laitinen LA, Jacobs L, Gold WM Nadel JAY (1976). Mechanisms of bronchial hyperreactivity in normal subjects after upper respiratory tract infection. Am Rev Resp Dis 113: 131-139.

Farmer SG, Fedan JS, Hay DWP, Raeburn D (1986). The effects of epithelium removal on the sensitivity of guinea-pig isolated trachealis to bronchodilator drugs. Br J Pharmac 89: 407-414.

Farmer SG (1987). Airway smooth muscle responsiveness: modulation by the epithelium. Trends Pharmacol Sci 8: 8-9.

Farmer SG, Hay DWP, Raeburn D, Fedan JS (1987). Relaxation of guinea-pig tracheal smooth muscle to arachidonate is converted to contraction following epithelium removal. Eur J Pharmac (Submitted for publication).

Fernandes LB, Preuss, JMH, Rigby PJ, Goldie RG (1987). Age-related changes in epithelium-induced modulation of guinea-pig tracheal responsiveness to spasmogens. Br J Pharmac (submitted for publication).

Flavahan NA, Aarhus LL, Rimele TJ, Vanhoutte PM (1985). Respiratory epithelium inhibits bronchial smooth muscle tone. J Appl Physiol 58: 834-838.

Furchgott RF, Zawadazki JV (1980). Acetylcholine relaxes arterial smooth muscle by releasing a relaxing substance from endothelial cells. Nature 288: 373-376.

Gleich GJ, Loegering DA, Frigas E, Filley WV (1983). The eosinophil granule major basic protein: biological activities and relationship to bronchial asthma. Monogr Allergy 18: 277-283.

Goldie RG, Papadimitriou JM, Paterson JW, Rigby PJ, Self HM, Spina D (1986a). Influence of the epithelium on responsiveness of guinea-pig trachea to contractile and relaxant agonists. Br J Pharmac 87: 5-14.

Goldie RG, Spina D, Henry PJ, Lulich KM, Paterson J.W. (1986b). In vitro responsiveness of human asthmatic bronchus to carbachol, histamine, beta-adrenoceptor agonists and theophylline. Br J clin Pharmac 22: 669-676.

Hargreaves FE, Dolovitch J, O'Byrne PM, Ramsdale EH, Daniel EE (1986). The origin of airway hyperresponsiveness. Allergy clin Immunol 78: 825-832.

Hers JFPH (1966). Disturbance of the ciliated epithelium due to influenza virus. Am Rev Resp Dis 93: 162-171.

Hay DWP, Farmer SG, Raeburn D, Robinson VA, Fleming WW, Fedan JS (1986). Airway epithelium modulates the reactivity of guinea-pig respiratory smooth muscle. Eur J Pharmac 129: 11-18.

Hudgel D, Langston L, Selner J, McIntosh K (1979). Viral and bacterial infections in adults with chronic asthma. Am Rev Resp Dis 120: 393.

Laitinen LA, Heino M, Laitinen A, Kava T, Haahtels T (1985). Damage of airway epithelium and bronchial reactivity in patients with asthma. Am Rev Resp Dis 131: 599-606.

Lee TP (1980). Virus exposure diminishes beta-adrenergic response in human leukocytes. Res Common Chem Path Pharmac 30: 469-476.

McFadden E (1984). Pathogenesis of asthma. J Allergy clin Immunol 73: 413-424.

Minor TE, Dick ER, Baker JW, Ouellette JJ, Cohen M, Reed CE (1976). Rhinovirus and influenza type A infections as precipitants of asthma. Am Rev Resp Dis 113: 149-153.

Page CP, Paul W, Archer CB, Macdonald DM, Morley J (1983). Platelet Activating Factor. In Benveniste J, Arnoux B (eds). INSERM Symposium. Elsevier pp 357-366.

Palmer RMJ, Ferrige AG, Moncada S (1987). Nitric oxide release accounts for the biological activity of endothelium-derived relaxing factor. Nature 327: 524-526.

Paterson JW, Lulich KM, Goldie RG (1982). The role of beta-adrenoceptors in bronchial hyperreactivity. In Morley J (ed): Perspectives in Asthma I. Acad Press Inc (London) Ltd. pp 19-37.

Peach MJ, Singer H, Loeb A. (1985). Biochem Pharmac 34: 1867-1874.

Raeburn D, Hay DWP, Farmer SG, Fedan JS (1986). Epithelium removal increases the reactivity of human isolated tracheal muscle to methacholine and reduces the effect of verapamil. Eur J Pharmac 123: 451-453.

Ranga V, Powers MA, Padilla M, Strope GL, Fowler L, Kleinerman J (1983). Effect of allergic bronchoconstriction on airway epithelial permeability to large polar solutes in the guinea-pig. Am Rev Resp Dis 128: 1065-1070.
Shimizu I, Toda N (1986). Alterations with age of the response to vasodilator agents in isolated mesenteric arteries of the beagle. Br J Pharmac 89: 769-778.
Tarlo S, Broder I, Spence L (1979). A prospective study of respiratory infection in adult asthmatics and their normal spouses. Clin Allergy 9: 293-301.
Tschirhart E, Landry Y (1987). Airway epithelium releases a relaxant factor: demonstration with substance P. Eur J Pharmac 132: 103-104.
Woolcock A, Salome C, Yan K (1984). The shape of the dose-response curve to histamine in asthmatic and normal subjects. Am Rev Resp Dis 13: 71-75.

Discussion on Paper by Roy Goldie

de Jongste: You showed that the hyperresponsiveness to inhaled histamine was best in animals 6 to 7 weeks old. Is the production of the relaxing factor related to the age of the animals or can you demonstrate the relaxing factor at all ages?

Goldie: Well at the moment we haven't looked at the younger or the older age group and in fact it was absolutely fortuitous that we ever saw this change in reactivity. We use as standard practice 6 to 7 week old animals. If we had used younger ones or older ones we may never have stumbled across this. In fact other groups have shown smaller shifts and it is because they are using wider weight ranges. To answer your question directly, I haven't looked at the younger or the older group. I hope that there is going to be a correlation between age and EpDRF production, there certainly is with blood vessels with respect to endothelial-derived relaxant factor (EDRF).

Black: The changes with epithelial removal are all small except for substance P. Do you think that is due to the removal of peptidases from the epithelium.

Goldie: Yes, I think that its quite likely they play a role.

Black: Rather than the removal of this EpDRF?

Goldie: Well that's possible. Other groups believe that it is due to the removal of the relaxing factor but I am dubious about this.

P. Barnes: Nellie Frossard in my lab has been looking at this and she has also found a big shift with substance P after removal of the epithelium. We have looked at the effect with phosphoramidon on that as well. As in the phosphoramidon studies of Jay Nadel we found that there is shift in sensitivity, (quite a big shift) to substance P with phosphoramidon. However the difference between this and epithelial removal, while reduced, is not abolished which brings it more in line with the other sort of spasmogens that we see. So probably all these things have a fairly similar effect but it is very much exaggerated with substance P presumably because you remove the endopeptidases.

Goldie: So in other words it is a multi-factorial thing as far as substance P is concerned.

P. Barnes: I think that the evidence is very good that EpDRF is not the same as EDRF. We have provided evidence for that in a paper that Francis Cuss wrote showing that nordihydroguaretic acid, which abolishes the action of EDRF, had no effect on this epithelial removal phenomenon.

Goldie: We have looked at methylene blue, a guanylate cyclase antagonist. While we get some inhibition of the EpDRF-induced response, it is only a partial inhibition. You would have noticed on both of the assay systems that I showed, that there is cross reactivity between EpDRF and vascular smooth muscle and also there is a species cross-over. But it doesn't work the other way, vascular EDRF does not relax airway smooth muscle or gastro-intestinal smooth muscle.

Anderson: That could be important in the control of bronchial circulation presumably.

Goldie: Yes.

Small: It is perhaps not surprising that your stripping procedure on guinea pig trachea potentiated some agonists and not others. What did surprise me though, was that you found a separation between acetylcholine and methacholine on the one hand and bethanachol and carbachol on the other. Do you have any pharmacological explanation as to why 2 of those should have been potentiated by the procedure and not the other 2?

Goldie: Yes but it is speculation. Carbachol and bethanachol have an amine loading on their molecules, acetylcholine and methacholine have a methyl loading. In fact that is the only clear difference that I can see maybe that the amine loading is critical for a turn-on of EpDRF production. If that is true, it suggests that the muscarinic receptor on the epithelial cell is a sub-class. We have these amine loadings on those molecules which did not change reactivity and methyl loadings on the drugs such as acetylcholine and methacholine, where you see a shift in reactivity. I don't know whether that is critical or not, it is the only thing I can come up with at the moment. Sub-classing of muscarinic receptors is a popular game and maybe we are looking at a new class.

Church: In the sensitised guinea pig work that we have been doing, we have looked at bronchial hyperreactivity, where it increases four-fold, a week after a fairly minimal antigen challenge. We have no evidence from microscopic examination that there is any damage at all to the epithelium. So in the guinea pig lack of EpDRF certainly does not explain all of the increased reactivity.

Goldie: I think that one of the problems is that it may only require quite subtle damage to the epithelium. We are ripping off the epithelium here, but it is possible that a metabolic damage may be all that is required. You may not pick that up at all microscopically, either at the electron microscopic level or the light microscope level.

Stephens: The vascular people have produced some rather variable evidence to indicate that there is also endothelium-derived excitatory factor. Have you had a chance to look at that yet in airway.

Goldie: No, I have got my hands full with the relaxant factor just at the moment.

Anderson: Do you have any evidence whether an increase in osmolarity could provoke the release of EpDRF?

Goldie: Well we had a look at that. Very briefly, the results are equivocal which is why I didn't include them in this particular talk. However I am now going to look at them in more detail. Essentially we were getting relaxation responses in both stripped and unstripped preparations with hyperosmolarity. We haven't done enough experiments to quantitate the extent of that relaxation nor have we determined whether or not there is a difference in the quality of the relaxation observed.

Mechanisms in Asthma: Pharmacology,
Physiology, and Management, pages 331–339

ROLE OF AIRWAY EPITHELIAL CELLS IN THE DEFENSE OF AIRWAYS

Jay A. Nadel

Cardiovascular Research Institute and Depts of Medicine and Physiology, University of California San Francisco, S.F., California, 94143, U.S.A.

The involvement of the airway epithelium in the pathogenesis of asthma is suggested by the finding of abnormal epithelium in airways of asthmatics. Thus, during asthma attacks, epithelial cells are desquamated and are found in the sputum as Creola bodies or Curschman's spirals. Postmortem examination of asthmatics who die show extensive shedding of epithelial cells and severe epithelial inflammation. Even subjects with stable asthma show evidence of airway epithelial desquamation.

Airway smooth muscle hyperresponsiveness is an important basic characteristic of asthma. The fact that a variety of clinical conditions causing airway hyperresponsiveness are associated with epithelial damage and airway inflammation lends further credence to the hypothesis that epithelial cells play a pathogenetic role in airway hyperresponsiveness. These conditions include viral infections (Empey et al., 1976) and exposure to irritants such ozone (Lee et al., 1977; Golden et al., 1987) and to toluene diisocyanate (Gordon, 1985).

Until recently, airway epithelial cells were considered to be simply an inert, physical lining that covers the airways. It is now apparent that these cells, with their key location at the interface between the external environment and the internal milieu, play an important role in the defense of the airways. These functions are discussed briefly.

A. EPITHELIAL CELL MEDIATOR RELEASE

Airway epithelial cells are capable of generating potent lipoxygenase products of arachidonic acid (Holtzman et al., 1983a; Hunter et al, 1985). Human airway epithelial cells produce 15-HETE and 8,15-di HETEs (Hunter et al., 1985) and dog epithelial cells produce LTB_4 and selected HETEs (Holtzman et al, 1983a). Both LTB_4 and 8,15-di HETEs (Shak et al., 1983; and Nadel, personal communication) are chemotactic for neutrophils, and this could explain the neutrophil infiltration of the airways that occurs with viral infection (Walsh et al., 1961), ozone (Holtzman et al,, 1983b; Fabbri et al, 1984), and other airway stimuli. The 15-HETEs are also of interest because they are reported to stimulate the release of mediators from mast cells (Phillips et al., 1983). Thus, epithelial cell stimulation by damage or by other mediators, produce lipoxygenase products which in turn stimulate other inflammatory cells.

B. SMOOTH MUSCLE MODULATION BY AIRWAY EPITHELIUM

Airway epithelium has multiple effects on airway smooth muscle. Intact epithelium inhibits muscle tone by releasing prostaglandin E_2 (PGE_2). PGE_2 has inhibitory effects directly in the muscle and also by inhibiting vagal neural transmission (Walters et al., 1984). Human and dog airway epithelial cells in culture produce low concentrations of PGE_2, but when they are stimulated by inflammatory mediators such as bradykinin (Leikauf et al., 1985), or by eosinophil major basic protein (Jacoby et al., in press 1987), these cells produce large amounts of PGE_2 which have profound effects on smooth muscle tone (Barnett et al., 1987). Removal of airway epithelium is reported to produce inhibitory effects on airway smooth msucle via an unknown mechanism (Flavahan et al., 1985). Contractile effects of tachykinins such as substance P are modulated by a membrane-bound enzyme, enkephalinase, which exists on airway epithelial cell membranes (Sekizawa et al, 1987). By cleaving and thus inactivating these neuropeptides, epithelial enkephalinase limits the action of tachykinins on airway smooth muscle. Removal of airway epithelium decreases the amount of enkephalinase in the airway and thus selectively increases the bronchoconstrictor effects of substance P. Enkephalinase is selective to tachykinins and does not affect contractions to other mediators such as acetycholine (Sekizawa et al., 1987; see also the chapter in this book entitled "Modulation of Tachykinin and Bradykinin by Enkephalinase").

Finally, as mentioned above, airway epithelial cells are capable of generating products of the 15-lipoxygenase pathway of arachidonate metabolism, and these products have indirect effects on smooth muscle (Holtzman et al., 1983a; Hunter et al., 1985): For example, 8,15-di HETEs are chemotactic for neutrophils (Shak et al., 1983) and the presence of activated neutrophils is associated with increased responsiveness of airway smooth muscle (Holtzman et al., 1983b; Irvin et al., 1984; Fabbri et al., 1984; O'Byrne et al., 1984). This could be the mechanism for the neutrophil chemotaxis and transient hyperresponsiveness that occurs with viral infections (Empey et al., 1976) and with ozone (Lee et al., 1977; Golden et al., 1978). These 15-lipoxygenase products of airway epithelium, the 15-HETEs, are also of interest because they stimulate selective release of mast cell mediators (Phillips et al., 1983). These 15-HETEs can also be converted to lipoxins, substances that contract airway smooth muscle (Serhan et al., 1984; 1986).

C. EPITHELIAL GLYCOCALYX

The luminal surface of the airway epithelium contains a glycocalyx consisting of high molecular weight glycoconjugates that contain specific types of carbohydrate chains of the poly(N-acetyl-lactosamine)-type (Varsano et al., 1987a). These high molecular weight materials are produced and secreted by the airway epithelium and thus contribute to the luminal secretions. As with other secretions, their exact function is unknown, but they may contain bonding sites for bacteria and other cells.

Under appropriate conditions, inflammatory cells such as mast cells, neutrophils, eosinophils and macrophages migrate to the airways. If these inflammatory cells adhere to airway epithelium, the actions of the inflammatory cells may be increased and prolonged. Studies of mast cells indicate that these inflammatory cells adhere to tracheal epithelial cells in culture and in tissue sections (Varsano et al., 1987b). This adhesion is selective and occurs preferentially with epithelial cells, with minimal adhesion to surfaces coated with basement membrane collagen (type IV), connective tissue matrix collagen (type I) or fibronectin. Adhesion to cultured epithelial cells was a characteristic of a subpopulation of mast cells, persisted for more than 48 hours, did not require energy or the presence of divalent cations, and was not mediated by a known family of leukocyte-associated adhesion glycoproteins. Adhesion was completely abolished by pretreatment of the mast cells with proteinase K or pronase E but not with trypsin. Pretreatment of the epithelial cells with proteinases was without effect. This latter fact suggests that the epithelial adhesion molecules are not proteins. Some epithelial cells carry glycolipid receptors (Andersson et al., 1983), and the airway epithelial binding sites for mast cells might also be lipids.

The existence of a population of adherent mast cells has important clinical implications. These adhesion properties may explain the localization of certain mast cell populations in the airway epithelium. Thus, in cigarette smokers (Lamb and Lumsden, 1982) and in asthmatics (Cutz et al., 1978), intraepithelial mast cells may be selectively adherent. This selective localization may play an important role in determining the phenotype of the intraepithelial mast cells. Adhesion may also form a microenvironment between the mast cells and epithelium by increasing local concentrations of mediators, thereby causing changes such as increased mucosal permeability to antigens and to other stimuli, increased secretions, ion transport and smooth muscle contraction, and influx of other inflammatory cells. This selectively adherent population of mast cells may differ in functional properties from non-adherent cells, such as those readily available to bronchoalveolar lavage.

D. ION TRANSPORT AND MUCUS SECRETION

This subject is reviewed elsewhere (Nadel et al., 1985) and will only be discussed briefly. Most of the fluid and mucus present in the airway lumen is believed to be derived from airway submucosal glands and can be stimulated to secrete mucus of different chemical and viscoelastic properties by different autonomic nervous and chemical mediators (Nadel et al., 1985). Active ion transport of chloride by airway epithelial cells (Olver et al., 1975) and secondary movement of fluid (Welsh et al., 1980) provides a mechanism for fine regulation of the sol layer in which the cilia move. Prostaglandin E_2 (PGE_2) produced by the epithelial cells stimulates Cl transport (Al-Bazzaz et al., 1981), and various inflammatory mediators stimulate PGE_2 production, thus increasing Cl transport. This autocrine function of the epithelium allows it to dilute inflammatory irritants in the microenvironment and thus lessen their deleterious effects.

Water is lost in the airway during breathing, and this loss is exaggerated during exercise and when breathing dry air. The water loss must first occur from the airway lumen and then from the interstititial space. Ultimately, the water loss must be made up from fluid supplied by the bronchial arteries or hyperosmolarity of the airway tissues must occur. Because exercise-induced asthma is believed to be triggered by hyperosmolarity, knowledge of the fluid reservoirs and limitations of fluid production in airways are important to the understanding and possibly the prevention of asthmatic attacks during exercise.

In summary, the airway epithelium is a dynamic tissue and plays an important, perhaps the most important, role in defense of the airways. In asthma and in other diseases of the airways, there are conspicuous alterations in the epithelium. The patho-physiologic implications of these changes remain to be elucidated.

Supported in part by NIH Program Project Grant HL-24136.

REFERENCES

Al-Bazzaz FJ, Yadava VP, Westenfelder C (1981). Modification of Na and Cl transport in canine tracheal mucosa by prostaglandins. Am J Physiol 240:F101-105.

Andersson B, Dahmen J, Frejd T, Leffler H, Magnusson G, Noore G, Eden CS (1983). Identification of an active disaccharide unit of a glycoconjugate receptor for pneumococci attaching to human pharyngeal epithelial cells. J Exp Med 158:559-570.

Barnett K, Jacoby DB, Lazarus SC, Nadel JA (1987). Bradykinin stimulates release of an epithelial cell product that inhibits smooth muscle contraction. Am Rev Respir Dis 135:A274.

Cutz E, Levison H, Cooper DM (1978). Ultrastructure of airways in children with asthma. Histopathology 2:407-421.

Empey DW, Laitinen LA, Jacobs L, Gold WM, Nadel JA (1976). Mechanisms of bronchial hyperreactivity in normal subjects following upper respiratory tract infection. Am Rev Respir Dis 113:131-139.

Fabbri LM, Aizawa H, Alpert SE, Walters EH, O'Byrne PM, Gold BD, Nadel JA, Holtzman MJ (1984). Airway hyperresponsiveness and changes in cell counts in bronchoalveolar lavage after ozone exposure in dogs. Am Rev Respir Dis 129:288-291.

Flavahan NA, Aarhus LL, Rimele TJ, and Vanhoutte PM (1985). Respiratory epithelium inhibits bronchial smooth muscle tone. J Appl Physiol 58:834-838.

Golden JA, Nadel JA, Boushey HA (1978). Bronchial hyperirritability in healthy subjects after exposure to ozone. Am Rev Respir Dis 118:287-294.

Gordon T, Sheppard D, McDonald DM, Distefano S, Scypinski L (1985). Airway hyperresponsiveness and inflammation induced by toluene diisocyanate in guinea pigs. Am Rev Respir Dis 132:1106-1112.

Holtzman MJ, Aizawa H, Nadel JA, Goetzl EJ (1983a). Selective generation of leukotriene B_4 by tracheal epithelial cells from dogs. Biochem Biophys Res Commun 114:1071-1076.

Holtzman MJ, Fabbri LM, O'Byrne PM, Gold BD, Aizawa J, Walters EH, Alpert SE, Nadel JA (1983b). Importance of airway inflammation for hyperresponsiveness induced by ozone in dogs. Am Rev Respir Dis 127:686-690.

Hunter JA, Finkbeiner WE, Nadel JA, Goetzl EJ, Holtzman MJ (1985). Predominant generation of 15-lipoxygenase metabolites of arachidonic acid by epithelial cells from human trachea. Proc Natl Acad Sci USA 82:4633-4637.

Irvin CG, Baltopoulos G, Henson P (1984). Airway hyperreactivity produced by products from phagocytizing neutrophils. Am Rev Respir Dis 131:A278.

Jacoby DB, Ueki IF, Widdicombe JH, Loegering DA, Gleich GJ, Nadel JA (in press 1987). Effect of Human eosinophil major basic protein on ion transport in dog tracheal epithelium. Am Rev Respir Dis.

Lamb D, Lumsden A (1982). Intra-epithelial mast cells in human airway epithelium: evidence for smoking-induced changes in their frequency. Thorax 37:334-342.

Lee L-Y, Bleecker ER, Nadel JA (1977). Effect of ozone on bronchomotor response to inhaled histamine aerosol in dogs. J Appl Physiol 43:626-631.

Leikauf GD, Ueki IF, Nadel JA, Widdicombe JH (1985). Bradykinin stimulates Cl secretion and prostaglandin E_2 release by canine tracheal epithelium. Am J Physiol 248:F48-F55.

Leikauf GD, Ueki IF, Widdicombe JH, Nadel JA (1986). Alteration of chloride secretion across canine tracheal epithelium by lipoxygenase products of arachidonic acid. Am J Physiol 250:F47-F53.

Nadel JA, Widdicombe JH, Peatfield AC (1985). Regulation of airway secretions, ion transport, and water movement. In Fishman AP, Fisher AB (eds): "Handbook of Physiology. The Respiratory System," Bethesda, MD: The American Physiological Society, Vol 1, pp419-445.

O'Byrne PM, Walters EH, Gold BD, Aizawa HA, Fabbri LM, Alpert SE, Nadel JA, Holtzman MJ (1984). Neutrophil depletion inhibits airway hyperresponsiveness induced by ozone exposure. Am Rev Respir Dis 130:214-219.

Olver RE, Davis B, Marin MG, Nadel JA (1975). Active transport of Na^+ and Cl^- across the canine tracheal epithelium in vitro. Am Rev Respir Dis 112:811-815.

Phillips MJ, Gold WM, Goetzl EJ (1983). IgE-dependent and ionophore-induced generation of leukotrienes by dog mastocytoma cells. J Immunol 131:906-910.

Sekizawa K, Tamaoki J, Nadel JA, Borson DB (in press 1987). Enkephalinase inhibitor potentiates substance P- and electrically induced contraction in ferret trachea. J Appl Physiol.

Serhan CN, Hamberg M, Samuelsson B (1984). Lipoxins: novel series of biologically active compounds formed from arachidonic acid in human leukocytes. Proc Natl Acad Sci USA 81:5335-5339.

Serhan CN, Nicolaou KC, Webber SE, Veal CA, Dahlen SE, Puustinen TJ, Samuelsson B (1986). Lipoxin A stereochemistry and biosynthesis. J Biol Chem 261:16340-16345.

Shak S, Perez HD, Goldstein IM (1983). A novel dioxygenation product of arachidonic acid possesses potent chemotactic activity for human polymorphonuclear leukocytes. J Biol Chem 258:14948-14953.

Varsano S, Basbaum CB, Forsberg LS, Borson DB, Caughey G, Nadel JA (1987a). Dog tracheal epithelial cells in culture synthesize sulfated macromolecular glycoconjugates and release them from the cell surface upon exposure to extracellular proteinases. Exp Lung Res 13:157-183.

Varsono S, Rosen SD, Lazarus SC, Gold WM, Nadel JA (1987b). Selective adhesion of mast cells to tracheal epithelial cells. Fed Proc 46:A992.

Walsh JJ, Dietlein LF, Low FN, Burch GE, Mogabgab WJ (1961). Bronchotracheal response in human influenza. Arch Intern Med 108:376-382.

Walters EH, O'Byrne PM, Fabbri LM, Graf PD, Holtzman MJ, Nadel JA (1984). Control of neurotransmission by prostaglandins in canine trachealis smooth muscle. J Appl Physiol 57:129-134.

Welsh MJ, Widdicombe JH, Nadel JA (1980). Fluid transport across the canine tracheal epithelium. J Appl Physiol 49:909.

Discussion on Paper by Jay Nadel

Burka: I was intrigued that you now put the epithelium into the metabolic functions of the lung. Mick Bakhle gave an excellent lecture on this subject at the IUPHAR meeting (1982), but he spoke mainly of the metabolic function of the endothelium. Does the epithelium play a function in breaking down histamine, prostaglandins, etc, similar to what the endothelium does. Should we now consider it as having a metabolic function?

Nadel: I gave a brief example of how the epithelium could work with drugs. They may metabolise antibiotics and other drugs. We simply don't know. I gave another example of the epithelium controlling smooth muscle through enkaphalinase. I think that is important. We know intuitively that airway epithelium has to mend itself or the body would drop out. When you go in with a bronchoscope, a million cells are destroyed. You have to have chemotaxis, differentiation, etc, to regenerate the cells, so in this respect that is a metabolic function.

Mapp: In the dog you took the supernatant and you were able to inhibit smooth muscle contractility and you relate this to a release of bronchodilator factor.

Nadel: Yes, release of PGE_2.

Mapp: Do you think, in this situation, that there is only release of PGE_2 or that more important bronchoconstrictor factors are released.

Nadel: I didn't actually set out to answer this precisely. We have known for a number of years that PGE_2 is modulating responses. We tried to demonstrate other bronchodilator factors and bronchoconstrictor factors and we have subsequently shown that lipoxins can be generated, but not alone. They are easiest to demonstrate in the presence of indomethacin. The huge effect that we get, almost without exception, is totally abolished by indomethacin. The exact amount of prostaglandins that we measure in the supernatent is the amount that would give the same pre-synaptic effect on the nerves in the muscle. So the answer is that we were disappointed. If these other relaxing and contracting factors are important and are there, they are very likely to be able to be up and down regulated. So I think the first step is to isolate it and know what it is, and then you have a much better shot at being able to up and down regulate it. Once we have gotten rid of the PGE_2 dilator fraction there isn't enough left for us in our hands right now to study it. We are not giving up there and I would welcome anybody who wants to come to work. We have dozens of transformer cell lines that do various things that preserve function.

Piper: A comment in answer to John Burka's question about the metabolism perhaps by the epithelium of the airways. A long while ago we perfused guinea-pig lungs by the trachea. At the time we were studying the metabolism of prostaglandins in the pulmonary circulation and we didn't lose biological activity when the perfusion was made by the airways. I think it was PGE_2 we were studying. We of course lost most of the activity when we perfused by the pulmonary vascular bed. Perhaps that throws some light that the epithelium isn't metabolising prostaglandins.

Mechanisms in Asthma: Pharmacology,
Physiology, and Management, pages 341–353

LEUKOCYTES AND MEDIATORS IN EXERCISE INDUCED ASTHMA AND HYPERTONIC CHALLENGE TO THE AIRWAYS

Stephen P O'Hickey, Jonathan P Arm, Nicholas G Belcher, Tak H Lee.

Departments of Medicine and Respiratory Medicine

United Medical and Dental Schools
Guy's Hospital, London SE1 9RT

INTRODUCTION

Airflow limitation occurs in 70 - 80 % of asthmatic subjects following vigorous exercise. The initiating mechanism is unknown and there is debate as to whether airway cooling or changes in the osmotic milieu of the bronchial mucosa causes exercise induced asthma (EIA) (Anderson 1984). Irrespective of the exact initiating event, there is evidence that EIA is associated with both mediator release and leucocyte activation .

MEDIATOR RELEASE

A neutrophil chemotactic factor (NCF) of high molecular weight is detectable in the circulation of 75 % of asthmatic subjects during EIA (Lee et al. 1982a). The release of NCF accompanies the development of asthma and is prevented by administration of disodium cromoglycate (DSCG) prior to exercise (Lee et al. 1982b). NCF is not released following methacholine induced bronchospasm despite the development of a similar magnitude of airflow obstruction as that observed during EIA, indicating that NCF release is not due to the bronchoconstriction *per se* (Lee et al. 1982a). The finding that an exercise task undertaken while breathing cold/dry air led to bronchoconstriction and NCF release, whereas inhalation of fully conditioned air during exercise did not produce asthma or release mediators (Lee et al. 1983a), suggests that the release of NCF during EIA is critically dependant upon the conditions of the inspired air.

If airway hypertonicity is an important initiating factor for EIA, it should be possible to reproduce many of the features of EIA with hypertonic challenge. We subjected 10 asthmatic subjects with EIA to pairs of challenges of exercise and ultrasonically nebulised hypertonic saline (3.6%) in different combinations(Belcher et al. 1987a). The protocol ensured that the magnitiude of the decrease in FEV1 induced by the initial hypertonic saline inhalation was matched to that elicited by an initial exercise challenge in each subject. Those subjects who were refractory to EIA after an initial exercise challenge were also refractory following initial hypertonic challenge to further challenge with hypertonic saline. Furthermore, there was cross refractoriness in that hypertonic saline challenge produced refractoriness to exercise, and exercise rendered the same individuals refractory to hypertonic challenge. In contrast, subjects who were not refractory to EIA following an initial exercise task, were not refractory to EIA or hypertonic challenge following initial provocation with 3.6% saline. In addition exercise did not render this group refractory to asthma initiated by hypertonic challenge. The demonstration that exercise and hypertonic challenge induced refractoriness interchangeably suggests that airway hypertonicity and exercise induce a refractory period by similar if not identical mechanisms.

In view of the suggestion that hypertonicity may be the initiating stimulus to exercise induced asthma , we have recently determined whether hyperosmolar challenge to the bronchi is associated with the release of mediators of hypersensitivity. Mediator release following hyperosmolar challenge was compared to that observed when the same subjects developed EIA (Belcher et al.1987b). NCF and plasma histamine concentrations were measured in nine asthmatic subjects with EIA following inhalation of ultrasonically nebulised hypertonic saline and following exercise which produced a decrease in FEV1 of 25% (± 4%) and 27% (± 3%) There was an approximate 300% maximal increase in NCF detected following both challenges. Gel filtration chromatography on columns of ultragel ACA 34 indicated that the NCF released after hyperosmolar challenge and exercise had a similar molecular size of 600 to 700 K daltons. Exercise but not hypertonic challenge was associated with a basophilia and a significant increase in plasma histamine from 3.5 ± 0.5 nmol/l to 6.5 ± 1.1 nmol/l (p=0.021) at five minutes. In contrast there was no basophilia and no significant increase in basophils or plasma histamine following hypertonic saline provocation. This finding is consistent with the view that increases in plasma histamine detected following exercise are related to the post-exertional basophilia. However, there are difficulties in accepting that basophils are the only cause of the rise in plasma histamine detected in EIA for several reasons. Spontaneous histamine release from basophils of asthmatic subjects decreases after exercise (Howarth et al. 1984) and while subjects with EIA have a post exercise basophilia similar to that of asthmatic subjects without EIA only the former individuals release histamine (Lee et al. 1984). An increase in plasma histamine can also occur following hyperventilation induced asthma in the absence of a basophilia (Lee et al. 1983b). Inhalation of terbutaline following EIA enhanced the release of histamine (Anderson et al. 1981), an effect which is unlikely to be related to basophilia. The mechanism for NCF release following hypertonic saline challenge may be an increase in the osmolarity of the airways epithelium and its constituent mediator containing cells; a stimulus which is known to cause mast cell degranulation <u>in vitro</u> (Eggleston et al. 1987).

MEDIATOR RELEASE IN THE REFRACTORY PERIOD

The cause of the refractory period following EIA is not known and at least three possible mechanisms have been suggested. First the refractory period may be due to mediator depletion; secondly catecholamines released following the first challenge may protect the airways from the subsequent bronchoconstrictor stimulus; thirdly there may be a reduction in airways smooth muscle responsiveness.

To examine further the role of mediator depletion, we have measured NCF and histamine during the refractory period in a group of 8 asthmatic subjects who were subjected to two bouts of cycle ergometer exercise and who demonstrated refractoriness to EIA (Belcher et al. 1988). At 5 minutes following the first and second challenge NCF increased by 349% and 327% respectively. In the same individuals there was a rise in plasma histamine from pre-challenge values of 3.2 ± 0.4 nmol/l to 4.7 ± 0.5 nmol/l ($p = < 0.05$) following the first exercise challenge and from 2.4 ± 0.4 nmol/l to 6.3 ± 2.3nmol/l following the second exercise challenge ($p < 0.05$). There were no significant differences in the levels or the time course of release of these mediators between the two exercise tasks. Gel filtration chromatography demonstrated that the NCF detected after both challenges had the same molecular size of 600 K dalton.

We have also examined the role of catecholamines in the development of the refractory period by measuring changes in the circulating levels of adrenaline and noradrenaline following EIA (Belcher et al. 1988) in these same individuals. There was no significant difference in the noradrenaline levels released between the two challenges even though the patients were still refractory to EIA. The recent demonstration that hypertonic saline challenge produces refractoriness but does not release catecholamines (Belcher et al. 1987b,1988) suggests that the refractory period cannot be explained by protection of the airways by catecholamine release.

Magnussen has recently suggested that the refractory period is due to smooth muscle hyporesponsiveness (Magnussen et al. 1986). This may be related to protection of the airways through the release of cyclo-oxygenase pathway products (O'Byrne and Jones 1986). Mattoli, studying the response to ultrasonically nebulised distilled water (UNDW) (Mattoli et al. 1987), also detected a relative hyporesponsiveness of the airways of refractory subjects relative to non-refractory subjects as assessed by methacholine challenge. However, previous work by Hahn et al demonstrated no alteration in histamine responsiveness following exercise in 8 refractory subjects (Hahn et al. 1984). Non refractory subjects were not considered. More recently Smith et al studied the methacholine response following UNDW, and hypertonic saline challenge in 14 asthmatic subjects. After UNDW there was a significant increase in methacholine sensitivity, but not after hypertonic saline challenge. However in this study, the refractory index of the subjects was not known. We have recently completed a study comparing the methacholine responsiveness at baseline and following hypertonic challenge in both refractory and non refractory subjects. There was a positive correlation ($r = 0.69$, $p = 0.017$) between refractory index (PD_{35} of 2nd hypertonic challenge ÷ PD_{35} of 1st hypertonic challenge) and the change in airway responsiveness to methacholine after the initial provocation.

LEUKOCYTE ACTIVATION.

Chemotactic factors have the capacity to activate inflammatory leukocytes. Since NCF is released into the circulation following EIA and hyperosmolar challenge, we have attempted to document evidence of leukocyte activation in peripheral blood leukocytes. This is not to suggest that leukocyte activation in EIA is due only to NCF, since the possibility exists that other chemotactic mediators for which we have no assay are also produced following exercise in asthmatic subjects. Studies on leukocyte activation have addressed the expression of membrane receptors (Papageorgiou et al. 1983), the generation of inflammatory mediators(Arm et al. 1987) and the capacity of cells to kill schistosomula (Moqbel et al. 1986).

Previous work has demonstrated an increase in the expression of neutrophil and monocyte complement receptors as assessed by the rosetting technique following EIA (Papageorgiou et al. 1983). These changes were preceded by an increase in serum NCF and inhibited by the prior administration of DSCG. Recent in vitro work however has suggested that the results obtained using the rosetting technique are discordant with those using more specific techniques for enumerating membrane receptors (Richerson et al. 1985). We have therefore studied the expression of complement receptors type 1 (CR1) and type 3 (CR3) using monoclonal antibodies with specificity for the receptors and flow cytometry (Lee et al. 1987). There was a maximal 34 ± 8% (Mean ± SEM, n=6) increase in granulocyte CR1 at 60 minutes following EIA (Walport et al.1987). There was no increase in granulocyte CR3 up to 6 hours following challenge. These changes were smaller than those previously observed using the rosetting techniques, and were small in comparison to the maximal 350 % and 450 % increases in granulocyte CR1 and CR3, respectively, elicited by 10^{-7} M formyl methionyl leucyl phenylalanine observed in the same study.

Moqbel et al. have used a functional test for assessing leucocyte activation (Moqbel et al. 1986). They measured the in vitro killing of schistosomula of Schistosoma mansoni and demonstrated that there was a significant increase in neutrophil and monocyte cytotoxicity up to 60 minutes following EIA . The increase in cytotoxicity was preceded by elevations in NCF and there was a significant correlation between the post-exercise reduction in FEV1 and increases in neutrophil cytotoxicity.

Following EIA peripheral blood neutrophils demonstrate an up-regulation of the 5-lipoxygenase pathway as indicated by a markedly enhanced capacity to generate Leukotriene B4 (LTB4), a potent pro-inflammatory mediator (Arm et al. 1987). In 10 asthmatic subjects PMN isolated at 3-6 hours after EIA and stimulated *in vitro* by $2x10^8$ and $4x10^8$ zymosan particles/$2x10^6$ PMN demonstrated a 12 and 4 fold enhancement, respectively, in the production of immunoreactive LTB4 as compared to PMN isolated before exercise. Enhanced generation of LTB4 was also observed in response to PMN stimulated with calcium ionophore under optimal conditions, and was accompanied by enhanced generation of 5 HETE and 6-*trans*-LTB4 diastereoisomers indicating up- regulation of the whole 5-lipoxygenase pathway. Enhanced generation of LTB4 was not demonstrated in PMN isolated from asthmatic individuals who did not develop EIA, or following methacholine challenge. This indicates that these changes were not due to exercise *per se* or to the non-specific effects of bronchoconstriction. This increase in the pro-inflammatory potential occurred independently of the late asthmatic response, indicating that PMN activation alone is not adequate to induce the late phase reaction and that other mechanisms must also be contributing to airways inflammation.

CONCLUSION

There is increasing evidence that the initiating stimulus for EIA is a transient hyperosmolarity of the airways epithelium caused by the respiratory water loss consequent upon the hyperventilation of exercise. We have demonstrated that both hyperosmolar challenge to the airways and EIA are associated with the release of NCF, a high molecular weight chemotactic peptide. Exercise, but not hypertonic challenge to the airways, releases histamine (Table 1). This would be consistent with the hypothesis that post-exertional histaminaemia is due to the associated basophilia. The release of mediators following hyperosmolar challenge may be related to the effect of hyperosmolarity on mediator containing cells in the airways, a stimulus which is known to cause mast cell activation.

There is no evidence at present to support the hypothesis that the refractory period may be due to either mediator depletion or to protection of the airways by catecholamine release. In contrast there appears to be a correlation between changes in smooth muscle responsiveness and the extent of the refractory period.

Mediators released into the airways following the initiating event in EIA may have direct effects on airway smooth muscle, mucous secreting glands, and blood vessels. In addition, there may be direct effects on circulating leukocytes. These effects include an increase in the expression of CR1 but not CR3, a substantial augmentation of the capacity of circulating neutrophils to generate LTB4 and the increased function of these leukocytes as assessed by their capacity to kill schistosomula in vitro. Nevertheless, despite clear enhancement in the pro-inflammatory potential of the neutrophil following EIA, this is not neccessarily associated with the development of a late phase asthmatic response. Thus other mechanisms must be contributing to the development of airways inflammation.

Table 1. The presence of a refractory period (REF), and the release of NCF, histamine catecholamines (CAT) and leukocyte activation (LA) following challenge with ultrasonically nebulised hypertonic saline (HS), or distilled water (UNDW), antigen (AG), exercise (EX), methacholine (METH), and histamine (HIST).

	REF	CAT	NCF	HIST	LA
HS	+	-	+	±	?
UNDW	+	?	+	±	?
AG	-	-	+	+	+
EX	+	+	+	+	+
METH	-	-	-	-	-
HIST	±	-	-	N/A	-

REFERENCES

Anderson SD, Bye PTP, Schoeffel RE, Seale JP, Taylor KM, Ferris L (1981). Arterial plasma histamine levels at rest, during and after exercise in patients with asthma; effects of Terbutaline aerosol. Thorax 36: 259-267.

Anderson SD (1984). Is there a unifying hypothesis for exercise-induced asthma? J Allergy Clin Immonol 73: 660-665.

Arm JP, Horton CE, Lee TH (1987). Enhanced leukotriene B_4 generation by circulating neutrophils following exercise induced asthma. J Allergy Clin Immunol 79: 129 (Abstract).

Belcher NG, Murdoch R, Dalton N, Rees PJ, Clark TJH, Lee TH (1988). Circulating concentrations of histamine neutrophil chemotactic activity and catecholamines during the refractory period in exercise induced asthma. J Allergy Clin Immunol (in press).

Belcher NG, Rees PJ, Clark TJ, Lee TH (1987a). A comparison of the refractory periods induced by hypertonic airway challenge and exercise in bronchial asthma. Am Rev Respir Dis 135: 822-825.

Belcher NG, Murdoch R, Clark TJH, Rees PJ, Lee TH (1987b). Serum neutrophil chemotactic activity and plasma histamine concentrations in asthma induced by hypertonic saline and exercise. J Allergy Clin Immunol 79: 128, (abstract).

Eggleston PA, Kagey-Sobotka A, Lichtenstein LM (1987) A comparison of the osmotic activation of basophils and human lung mast cells. Am Rev Resp Dis 135: 1043-1048.

Howarth PH, Pao G J-K, Church MK, Holgate ST (1984). Exercise and isocapnic hyperventilation-induced bronchoconstriction in asthma: relevance of circulating basophils to measurement of plasma histamine. J Allergy Clin Immunol 73: 391-399.

Lee TH, Nagy L, Nagakura T, Walport MJ, Kay AB (1982a). Identification and partial characterization of an exercise-induced neutrophil chamotactic factor in bronchial asthma. J Clin Invest 69: 889-899

Lee TH, Brown MJ, Nagy L, Causon R, Walport MJ, Kay AB (1982b). Exercise-induced release of histamine and neutrophil chemotactic factor in atopic asthmatics. J Allergy Clin Immunol 70: 73-81.

Lee TH, Assoufi BK, Kay AB (1983a). The link between exercise, respiratory heat exchange, and the mast cell in bronchial asthma. Lancet i: 520-522

Lee TH, Assoufi BK, Cromwell O, Kay AB (1983b). Exercise-induced asthma and the mast cell. Lancet 2: 164-165.

Lee TH, Nagakura T, Cromwell O, Brown MJ, Causon R, Kay AB (1984). Neutrophil chemotactic activity and histamine in atopic and non-atopic subjects after exercise-induced asthma. Am Rev Respir Dis 129: 409-412.

Lee TH, Sethi T, Crea AE, Peters W, Arm JP, Horton CE, Walport MJ, Spur BW. Characterization of leukotriene B3. Comparison of its biological activities with leukotriene B4 and leukotriene

B5 in complement receptor enhancement, lysozyme release and chemotaxis of human neutrophils. Clin. Sci (in press).
Hahn AG, Nogrady SG, Tumilty DM, Lawrence SR, Morton AR (1984). Histamine reactivity during the refractory period after exercise induced asthma. Thorax 39: 919-923.
Magnussen H, Reuss G, Jorres R (1986). Airway response to methacholine during exercise induced refractoriness in asthma. Thorax 41: 667-70.
Mattoli S, Forest A, Corbo GM, Valente S, Culla G, Toscano L, Bevignani G, Porcarelli MG, Patalano F, Ciappi G (1987). Refractory period to ultrasonic mist of distilled water: relationship to methacholine responsiveness, atopic status and clinical characteristics. Ann Allergy 58: 134-140.
Moqbel R, Durham SR, Shaw RJ, Walsh GM, MacDonald AJ, Mackay JA, Carroll MP, Kay AB (1986). Enhancement of leukocyte cytotoxicity after exercise induced asthma. Am Rev Respir Dis 133: 609-613.
Nagakura T, Lee TH, Assoufi BK, Denison DM, Newman-Taylor AJ, Kay AB (1983). Neutrophil chemotactic factor in exercise and hyperventilation induced asthma. Am Rev Resp Dis 128: 294-296.
O'Byrne P, Jones G (1986). Effect of Indomethacin on exercise-induced bronchoconstriction and refractoriness after exercise. Am Rev Respir Dis 134: 69-72.
Papageorgiou N, Carroll M, Durham SR, Lee TH, Walsh GM, Kay AB (1983). Complement receptor enhancement as evidence of neutrophil activation following exercise-induced asthma. Lancet 2: 1220-1222.
Richerson HB, Walsh GM, Walport MJ, Moqbel R, Kay AB (1985). Enhancement of neutrophil complement receptors: a comparison of the Rosette technique with the uptake of radio labelled and CR1 monoclonal antibodies. Clin Exp Immunol 62: 442-448.
Smith CM, Anderson SD, Black JL (1987). Methacholine responsiveness increases after ultrasonically nebulised water but not after ultrasonically nebulised hypertonic saline in

patients with asthma. J Allergy Clin Immunol 79: 85-92.
Walport MJ, Arm JP, Sethi TJ, Lee TH (1987). Neutrophil (PMN) complement receptor enhancement in experimentally provoked asthma. J Allergy Clin Immunol 79: 258 (abstract).

Discussion on Paper by Tak Lee

Fuller: We had the opportunity to study LTB_4 release from ionophore challenge of whole blood in patients who had allergen challenges with late reactions. We were unable to see any changes in releasibility through 1, 4, and 24 hours after the allergen challenge. I just wonder whether there might be more differences between antigen and exercise rather than just the expression of complement receptors.

Lee: Well that is certainly possible. We've also just completed a study on antigen challenge. We did find a small enhancement in LTB_4 generation by the neutrophils stimulated by zymosan, but this was much less marked than after exercise. Furthermore, the effect was apparent only with zymosan, but not with calcium ionophore activation. It seems likely that the 5-lipoxygenase pathway is already maximally stimulated by the ionophore and any further small enhancement is masked. In fact, even with EIA, the enhancement of LTB_4 generation by neutrophils stimulated with zymosan was greater than that seen when the cells were activated by ionophore.

Nadel: Whatever else it means you have something that activated neutrophils in the blood. I'm more interested in the mechanism that the activation. Is it a plasma transferable phenomena?

Lee: I can't answer that at the moment. The interesting thing is that the extent of leukocyte activation correlates with the acute bronchospastic response suggesting that the two events are related. The kinetics of enhancement are very intriguing because it takes 3 to 6 hours before the augmentation is statistically significant. I can only presume that other signals, quite possibly intracellular, are needed to transduce the priming signal during this time.

Seale: Recognising the fact that there are a range of medications that we can use to block exercise-induced asthma, have you looked at any of those in terms of whether or not they are working at the level of impairing this activation of neutrophils by zymosan?

Lee: Yes we are studying that right now. The first drug we are studying is Nedocromil in a double blind manner.

Seale: Beta-agonists?

Lee: We will be studying these in the future.

Woolcock: You mentioned that there was no correlation between the activation of neutrophils and late-reactions but did you actually have any late-reactions and did you look for them carefully?

Lee: We had three people who had a biphasic fall in SGaw. However we did not have a control day so I do not know if the late decrease in SGaw would have occurred on the control day as well. There was no correlation between the enhancement in LTB_4 generation in these individuals with their lung function at 3 and 6 hours.

Benveniste: Tak, I thought that the receptor for the C_3 converting particle was not present on the PMN. We cannot activate the PMN by zymosan at all. So there are 2 questions, first, why did you use opsonised zymosan and second, can you find any anomolous behaviour of the whole factor or are you planning to study the monocytes too.

Lee: We are also studying monocytes, but the data is preliminary. There are a number of studies which have demonstrated the presence of CR_3. The reason we didn't used opsonised zymosan is that with opsonised zymosan there is also involvement of other receptors such as CR_1 and the IgG-Fc receptors. I wanted to use a probe which only works through one receptor.

Mechanisms in Asthma: Pharmacology,
Physiology, and Management, pages 355–363

MEDIATOR RELEASE AFTER LOCAL OSMOLAR CHALLENGE TO THE AIRWAYS

William L. Eschenbacher and Thomas R. Gravelyn

Department of Internal Medicine/Pulmonary
University of Michigan Medical Center, Ann Arbor, Michigan, 48109

INTRODUCTION

Alterations in the osmolarity of the fluid lining the airways may occur during inhalation of aerosols (distilled water or hypertonic solutions), exercise, or hyperventilation (respiratory water loss leading to hyperosmolarity). Changes in osmolarity could in turn lead to mediator release from cells present in the airway. Hyperosmolar stimulation of mast cells from human lung fragments (Eggleston, 1984; Eggleston, 1987) and from bronchoalveolar lavage (Flint, 1985a) results in histamine release *in vitro*. We hypothesized that osmolar challenge (hyperosmolar and hypo-osmolar) *in vivo* would result in histamine release and that there would be differences between subjects with and without asthma.

METHODS

We have developed a technique for isolated airway segment lavage (IASL) that allows the introduction into and withdrawal of fluids from into a segment of airway in human subjects (Eschenbacher, 1987). With this technique we can challenge the airway segment *in vivo* with different agents (e.g., osmolar stimuli) and analyze the recovered lavage fluid from the same segment before and after challenge for changes in mediator concentrations.

The IASL was performed using a specially modified pulmonary artery catheter with two balloons at the distal end which are separated by 2 cm. Within the interballoon segment, there are openings into separate channels for the infusion and withdrawal of fluids. During our challenge protocol, the catheter was inserted through the nose and positioned in the left mainstem bronchus using a fiber-optic bronchoscope for visual guidance. The balloons of the catheter were inflated creating the isolated airway segment. Two milliliter aliquots of fluid were then introduced into the airway segment and withdrawn immediately. The lavage fluid was then centrifuged and the supernatant frozen for subsequent mediator analyses.

The histamine assay, similar to the technique described previously (Dyer, 1982), used a modified isotopic-enzymatic procedure. Prostaglandin, thromboxane, and leukotriene concentrations were determined by radioimmunoassay as performed by the Ligand Core Laboratory at the University of Michigan.

Thirty-two non-smoking volunteer subjects between the ages of 18 and 34 were challenged. Eighteen subjects (six atopic asthmatics, six atopic non-asthmatics, and six non-atopic, non-asthmatic controls) were given a hyperosmolar salt solution (900 milliosmolar sodium chloride) as the challenge stimulus and fourteen subjects (six atopic asthmatic, four atopic non-asthmatics, and four non-atopic, non-asthmatic controls) were given distilled water as the hypo-osmolar challenge stimulus. Each subject was premedicated with 1 mg of atropine sulfate IM followed by routine nasal, pharyngeal, laryngeal and upper airway anesthesia with 2% and 4% lidocaine. Measurements of specific airway resistance (SRaw) using a body plethysmograph were made before medication, after medication and after the procedure with the catheter. The procedure itself began with the introduction of a fiberoptic bronchoscope through one nares and into a subsegment of the right middle lobe for conventional bronchoalveolar lavage (BAL). This was followed by the placement of the catheter in the left mainstem bronchus and inflation of catheter balloons to create the isolated airway segment. Isotonic saline was first used for IASL to obtain baseline values of mediator concentrations (IASL-NS1). A total of 5-7 2 ml lavages were used. The challenge osmolar solution was then introduced into the airway segment in a similar fashion (5-7 2 ml aliquot lavages: IASL-DW [distilled water] or IASL-HT [hypertonic saline]). Finally, a third series of lavages were performed again with isotonic saline to obtain the mediator concentrations after the challenge stimulus (IASL-NS2). Each IASL series took 4-6 minutes to complete.

RESULTS

All thirty-two subjects completed the entire procedure without difficulty. The measurements of SRaw for each subject group are shown in Table 1.

Table 1. Changes in Specific Airway Resistance (L x cmH_2O/L/s) during the Protocol*

Subject Group	Baseline	After Medication	After Procedure
Atopic Asthmatics	7.1±4.2	4.1±2.5	6.2±3.0
Atopic Non-asthmatics	4.8±1.5	2.9±1.2	3.4±1.4
Non-atopic Non-asthmatics	4.4±1.4	3.1±1.1	3.2±1.3

* Values are mean ± SD

No subject with asthma had greater than a 50% increase in SRaw when the initial baseline measurement was comprared with the value after the procedure.

The concentrations of histamine in the supernatants from the different lavage samples for each subject group are shown in Table 2.

Table 2. Histamine Concentrations (pg/ml) in the Lavage Samples*

	BAL	IASL-NS1	IASL-NS2 ($\bar{p}$ DW)†	IASL-NS2 ($\bar{p}$ HT)†
Atopic Asthmatics	761±224 (n=12)	568±192+ (n=12)	1892±783+ (n=6)	1037±237+ (n=6)
Atopic Non-asthmatics	44±43 (n=10)	165±75 (n=10)	554±250 (n=4)	156±80 (n=6)
Non-atopic Non-asthmatics	7±7 (n=10)	41±23 (n=10)	173±173 (n=4)	63±31 (n=6)

* Values are mean ± SEM
† $\bar{p}$ DW = after the distilled water challenge and $\bar{p}$ HT = after the hypertonic salt solution challenge.
+ Difference between IASL-NS2 and IASL-NS1 is significant ($p < 0.05$).

The histamine concentrations of the baseline lavages (BAL and IASL-NS1) for the subjects with asthma were significantly greater than the respective concentrations for either the atopic, non-asthmatic subjects or the non-atopic, non-asthmatic controls ($p < 0.05$). There was a trend in all three subject groups for increases in histamine concentrations after either osmolar challenge; however, only the subjects with asthma had a significant increase in histamine concentration after both the distilled water and the hypertonic salt solution challenge ($p < 0.05$).

Of the products of arachidonic acid metabolism, PGD_2 was significantly increased after both the hypo-osmolar and the hyperosmolar challenges only in the subjects with asthma. $PGF_2\alpha$ was also significantly increased in the subjects with asthma after the hyperosmolar challenge.

DISCUSSION

We have been able to successfully challenge an isolated segment of airway in subjects with and without asthma and to recover lavage fluid from this airway segment before and after the introduction of an osmolar stimulus. We have found that the histamine concentrations of the airways at baseline before challenge was significantly greater in the subjects with asthma when compared to the other two subject groups. We have also found that histamine and PGD_2 were significantly increased in the airway lavage fluid after both types of osmolar challenge (distilled water and hypertonic salt solution) although there was a trend towards increases in histamine concentrations in the other two subject groups.

It is perhaps not surprising that we found an increase in baseline histamine concentrations in the subjects with asthma. Some authors have shown that there are increased number of mast cells in the airways of patients with asthma (Tomioka, 1984, Flint, 1985b) and that these mast cells from asthmatics may have greater releasability of histamine (Flint, 1986).

We did find a significant increase in histamine concentration in the airway lavage fluid in the subjects with asthma after the two osmolar challenges. This would suggest that mast cells are being stimulated by the local challenge. Also finding that PGD_2 was increased in the lavage fluids after challenge lends further support that airway mast cells are being stimulated (Peters, 1984). The mechanism of distilled water stimulated release mast cell histamine is unknown but a component of the release may have been due to cytolysis (Kaliner, 1974). Hyperosmolar stimulated release of histamine from lung mast cells is also unknown but it is felt to be a non-cytolytic process (Eggleston, 1984; Eggleston, 1987). It is possible we could have found even a greater increase in histamine in the lavage fluid after the hyperosmolar challenge had we used a solute that was not as permeable as sodium chloride; e.g., sucrose or mannitol (Eggleston, 1987).

These results provide further evidence for the hypothesis that changes in the osmolarity of the fluid lining the airways can result in mediator release (mast cells being one source) and that the mediators can in turn lead to the acute bronchoconstriction that occurs in exercise-induced bronchoconstriction or as the response to inhalation challenges with aerosols of hypo- and hyperosmolar solutions.

Further studies to evaluate the local release of mediators to different stimuli will include the measurement of changes in the local airway diameter while the challenge stimulus is introduced into the isolated airway segment. In this way a physiological counterpart to the mediator release can be measured. In studies now underway, we are using antigen as the challenge stimulus and specific blocking agents of mediator release or production.

REFERENCES

Dyer J, Warren K, Merlin S, Metcalfe DD, Kaliner M (1982). Measurement of plasma histamine: description of an improved method and normal values. J Allergy Clin Immunol 70:82-87.

Eggleston PA, Kagey-Sobotka A, Schleimer RP, Lichtenstein LM (1984). Interaction between hyperosmolar and IgE-mediated histamine release from basophils and mast cells. Am Rev Respir Dis 130:86-91.

Eggleston PA, Kagey-Sobotka A, Lichtenstein LM (1987). A comparison of the osomotic activation of basophils and human lung mast cells. Am Rev Respir Dis 135:1043-1048.

Eschenbacher WL, Gravelyn TR (1987). A technique for isolated airway segment lavage. Chest 92:105-109.

Flint KC, Hudspith BN, Leung KBP, Pearce FL, Johnson NMcI (1985a). The hyperosmolar release of histamine from bronchoalveolar mast cells and its inhibition by sodium cromoglycate. Thorax 40:717.

Flint KC, Leung KBP, Hudspith BN, Pearce FL, Brostoff J, Johnson NMcI (1985b). Bronchoalveolar mast cells in extrinsic asthma. A mechanism for the initiation of antigen specific bronchoconstriction. Br Med J 291:923-927.

Flint KC, Leung KBP, Hudspith BN, Pearce FL, Brostoff J, Johnson NMcI (1986). The function and properties of human lung mast cells. Respiration 50:Suppl 2:31-41.

Kaliner M, Austen KF (1974). Cyclic AMP, ATP, and reversed anaphylactic histamine release from rat mast cells. J Immunol 112:664-674.

Peters SP, MacGlashan DW, Schulman ES, Schleimer RP, Hayes EC, Rokach J, Adkinson NF, Lichtenstein LM (1984). Arachidonic acid metabolism in purified human lung mast

cells. J Immunol 132:1972-1979.
Tomioka M, Ida S, Shindok Y, Ishihara T, Takishima T (1984). Mast cells in bronchoalveolar lumen of patients with bronchial asthma. Am Rev Respir Dis 129:1000-1005.

Discussion on Paper by William Eschenbacher

Fuller: Sandy Anderson showed on her slides only small increases in omsolarity up to 370 millisomoles. How do you think that the osmolarity changes during evaporative water loss compare with your study when you added 900 milliosomole saline?

Anderson: Those values were obtained at rest in laryngectomy patients, not during exercise at high ventilation. The 900 milliosmoles would be very similar to the osmolarity we achieve by giving 4.5% saline, which has an osmolarity of 1500 milliosmoles.

Eschenbacher: We don't know what is going on locally in the airway in terms of changes in osmolarity. We picked that osmolarity based on the *in vitro* work with mast cells. That seemed to be the optimal osmolarity for mast cell release of histamine.

Pare: I just wondered if you could comment on why you don't get mediator release in normal subjects. As far as I know, it has been shown that osmolar effects occur with mast cells and basophils from normal subjects as well as from asthmatic subjects. Is there any difference in osmolar releasibility of mediators between normals and asthmatics, or are your results simply based on the fact that you have more mast cells in the lavage of asthmatic subjects? Finally, did you count the mast cells in the lavage fluid?

Eschenbacher: The answer to the last part - no we didn't, we tried to but they are in very low concentration in most instances, being less than 0.1%. I think that what you suggested is true, that it just has to do with the number of mast cells. People with asthma have been shown to have more mast cells and therefore it is likely they will have more change in the concentration of mediators measured during isolated airway segment lavage.

Smith: There has been some debate as to the relative importance of heat exchange and water flux with exercise-induced asthma. Do you think you could use this technique by changing the temperature of the lavage fluid to look at the importance of temperature in mediator release?

Eschenbacher: That's something that we could look at directly. If we gave very cold saline we would need to know the actual temperature at the point we delivered it which means we have to have some elaborate temperature measuring device.

Anderson: A Yellow Springs Thermistor probe No 500 would easily fit into your catheter.

Benveniste: Not being a lung physiologist I have some difficulty in intepreting all studies dealing with the presence of prostaglandin in the lung. In my lab, Charles Brink has shown that by stimulating lung tissue from guinea pig or man with various agonists you can get similar release of prostaglandins. It is also very easy to show that these prostaglandins have profound regulatory influences on the guinea pig tissue, both positive and negative, whereas they have absolutely no influence whatsoever in man, even when human tissue is contracted or relaxed. In your opinion what is the exact role that we can ascribe to these mediators when we have difficulty showing that both their presence or their blockade doesn't affect the function of the lung.

Eschenbacher: Yes, just by showing the presence, it still doesn't tell us anything about mechanisms as to what is going on and provides only circumstantial evidence. Further studies will be done looking at physiologic correlates. We will try to make measurements of changes in airway diameter and then by using more specific blocking agents be able to see if that makes any difference in terms of the physiologic counterpart. I agree with you that just finding it doesn't tell us what is going on.

Walters: I can't resist the temptation of responding to Dr. Benveniste's statement. It seems quite an absurd thing to say. If normals or asthmatics inhale things like PGD_2 or PGE_2 you have a very dramatic effect on the airways. If you give people aspirin or indomethacin, particularly in some asthmatics you get a very dramatic effect. Now it happens that some of those effects are very negative but you certainly have effects and in some asthmatics actually good effects.

Nadel: You have a beautiful study. I wouldn't be modest about it. I think if you see a pattern of PGD_2 and histamine release, until proven otherwise, it says that you have activated mast cells. Do you believe that?

Eschenbacher: Yes I do.

Nadel: There may be a whole bunch of other cascades involved in mast cells but that in itself is interesting and whether there are more mast cells or they more releasible is something that is testable. Elliott Phillipson had a neat preparation where he could look at the bronchomotor tone of dogs using the pressure in the balloon. Have you taken a crack at that yet?

Eschenbacher: Yes, I've tried that already, both in animals and intubated patients. I have been able to see changes in animals as a result of the introduction of methacholine so I will be able to look at that in subsequent studies.

Stephens: It seems to me that this might provide an opportunity to look at epithelial-derived relaxing factor. If you did it in the dog you could do it before and after destruction. Just recently somebody has described an <u>in vivo</u> method of interfering with the function of the endothelial cells showing that there are changes in the responsiveness and then later on taking out the segment and looking at the <u>in vitro</u> responsiveness.

Eschenbacher: The setup does provide a lot of possibilities for looking at other things too so that would be possible.

Pharmacological Treatment of Asthma

Mechanisms in Asthma: Pharmacology,
Physiology, and Management, pages 367–377

WHITHER β-ADRENOCEPTOR AGONISTS IN THE TREATMENT OF ASTHMA

J. Paul Seale

Department of Pharmacology, University of Sydney and Department of Thoracic Medicine, Royal Prince Alfred Hospital, Camperdown 2050.

INTRODUCTION

Adrenergic agonists have maintained a pre-eminent position in the management of asthma for more than 80 years. Adrenaline, given subcutaneously, was first described as effective treatment for bronchospasm in 1903 (Bullowa & Kaplan, 1903). Thereafter, it remained standard therapy for acute asthma until the advent of isoprenaline in 1940 (Konzett, 1940). This development of a β-adrenoceptor agonist, which was devoid of α stimulatory activity, represented a major advance in the evolving story of adrenergic bronchodilators. However, its short duration of action (1-2 hours) and its non-selective action on both β_1 and β_2 receptors were considered disadvantages in some clinical situations.

Modifications to the catechol ring structure rendered compounds with longer durations of action because they were no longer substrates for catechol-o-methyltransferase. One approach was the placement of hydroxyl groups on the 3 and 5 carbon atoms to form compounds called resorcinols (Engelhardt et al., 1961). Orciprenaline was the first resorcinol to gain wide clinical usage and others were terbutaline and fenoterol. Another approach was the substitution of a methyl alcohol for the hydroxyl group on the 3 carbon atom yielding compounds (such as salbutamol) which were also resistant to catechol-o-methyltransferase (Brittain et al., 1968). Increased specificity for β_2-adrenoceptors has been achieved by addition to the terminal nitrogen of tertiary butyl groups (e.g. salbutamol, terbutaline) or cyclically substituted isopropyl groups (e.g. fenoterol).

Thus, 40 years of research, concentrated on modifications to the basic phenylethylamine structure of catecholamines has resulted in a family of drugs, called the β_2-adrenoceptor agonists which constitute the most effective bronchodilators currently available for the treatment of asthma and other causes of airflow limitation.

PHARMACOLOGY

The β-adrenoceptor agonists have various pharmacological actions which may contribute to their beneficial effects in the treatment of asthma.

i) Airway smooth muscle

In vitro experiments with isolated preparations of human bronchus indicate that β-agonists have potent relaxant effects on human airway smooth muscle. EC_{50} values for fenoterol approximate 8 nM (Goldie et al., 1984). Based on the rapid time course of bronchodilation following inhalation of agonists it is probable that these agents also relax airway smooth muscle in vivo. By using selective receptor antagonists in vitro it has been possible to demonstrate that β_2-adrenoceptors mediate the relaxation in human bronchial preparations (Goldie et al., 1984).

ii) Mediator release

The release of slow-reacting substance of anaphylaxis, now known to comprise a mixture of leukotrene C_4, D_4 and E_4 (Lewis et al., 1981) and histamine from human lung tissue in vitro is inhibited by β-adrenoceptor agonists(Orange et al., 1971). This inhibitory effect on mediator release is also mediated via β_2-adrenoceptors (Butchers et al., 1980; Hughes et al, 1983). Furthermore, the EC_{50} for fenoterol (6 nM, Hughes et al., 1983) for the inhibition of leukotriene release is similar to the EC_{50} for relaxation of human bronchus in vitro (Goldie et al., 1984). Thus, it is possible that the doses of β-adrenoceptor agonists which produce bronchodilation in patients are adequate for inhibition of histamine and leukotriene release. Moreover, inhalation of nebulized terbutaline abolished the rise of arterial plasma histamine associated with exercise-induced asthma (Anderson et al., 1981) and inhaled salbutamol inhibited the rise in plasma histamine and neutrophil chemotactic factor induced by allergen challenge (Howarth et al., 1985). Since mast cells are the only source of histamine in the lung, these results show that β-adrenoceptor agonists inhibit immunologically-induced release of histamine and leukotrienes from lung mast cells. However, the extent to which this inhibitory effect contributes to the clinical efficacy of β-adrenoceptor agonists is unknown.

Alveolar macrophages (AM) are potential effector cells in allergic lung disease since they possess immunoglobulin E (IgE) receptors (Joseph et al., 1980) and they release thromboxane B_2 following immunological stimulation (Fuller et al., 1986). Whilst the phagocytic function of guinea-pig AM can be suppressed by β-adrenoceptor agonists (Henricks et al., 1986) via a non-receptor mechanism (see Discussion), the release of glucosaminidase and thromboxane B_2 from human AM, stimulated by opsonised zymosan or anti-IgE, was not affected by isoprenaline (Fuller et al., 1987). These findings show that if AM do possess β-adrenoceptors they do not modulate immunological or zymosan-induced activation.

iii) Mucociliary function

The normal clearance of inhaled particles and cellular debris from the respiratory tract requires the co-ordinated beating of adequate numbers of cilia, which interact with viscid mucus overlying a periciliary fluid layer of low viscosity (Editorial, 1982). Measuring the transit time of inhaled markers provides the current basis for assessing mucociliary function. However, such techniques cannot distinguish between the various components of clearance. Despite the relative crudity of these measures it has been possible to demonstrate β-adrenergic stimulation of tracheal mucus velocity in normal subjects (Camner et al., 1976) and in patients with a variety of lung diseases (Editorial, 1982), although other studies have not supported these findings (Santa Cruz et al., 1974). <u>In vitro</u> studies with respiratory epithelium have indicated that β-adrenoceptor agonists stimulate cilial beat frequency (Van As, 1974) but their effects on the physicochemical properties of mucus have not been investigated fully. The clinical significance of these effects are questionable because terbutaline, given by the most common route of adminstration (i.e. metered dose aerosol) in a large dose of 1mg which produced adequate bronchodilation, did not enhance mucociliary clearance in patients with mild asthma (Bateman et al., 1983).

iv) Microvascular permeability

When guinea-pigs inhale low concentrations of histamine aerosol there is an increase in lung weight which has been attributed to microvascular leakage of protein and fluid. This effect of histamine is inhibited by pretreatment with isoprenaline and terbutaline (Persson et al., 1979). In addition, β-adrenoceptor agonists were found to suppress the microvascular permeability effects of local chemical mediators released by antigen challenge of air pouches in rats (Ohuchi et al., 1987). More direct studies in experimental animals have shown that β-adrenoceptor agonists inhibit postcapillary venular leakage induced by certain stimuli (see Persson et al., 1985). The relevance of these findings to the clinical efficacy of these drugs in patients with asthma requires further investigation.

v) Inhibition of phospholipase A_2

Pretreatment of rats with fenoterol inhibited phospholipase A_2 activity, which was determined in lung microsomal enzyme preparations in vitro (Wichert & Meyer, 1983). In guinea-pig isolated perfused lungs, histamine and leukotrienes activate arachidonic acid metabolism resulting in the release of cyclo-oxygenase products, predominantly thromboxane A_2 (Blackwell et al., 1978). Using double-isotope assays, Blackwell et al.(1978) demonstrated that histamine activates phospholipase A_2, liberating arachidonic acid from endogenous lipid pools. β-adrenoceptor agonists inhibit the histamine-induced release of thromboxane A_2 from guinea-pig lungs and this effect is antagonised by propranolol (Compton et al., 1985). Since this inhibition occurs without affecting the conversion of exogenous arachidonic acid to thromboxane A_2 it suggests that the β-adrenoceptor agonists directly inhibit phospholipase A_2. From these experiments in perfused lungs, it is not possible to determine in which cell types the phospholipase A_2 is susceptible to inhibition by β-adrenoceptor agonists.

Further studies are necessary to investigate the relevance of this finding to human asthma.

TACHYPHYLAXIS

There are theoretical grounds for suspecting diminished responsiveness (or tachyphylaxis) in patients using β-adrenoceptor agonists regularly because extensive studies of intact cells from a variety of tissues have shown that the β-adrenoceptor adenyl cyclase-linked system is susceptible to agonist-induced desensitisation (Harden et al., 1983). This phenomenon of tachyphylaxis can be demonstrated quite easily in human airway smooth muscle <u>in vitro</u> (Davis & Conolly, 1980). In contrast, attempts to demonstrate down-regulation of the inhibitory effects of β-adrenoceptor agonists on mediator release from human lung fragments have not been successful. Based on the data of Orange et al (1971) that pre-incubation with noradrenaline and propranolol enhanced antigen-induced histamine and leukotriene release from human lung, if prolonged agonist stimulation induced a change analogous to β-blockade then overnight incubation of lung fragments with isoprenaline, followed by acute noradrenaline (NA) before antigen challenge, should enhance mediator release. However this was not the case (see figure). Neither histamine release nor leukotriene release was greater in isoprenaline and NA treated lung fragments compared with NA alone (bottom panels of figure). In fact the overnight incubation with isoprenaline further reduced release of histamine and leukotrienes ($P < 0.007$ and $P < 0.004$ respectively compared with NA alone) indicating a protracted β receptor stimulation despite repeated washing of lung fragments after overnight incubation (see legend to figure).

In normal human subjects acute airway responses to salbutamol waned over a 4 week period in which regular inhalations of salbutamol were used (Holgate et al., 1977). However, it has been quite difficult to find any convincing evidence of tachyphylaxis with long-term usage of β-adrenoceptor agonists in the clinical setting of asthma. Patients taking oral terbutaline for 12 months retained their acute bronchodilator responsiveness to intravenous isoprenaline (Larsson et al., 1977) and aerosol salbutamol, taken in the recommended dose of 200 μg four times daily for

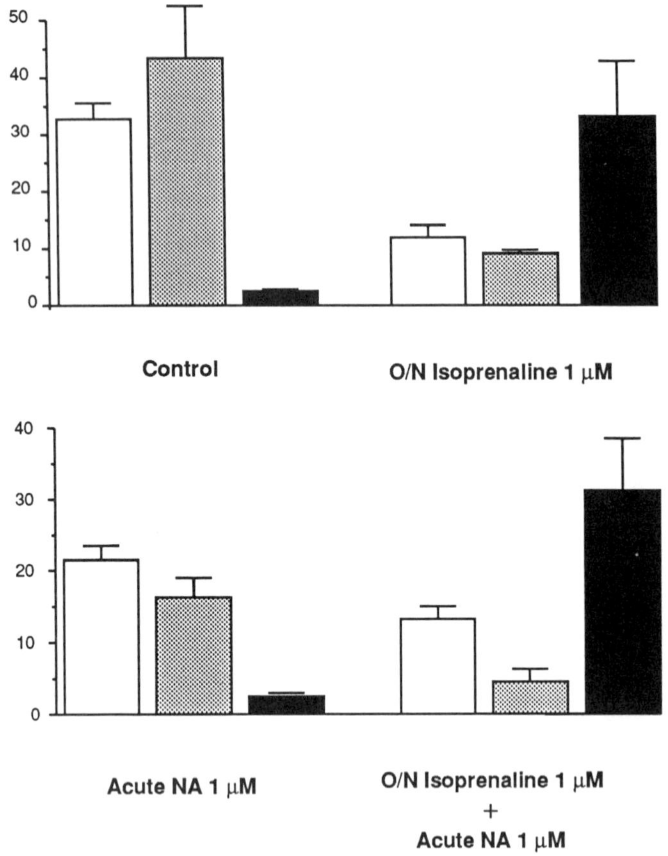

FIGURE 1

Human lung fragments were passively sensitized in serum with a high IgE titre and incubated overnight (O/N) in 0.9% Saline (Control) or isoprenaline for 20h. The next day lung fragments were washed thoroughly x 3 and noradrenaline (NA) or vehicle was added 10min before antigen challenge. Height of columns (±SE) show histamine % release (open), ng equivalents LTE_4 (stippled) and pmol/mg protein cyclic AMP (solid).

one month did not aggravate bronchial hyperreactivity as determined by histamine bronchoprovocation (Peel and Gibson, 1980). Even higher doses of metered dose aerosol (up to 500 μg four times daily) failed to diminish acute bronchodilator responsiveness to salbutamol over a 4 week period (Harvey & Tattersfield, 1982). On the other hand, some studies have found subsensitivity in patients who are withdrawn from all β -agonists for 3 months (Weber et al, 1982).

From all the studies which have addressed the question of tachyphylaxis the present evidence suggests that is this not a clinical problem (Tattersfield, 1985). The apparent resistance of asthmatic airways to desensitization may be a consequence of the basic receptor abnormality in asthma such that its structural or functional deficiency results in a conformational change which is no longer conducive to down-regulation. Further experiments will be necessary to investigate this intriguing possibility.

FUTURE DIRECTIONS

The currently used β-adrenoceptor agonists have predominant effects in the lung. This functional selectivity, which is the most relevant consideration for clinical acceptability, is the net result of drug characteristics (i.e. receptor affinity and efficacy), tissue characteristics (i.e. distribution of receptors and the nature of receptor-coupling to biological response) and the route of drug administration. The tissue characteristics cannot be altered but structural modification of drugs with respect to receptor selectivity has been the major basis of drug development to date. Another approach to functional selectivity is to synthesise effective bronchodilators which are inhaled into the lungs and rapidly inactivated in the systemic circulation (Albrecht et al., 1985).

More recent endeavours have been directed towards increasing the duration of drug action. A lipophylic carrier group, which binds to postulated exoreceptor sites, can be attached to β-adrenoceptor agonists via a spacer arm, leaving the active part of the molecule free to interact with β-receptors for prolonged periods.

The concept of a "prodrug", which requires metabolic

conversion before it becomes biologically active, has not been used yet for bronchodilators. However, such an approach offers great potential with respect to duration of action. Thus, bambuterol, which is sequentially metabolised to terbutaline, achieves therapeutic plasma concentrations for at least 24 hours (Nyberg, 1986).

Given the energy and time being devoted to exploring these new possibilities by research scientists it is likely that novel β-adrenoceptor agonist bronchodilators will emerge over the next decade.

REFERENCES

Albrecht R, Heindl J, Loge O (1985). β_2-agonists containing metabolically labile groups. II. The influence of ester groups in the aryl system. Eur J Med Chem -Chim Ther 20:57-60.

Anderson SD, Bye PTP, Schoeffel RE, Seale JP, Taylor KM, Ferris L (1981). Arterial plasma histamine levels at rest, and during and after exercise in patients with asthma: effects of terbutaline aerosol. Thorax 36:259-267.

Bateman JRM, Pavia D, Sheahan NF, Newman SP, Clarke, SW (1983). Effects of terbutaline sulphate aerosol on brochodilator response and lung mucociliary clearance in patients with mild stable asthma. Br J clin Pharmac 15:695-700.

Blackwell GJ, Flower RJ, Nijkamp FP, Vane JR (1978). Phospholipase A_2 activity of guinea-pig isolated perfused lungs: stimulation and inhibition by anti-inflammatory steroids. Br J Pharmac 62:79-89.

Brittain RT, Farmer JB, Jack DJ (1968). α-(t-butylamino)-methyl-4-hydroxy-m-xylene-α^1,α^3-diol (AH 3365): a selective β-adrenergic stimulant. Nature 219:862-863.

Bullowa JGM, Kaplan DM (1903). On the hypodermic use of adrenalin chloride in the treatment of asthma attacks. Med News 83:787-790.

Butchers PR, Fullarton JR, Skidmore IF, Vardey CJ, Wheeldon A (1980). Characterisation of the receptor mediating the anti-anaphylactic effects of adrenoceptor agonists in human lung _in vitro_. Br J Pharmac 71:663.

Camner P, Strandberg K, Philipson K (1976). Increased mucociliary transport by adrenergic stimulation. Arch Environ Health 39:79-82.

Compton MR, Seale JP, Shaw J (1985). A possible mechanism in the anti-anaphylactic effect of beta adrenoceptor agonists in guinea-pig lungs. Arch int Pharmacodyn 276:112-119.

Davis C, Conolly ME (1980). Tachyphylaxis to β-adrenoceptor agonists in human bronchial smooth muscle: studies in vitro. Br J Clin Pharmac 10:417-423.

Editorial (1982). Pulmonary mucociliary clearance. Lancet 1:203-204.

Engelhardt A, Hoefke W, Wick H (1961). Zum pharmacology des sympathomimeticums 1-(3,5-dihydroxy-phenyl)-1-hydroxy-2-150-propylaminoathan. Arzneimittelforsch 11:521-525.

Fuller RW, Kemeny DM, Holgate ST, MacDermot J, Morris PK, Sykes D (1986). IgE-dependent stimulation of human alveolar macrophages. Br J Pharmac 87:13P.

Fuller RW, O'Malley G, Baker AJ, MacDermot J (1987). β-adrenoceptor agonists do not inhibit human macrophage activation. Proceedings IUPHAR Congress P 1339.

Goldie RG, Paterson JW, Spina D, Wale JL (1984). Classification of β-adrenoceptors in human isolated bronchus. Br J Pharmac 81:611-615.

Harden TK (1983). Agonist-induced desensitization of the β-adrenergic receptor-linked adenylate cyclase. Pharmacol Rev 35:5-32.

Harvey JE, Tattersfield AE (1982). Airway response to salbutamol: effect of regular salbutamol inhalations in normal, atopic and asthmatic subjects. Thorax 37:280-287.

Henricks PAJ, Van Esch B, Nijkamp FP (1986). β-agonists can depress oxidative metabolism of alveolar macrophages. Agents Actions 19:353-354.

Holgate ST, Baldwin CJ, Tattersfield AE (1977). β-adrenergic agonist resistance in normal human airways. Lancet ii:375-377.

Hughes JM, Seale JP, Temple DM (1983). Effect of fenoterol on immunological release of leukotrienes and histamine from human lung in vitro: selective antagonism by β-adrenoceptor antagonists. European J Pharmacol 95:239-245.

Howarth PH, Durham SR, Lee TH, Kay AB, Church MK, Holgate ST (1985). Influence of albuterol, cromolyn sodium and ipratropium bromide on the airway and circulating mediator responses to allergen bronchial provocation

in asthma. Am Rev Respir Dis 132:986-992.
Joseph M, Tonnel AB, Capron A, Voisin C (1980). Enzyme release and superoxide anion production by human alveolar macrophages stimulated with immunoglobulin E. Clin Exp Immunol 40:416-422.
Konzett H (1940). Neue broncholytisch hochwirksame Korper der adrenalinreihe. Arch Exp Path Pharm 197:27-40.
Larsson S, Svedmyr N, Thiringer G (1977). Lack of bronchial beta adrenoceptor resistance in asthmatics during long-term treatment with terbutaline. 59:93-100.
Lewis RA, Drazen JM, Corey EJ, Austen KF (1981). Structural and functional characteristics of the leukotriene components of slow-reacting substance of anaphylaxis (SRS-A). In: SRS-A and leukotrienes, pp. 101-117, Piper PJ (ed), John Wiley & Sons, England.
Nyberg L (1986). Pharmacokinetic properties of bambuterol in solution and tablet - basis for once-daily dosage in asthma. Acta Pharmcol et Toxicol, 59, suppl V.
Ohuchi K, Hirasawa N, Takeda H, Asano K, Watanabe M, Tsurufuji S (1987). Mechanism of antianaphylactic action of β-agonists in allergic inflammation of air pouch type in rats. Int archs Allergy appl Immun 82:26-32.
Orange RP, Kaliner MA, Laraia PJ, Austen KF (1971). Immunological release of histamine and slow reacting substance of anaphylaxis from human lung. II. Influence of cellular levels of cyclic AMP. Fed Proc 30:1725-1729.
Peel ET, Gibson GJ (1980). Effects of long term salbutamol therapy on the provocation of asthma by histamine. Am Rev Respir Dis 121:973-978.
Persson CGA, Ekman M, Erjefalt I (1979). Vascular anti-permeability effects of β-receptor agonists and theophylline in the lung. Acta pharmacol et toxicol 44:216-220.
Persson CGA, Erjkalt I, Karlsson JA (1985). Effects of tachykinins and tachykinin antagonists on the tracheobronchical micrcirculation. In: Tachykinin Antagonists. Hakanson R, Sundler F, (eds) Elsevier, Amsterdam pp. 171-179.
Santa Cruz R, Landa J, Hirsch J, Sackner MA (1974). Tracheal mucous velocity in normal man and patients with obstructive lung disease; effects of terbutaline. Am Rev Respir Dis 109:458-463.

Tattersfield AE (1985). Tolerance to beta-agonists. Bull Eur Physiopathol Respir 21:1s-5s.

Van As A (1974). The role of selective β_2-adrenoceptor stimulants in the control of cilial activity. Respiration 31:146-151.

Weber RW, Smith JA, Nelson HS (1982). Aerosolized terbutaline in asthmatics: development of subsensitivity with long-term administration. J Allergy Clin Immunol 70:417-422.

Wichert PV, Meyer W (1983). In vivo inhibition of phospholipase A_2 in rat lung by a β-adrenergic agonist. Agents Actions 13:233-234.

Mechanisms in Asthma: Pharmacology, Physiology, and Management, pages 379–391

ANTI-CHOLINERGIC AGENTS AND THEIR USE IN ASTHMA

David H. Bryant,

Department of Thoracic Medicine, St. Vincent's Hospital, Sydney, N.S.W. 2010, Australia

Anti-cholinergic alkaloids exist in a variety of plants, especially the Datura genus, and their use for the relief of respiratory symptoms originated thousands of years ago in India (Gandevia, 1975). The use of these substances for the relief of respiratory disorders was gradually incorporated into Western Medicine during the early nineteenth century and smoke from the leaves of the stramonium plant became the preparation of choice for the relief of bronchospasm. They were surplanted only by the development of adrenaline and ephedrine in the first half of this century. However since the early 1970's there has been a reawakening of interest in anti-cholinergic bronchodilators. In part this has been due to studies clarifying the role of the parasympathetic nervous system in obstructive airways diseases and in part due to the introduction of ipratropium bromide.

CLINICAL PHARMACOLOGY OF IPRATROPIUM BROMIDE

Ipratropium bromide, a quaternary ammonium derivative of atropine, is largely excluded from the central nervous system and has only very limited gastric absorption. What little ipratropium is absorbed after aerosol administration is broken down to metabolites with essentially no pharmacological effect (Bauer et al, 1979). The most sensitive side effect of anti-cholinergic drugs is the inhibition of salivary secretions. The wide margin of safety of ipratropium is demonstrated by the finding that 300 times as much ipratropium by the aerosol route is needed to inhibit salivary secretions as to inhibit acetylcholine-induced bronchoconstriction. The safety margin for tachycardia is even greater (Bauer et al, 1979).

Acetylcholine is the vagal neuro-transmitter and anti-cholinergic drugs probably produce bronchodilatation by antagonising the action of acetylcholine at its receptor site (Pakes et al, 1980). The extent to which they may also inhibit bronchoconstriction by blocking the cholinergic receptors on the surface of Mast cells, thus inhibiting release of bronchoconstrictor mediators, such as histamine, remains uncertain. (Cugell, 1986).

The exact site within the airways where ipratropium acts is uncertain. Post-ganglionic cholinergic fibres innervate respiratory smooth muscle down to the small bronchioles (Richardson, 1979). The majority of studies show that the site of major bronchodilator effect of ipratropium within the tracheo-bronchial tree is in the central airways (reviewed by Schlueter, 1986). However other investigators have concluded that large and small air-ways are effected and that methodological differences between studies may account for these disparate findings (Partridge and Saunders, 1981; Frith et al, 1982). It has subsequently been reported (jardim et al, 1987) that there is equal probability of ipratropium acting predominantly at central or peripheral airways and that the site of action may change with patients over periods of time independently of the severity of asthma. Indeed there may be heterogeneity in the responses of individuals to anti-cholinergic agents caused by variations in baseline cholinergic tone in the airways as well as differences related to the route of delivery and the dose of the agent used (Bleecker, 1986).

EFFICACY OF ANTI-CHOLINERGIC AGENTS AGAINST BRONCHOCONSTRICTION PRODUCED BY SPECIFIC STIMULI

Comparisons of the effects of ipratropium on air flow obstruction induced by specific stimuli should provide precise information of the mechanisms of action of this drug and its therapeutic profile. However in practice it has proved difficult to obtain comparable data despite the large number of published studies in this field. This reflects a lack of uniformity in the provocation tests used, lack of information concerning the characteristics of the subjects tested, together with the wide variety of techniques used to assess responses. Furthermore the doses of ipratropium used in these studies range from 20 to 2,000 ugs. with widely differing time intervals between the administration of ipratropium or other bronchodilators and the start of the challenge procedure. Bearing these difficulties in mind certain generalised conclusions can be reached concerning the effects of inhaled ipratropium on specific airways responses.

RESPONSE TO METHACHOLINE

As might be expected anti-cholinergic agents are highly protective against bronchospasm caused by the administration of cholinergic agents, (see Table 1) protective effects in various studies ranging from a 97% reduction in the drop in FEV_1 after Methacholine (Cockcroft et al, 1978) up to 6 to 50-fold increases in the provocation doses of Methacholine required to induce a 20% change in FEV_1 (Bandouvakis et al, 1981). There are some indications that anti-cholinergic agents are less effective when given after the cholinergic spasmogen rather than before it and this could be explained by the release of secondary mediators when bronchospasm has been allowed to occur (Atkins et al, 1980).

TABLE 1. Effects of Ipratropium on responses to Methacholine, Histamine and Allergen.

	Degree of Protection	
Stimulus	%Reduction in Fall in FEV_1	%Increase in Provocation Dose
Methacholine	97%	400%
Histamine	57%	200%
Allergen	30%	0%

Cockcroft et al, 1978

RESPONSE TO HISTAMINE

Ipratropium shifts the dose-response curve to inhaled

histamine to the right (Morris, 1986). However in comparison with the effects on Methacholine-induced bronchospasm, ipratropium has a smaller and more variable effect on the response to histamine and the protective effects are more apparent when the airways response is centrally located.

RESPONSE TO EXERCISE

Nearly all studies show that anti-cholinergic agents reduce the severity of exercise induced asthma but do not prevent it entirely (Reviewed by Morris, 1986). A summary of three such reports is shown in Table 2. Two important points are repeatedly made in these studies.

Table 2. Comparison of Drug Effects on Exercise-Induced Asthma in Three Patient Groups

	%FALL IN FEV_1 FROM BASELINE		
DRUG	GROUP 1	GROUP 2	GROUP 3
Placebo	47%	38%	36%
Cromoglycate	7%	11%	-
Fenoterol	-	-	12%
Ipratropium	23%	19%	27%
Lignocaine	-	35%	-
Ketotifen	39%	-	-

When anti-cholinergic agents are compared with other agents they are invariably found to be weaker in their protective effects than are adrenergic agonists and often weaker than sodium cromoglycate (Neijens et al, 1981; Tullett et al, 1982). Secondly anti-cholinergic agents, like adrenergic agonists, alter the baseline and this complicates the interpretation of the results. Indeed in several studies it was suggested that the benefits of treatment were entirely due to the improvement in baseline function (Wolkove et al, 1981). Others have reported that patients responding to ipratropium (those exhibiting at least a 50% reduction in the magnitude of the decrease in FEV_1) were characterised by having less severe asthma, milder exercise-induced bronchospasm, and largely central (rather than peripheral) airways responses to exercise (Thomson et al, 1978; Horie et al, 1983).

RESPONSE TO INHALED ALLERGENS

Despite numerous reports no consistent picture of the effects of anti-cholinergic agents on antigen induced asthma has emerged (Gross & Skorodin, 1984). Some groups have found that ipratropium or related compounds provided excellent protection while an equal number have found an inconsistent or little such effect (Cockcroft et al, 1978; Ruffin et al, 1978). There are clearly a large number of methodologic and interpretive variables in these studies and these questions have not yet been resolved. Whatever the extent and protection afforded by anti-cholinergic agents (see Table 1) it is not complete as subsequent adrenergic agonist administration can improve airways function after cholinergic blockade (Ruffin et al, 1978).

However in considering the effects of anti-cholinergic agents on bronchoconstriction produced by specific stimuli there are several questions that have received little attention. One of these is the possibility that pre-treatment with ipratropium and a beta-adrenergic agonist might be more effective than either agent by itself. Clinical reports (see later) suggest that these two classes of medication have additive effects and that combined therapy may provide greater and more sustained broncho-dilatation than when either drug is administered alone. The possibility of a similar addictive effect against the responses to induced bronchospasm warrants further consider-ation.

In summary inhaled anti-cholinergic agents have some efficacy protecting patients with asthma from most forms of induced bronchospasm. However the degree of protection is variable. Although the data do not support the use of ipratropium as the preferred form of treatment for prevent-ing most types of induced bronchospasm in asthma these studies have broadened our understanding of the pathogenic mechanisms of asthma, they have reemphasised the hetero-geneity of airways responses to all stimuli, and indicate that effective prophylaxis may involve the use of drugs from more than one pharmacological group.

CLINICAL EFFICACY

Since the introduction of ipraptropium over 1,000 clinical articles on the drug have been published many of these describing the results with patients having asthma. The majority of these studies on asthmatic patients involve double blind controlled protocols in patients whose condition was stable. However in most instances the number of experimental subjects was very small giving a high potential for a type 2 statistical error. Furthermore, in many of the studies dealing with combined therapy, sub-maximal doses of one or both agents have been used so that results purporting to show that the combined effect is better than either agent given alone may only be showing that dose dependent bronchodilatation is occurring. A further problem which has not been generally addressed is the optimal way to assess drug response. Invariably this has been done by measurement of air flow obstruction. However it has been shown that Methacholine responsiveness may be inhibited long after any effect on airways calibre has disappeared (Sly et al, 1987). It may therefore be appropriate to include tests of bronchial reactivity as well as measurements of air flow in an assessment of drug response. Bearing in mind these potential difficulties several overall conclusions can be reached concerning the clinical efficacy of ipratropium bromide in asthma.

Although ipratropium is an effective bronchodilator its onset of action is less rapid than with adrenergic agonists and the peak effect is usually achieved in between one to two hours. It is difficult to compare the bronchodilator responses to atropine and adrenergic agonists due to differences in the dosage schedule in most clinical studies. Some studies have shown that ipratropium has almost the same peak effect as salbutamol and terbutaline (Leahy et al, 1983; Grandordy et al, 1984) while other studies showed that it was about 75% as effective as metaproterenol or fenoterol (Ruffin et al, 1982; Bruderman et al, 1983). When mean data is examined more closely it is apparent that numbers of patients have no bronchodilator response and that this obscures the interpretation of responses. Storms et al,(1986) studied 164 patients with asthma all of whom had a 15% or greater improvement in FEV_1 after inhalation of two puffs (0.15 mgs) of isoproterenol. The patients response to two puffs of ipratropium (40 ugs.) and two puffs of metaproterenol (1.5 mgs.) was then determined. Although the mean data showed a significant improvement in

FEV_1 after each drug 49% of the patients receiving ipratropium and 27% of the patients receiving metaproterenol did not achieve a 15% or more increase in baseline FEV_1. Statistical analysis did not reveal any physical or clinical characteristic that could predict response to ipratropium. Some studies have suggested that ipratropium may be more effective in patients over 40 years of age and those with a longer history of asthma (Ullah and Saunders, 1980: Frith, et al, 1982) but overall, ipratropium has been equally effective in asthmatic patients having atopic disease as having cryptogenic asthma (Ruffin et al, 1982; Ullah and Saunders, 1980). It has not proved possible to characterise those patients most likely to respond to ipratropium and this can only be achieved by a satisfactory therapeutic trial in each patient.

Various combinations of ipratropium, adrenergic agonist, and theophylline have been investigated. In acute asthma in adults these studies have uniformly shown (see figure 1) that combinations of ipratropium and adrenergic agonists produce significantly more bronchodilatation than either drug give alone (Bryant, 1985; Ward et al, 1985; Roesler and Reynaert, 1987; Rebuck et al, 1987).

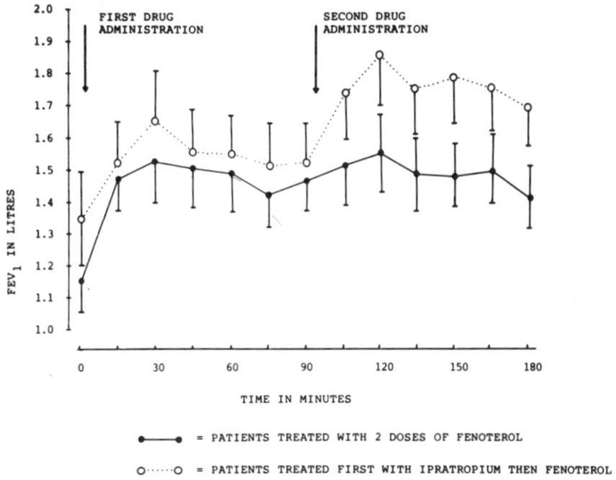

Figure 1. Changes in FEV_1 (mean + SEM) after initial treatment in two groups of patients with acute asthma. Reproduced from Bryant (1985) with permission

Furthermore these experiments have shown that the increased response to the two drugs cannot be attributed to the use of suboptimal doses of adrenergic agonists. With one exception (Petrie and Palmer, 1975) studies in adults with stable asthma have shown that combinations of ipratropium and a adrenergic agonist drug produce significantly more bronchodilatation than either drug given alone (Morton, 1984; Fischbacher et al, 1984; Chakravarti et al, 1987). Furthermore studies of the combination of ipratropium, adrenergic agonist and theophylline have shown (See figure 2) that the bronchodilator effects of all three agents given together was greater and more prolonged than any two agents given together (Rebuck et al, 1983; Krivoy et al, 1987).

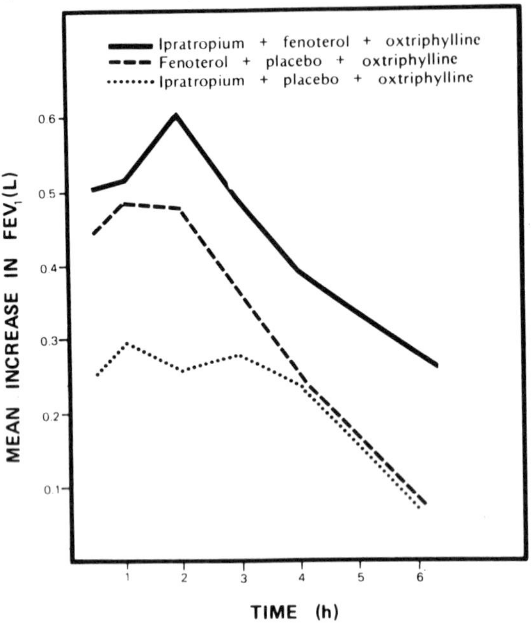

Figure 2. Efficacy of ipratropium in combiination with other drugs in patients with asthma. Reproduced from Rebuck et al, (1983) with permission

It is possible that the sequence of administration of ipratropium and adrenergic agonist may effect the response as it has been noted that the response is more positive and more prolonged when ipratropium is given first (Bruderman et al, 1983; Leahy et al, 1983). However this phenomenon has not been closely studied.

Responses to ipratropium in children with asthma have not been so clear cut as the studies in adults. Several studies have shown that a combination of ipratropium and an adrenergic agonist is more effective than a adrenergic agonist given alone (Beck et al, 1985; Bratteby et al, 1986; Boner et al, 1987) while other studies have failed to show any benefit from the addition of ipratropium (Cook et al, 1985; Lenney and Evans, 1986).

SIDE EFFECTS

Ipratropium is remarkably free of significant side effects, noteably the tremor, nervousness, and tachycardia associated with adrenergic agonist administration. The side effects most frequently encounted are dry mouth and cough. There are no significant cardiovascular effects of inhaled ipratropium and studies of muco-ciliary function and tracheo-bronchial clearance have shown either no effect or a slight increase in the rate at which radioactive particles are cleared from the lungs following a single dose of ipratropium (Cugell, 1986). There have been reports of paradoxical responses to inhaled ipratropium solution resulting in bronchospasm. Initially this was caused by hypotonicity of the aerosol solution (Mann et al, 1984) but there has been a subsequent report of occasional bronchoconstriction due to preservative agents in ipratropium nebuliser solution (Beasley et al, 1987). The prevalence and significance of this reaction is currently the subject of investigation.

CONCLUSION

Ipratropium bromide has been shown to be a safe and effective bronchodilator in many adults with either acute or chronic asthma. It appears to be most effective in older patients and in those with asthma of long duration but there are no clinical variables which enable one to predict with accuracy which patients are most likely to respond and the efficacy of the drug can only be assessed by therapeutic trial in individual patients. For certain specific trigger factors (exercise and allergen induced asthma) ipratropium is a less effective prophylactic agent than either adrenergic agonists or sodium cromoglycate. However its additive effect in combination with adrenergic agonists and theophylline has been established in a large number of clinical studies and it is likely to find its place as an adjunct to the use of these two agents in the management of sub-acute and acute asthma in adults. Its place in the treatment of asthma in children is less clearly established.

One major strength of ipratropium is its safety. Since beta agonists and theophylline have sometimes to be used to the extent that side effects occur, the addition of ipratropium may allow for increased bronchodilatation while permitting the individual asthmatic patient to reduce the dose of these other drugs. Thus although the onset of bronchodilatation with ipratropium is not as rapid as that with adrenergic agonists it has a very wide margin of safety and a tendency for a longer duration of bronchodilatation and it should be useful as an adjunct in our current therapy for asthma.

REFERENCES

Atkins PC, Rosenblum F, Dunsky EG, Coffey R, Zweiman B (1980). Comparison of plasma histamine and cyclic nucleotides after antigen and methacholine inhalation in man. J Allergy Clin Immunol 66:478-485.

Bankouvakis J, Cartier A, Ryan G, Hargreave FE (1981). The effects of ipratropium bromide and fenoterol on methacholine and histamine-induced bronchoconstriction. Br J Dis Chest 75:295:305.

Bauer R, Banholzer R, Griben C (1979). Ipratropium bromide. Pharmacol Biochem Prop Drug Subst 2:489-515.

Beasley CR, Rafferty P, Holgate ST (1987). Bronchoconstrictor properties of preservatives in ipratropium bromide (atrovent) nebuliser solution. Br Med J 294:1197-1198.

Beck R, Robertson C, Galdes-Sebalt M, Levison H (1985). Combined salbutamol and ipratropium bromide by inhalation in the treatment of severe acute asthma. J Pediat 107:605-608.

Bleecker ER (1986). Cholinergic and neurogenic mechanisms in obstructive airways disease. Am J Med 81 (Suppl 5A):93-102.
Boner AL, De Stefano G, Niero E. Vallone G, Gaburro D (1987). Salbutamol and ipratropium bromide solution in the treatment of bronchospasm in asthmatic children. Ann Allergy 58:54-58.
Bratteby LE, Foucard T, Lonnerholm G (1986). Combined treatment with ipratropium bromide and beta-2-adrenorecptor agonists in childhood asthma. Eur J Respir Dis 68:239-247.
Bruderman I, Cohen-Aronovski R, Smorzik J (1983). A comparative study of various combinations of ipratropium bromide and metaproterenol in allergic asthmatic patients. Chest 83:208-210.
Bryant DH (1985). Nebulised ipratropium bromide in the treatment of acute asthma. Chest 88:24-29.
Chakravarti A, Pratley M, Barcharb M, Musiosky F, McDonald F, Vickerson F, Kazim F (1987). Postgrad Med J 63 (Suppl 1):5.
Cockcroft DW, Ruffin RE, Hargreave FE (1978). Effect of Sch 1000 in allergen-induced asthma. Clin Allergy 8:361-372.
Cook JJ, Fergusson DM, Dawson KP (1985). Ipratropium and fenoterol in the treatment of acute asthma. Pharmatherapeutica 4:383-386.
Cugell DW (1986). Clinical pharmacology and toxicology of ipratropium. Am J Med 81 (Suppl 5A):18-22.
Fischbacher CM, Milroy R, Giannini D, Monie RD (1984). Comparison of Douvent and salbutamol inhalers in chronic stable asthma. Postgrad Med J 60 (Suppl 1)28-31.
Frith PA, Thomas PD, McEvoy RD, Antic R (1982). Factors contributing to bronchodilation induced by ipratropium bromide in asthmatics. Aust NZ J Med 12:686.
Gandevia B (1975). Historical view of the use of parasympatholytic agents in the treatment of respiratory disorders. Postgrad M J 51 (Suppl 7):13-20.
Grandordy B, Thomas V, Marsac J (1984). Compared bronchodilation after inhaled salbutamol and ipratropium bromide in asthma. Am Rev Resp Dis 129 (part 2):A-91.
Gross NJ, Skorodin MS (1984). Anticholinergic, antimuscarinic bronchodilators. Am Rev Resp Dis 129:856-870.
Horie T, Enomoto S, Inazawa T (1983). Effect of disodium cromoglycate and Sch 1000 on exercise-induced asthma. Nihon Univ J Med 25:207-216.
Jardim JR, De Oliveira JA, Nery LE (1987). The changing site of bronchial obstruction in asthmatic patients and the site of action of ipratropium bromide. Postgrad Med J 63(Suppl 1):12

Krivoy N, Jubarin A, Gaitini L, Rubin A, Alroy G (1987). Combination therapy of ipratropium bromide, terbutaline and slow release theophylline in asthma and chronic airways obstruction. Postgrad Med J 63 (Suppl 1):21.
Leahy BC, Gomm SA, Allen SC (1983). Comparison of nebulised ipratropium bromide in acute asthma. Br J Dis Chest 77:159-163.
Lenney W, Evans NA (1986). Nebulised salbutamol and ipratropium bromide in asthmatic children. Br J Dis Chest 80:59-65.
Mann J, Howarth P, Holgate ST (1984). Bronchoconstriction induced by ipratropium bromide in asthma: relation to hypotonicity. Br J Med 289:469-
Morris HG (1986). Review of ipratropium bromide in induced bronchospasm in patients with asthma. Am J Med 81 (Suppl 5A): 36-44
Morton O (1984). Response to Duovent of chronic reversible airways obstruction - a controlled trial in general practice. Postgrad Med J 60 (Suppl 1):32-35.
Neijens HJ, Wesselius T, Kerrebijn K (1981). Exercise-induced bronchoconstriction as an expression of bronchial hyperreactivity. A study of its mechanisms in children. Thorax 36:517-522.
Pakes G, Brogden R, Heel R, Speight T, Avery G (1980). Ipratropium bromide: a review of its pharmacological properties and therapeutic efficacy in asthma and chronic bronchitis. Drugs 20:237-266
Partridge MR, Saunders KB (1981). Site of action of ipratropium bromide and clinical physiologic determinants of response in patients with asthma. Thorax 36:530-533.
Petrie GR, Palmer KNV (1975). Comparison of ipratropium bromide and salbutamol in chronic bronchitis and asthma. Br Med J 1:430-432.
Rebuck AS, Gent M, Chapman KR (1983). Anticholinergic and sympathomimetic combination therapy of asthma. J Allergy Clin Immunol 71:317-323.
Rebuck AS, Chapman KR, Aboud R, Pare PD, Kreisman H (1987). Nebulised anticholinergic and sympathomimetic treatment of asthma and chronic obstructive airways disease in the emergency room. Am J Med 82:59-64.
Richardson JB (1979). Nerve supply to the lungs. Am Rev Resp Dis 119:785-802.
Roesler J, Reynaert M (1987). Aerosols of fenoterol and association of fenoterol-ipratropium: a comparative study of efficacy in acute asthma. Postgrad Med J 63 (Suppl 1):2.

Ruffin RE, Cockcroft DW, Hargreave FE (1978). A comparison of the protective effect of fenoterol and Sch 1000 on allergen-induced asthma. J Allergy Clin Immunol 61:42-47.
Ruffin RE, McIntyre E, Crockett AJ, Zeilonka K, Alpers JH (1982). Combination bronchodilator therapy in asthma. J Allergy Clin Immunol 69:60-65.
Schleuter DP (1986). Ipratropium bromide in asthma. Amer J Med (Suppl 5A) 81:55-59.
Sly PD, Landau LI, Olinsky A (1987). Failure of ipratropium bromide to modify the diurnal variation of asthma in asthmatic children. Thorax 42:357-360.
Storms WW, Bodman SF, Nathan RA, Busse WW, Bush RK, Falliers CJ, O'Hollaren JD, Weg JG, (1986). Use of ipratropium bromide in asthma. Am J Med 81 (Suppl 5A):61-65.
Thomson NC, Patel KR, Kerr JW (1978). Sodium cromoglycate and ipratropium bromide in exercise-induced asthma. Thorax 33: 694-699.
Tullett WM, Patel KR, Berkin KE, Kerr JW (1982). Effect of lignocaine, sodium cromoglycate and ipratropium bromide in exercise induced asthma. Thorax 37:737:740.
Ullah M, Saunders KB (1980). Influence of age on response to ipratropium bromide and salbutamol in asthmatic patients. Prof Respir Res 14:150-154.
Ward MJ, MacFarlane JT, Davies D (1985). A place for ipratropium bromide in the treatment of acute severe asthma. Br J Dis Chest 79:374-378.
Wolkove N, Kreisman H, Frank H, Gent M (1981). The effect of ipratropium bromide on exercise-induced bronchoconstriction. Ann Allergy 47:311:315.

Mechanisms in Asthma: Pharmacology,
Physiology, and Management, pages 393–403

STUDIES OF LEUKOTRIENE ANTAGONISTS AND SYNTHESIS INHIBITORS IN MAN

Neil Barnes, Jane Evans, Jerzy Zakrzewski,
Priscilla Piper and John Costello

London Chest Hosp., Bonner Road, London E2, (N.B.), Dept. of Thoracic Medicine, King's College School of Medicine and Dentistry, Denmark Hill, London SE5, (J.E., J.Z., J.C.) and Dept. of Pharmacology, Royal College of Surgeons, Lincoln's Inn Fields, London WC2, England (P.P.).

INTRODUCTION

The known actions of the cysteinyl-leukotrienes and the fact that they are released from sensitised lung tissue following antigenic stimulation has led to the suggestion that leukotrienes (LTs) may be important chemical mediators of human asthma. Since the elucidation of the structure of slow-reacting substances (SRS's) as LTs (Hammarström et al, 1979; Morris et al, 1980; Lewis et al, 1980) there has been enormous interest in developing LT receptor antagonists and synthesis inhibitors in the hope that they may represent novel therapies in asthma. Such drugs will also be powerful tools to help determine the contribution of LTs to the bronchoconstriction caused by inhaled antigen in atopic asthmatic patients, the role of LTs in airways hyperresponsiveness and the importance of LTs in clinical asthma. In this respect, though not necessarily as treatments in asthma, LT receptor antagonists are in many ways preferable to drugs preventing LT synthesis. Leukotriene antagonists can be specific for the cysteinyl-LTs rather than also preventing the production of the chemotactic agent LTB_4. Furthermore with drugs preventing LT synthesis there is the theoretical possibility of the substrate arachidonic acid being redirected to the cyclo-oxygenase pathway in a situation analagous to that which occurs in the reverse direction with aspirin-like drugs (Walker, 1973).

With such a new class of drugs the first requirement when assessing any compound acting against LTs must be to prove the efficacy and potency of the drug as an LT antagonist (or synthesis inhibitor) in man. Following this clinical trials in controlled models of asthma such as antigen and exercise challenge and in clinical asthma can be undertaken with the knowledge that the drug is effectively preventing the actions (or production) of LTs in man.

STUDIES OF LEUKOTRIENE ANTAGONISTS

The first LT antagonist to be reported was FPL 55712 (Augstein et al, 1973) a chromone-2-carboxylic acid. It is interesting to note that this compound was synthesised before the structure of slow-reacting substance of anaphylaxis (SRS-A) was elucidated as being LTs, and that several of the LT antagonists now being evaluated are structurally related to FPL 55712. Only a limited number of studies with FPL 55712 were performed in man because of a short half life and poor oral absorption. Holroyde et al (1981) demonstrated that prior inhalation of FPL 55712 or the related compound FPL 59257 could particularly inhibit the bronchoconstriction caused by inhalation of LTC_4 and LTD_4 in two normal subjects. In a limited open study two out of four asthmatic patients administered aerosolized FPL 55712 four times a day for one week showed a slight improvement in forced expiratory volume in one second (FEV_1) (Lee et al, 1981). The effect of inhaled FPL 55712 on the immediate response to antigen challenge was studied in six ragweed sensitive asthmatics (Ahmed et al, 1981). This study primarily investigated the effect of FPL 55712 on the decrease in tracheal mucous velocity (TMV) which occurs after antigen inhalation. Inhaled FPL 55772 after antigen challenge prevented the decrease in TMV. Although it was not statistically significant there was a trend for the drop in pulmonary function caused by antigen challenge to be less after inhalation of FPL 55712.

Several new LT receptor antagonists have now been evaluated in man. L649,923 is structurally related to FPL 55712 but is orally active (Jones et al, 1986a). L649,923 is a receptor antagonist of the cysteinyl-LTs and has been shown to be active on the guinea pig ileum and trachea. Studies in anaesthetised guinea pigs have demonstrated the drug to be active against LTD_4-induced bronchoconstriction at doses of 5 and 10 mg/kg intraduodenally (Jones et al, 1986a).

We have investigated the effect of L649,923 on histamine and LTD_4-induced bornchoconstriction in normal man (Barnes, Piper and Costello, 1987). Eleven normal subjects completed a double blind, placebo-controlled, cross-over design study. On four days, each separated by at least a week, subjects took 1g L649,923 or matching placebo orally and then underwent a histamine or LTD_4 challenge. Subjects inhaled increasing concentrations of histamine or LTD_4 until the highest concentration of agonist was reached (10^{-1} moles/l for histamine, 2×10^{-4} moles/l for LTD_4) or until a 35% fall in specific airways conductance (sGaw) occurred. Pulmonary function was monitored using sGaw and the flow at 30% of vital capacity above residual volume from a partial flow volume curve ($\dot{V}max_{30}$). The provocation concentration (PC) of each agonist necessary to cause a 35% fall in sGaw (PC_{35}) or a 30% fall in $\dot{V}max_{30}$ (PC_{30}) was determined. L649,923 had no effect on the baseline pulmonary function or on histamine-induced bronchoconstriction. The drug shifted the LTD_4 dose-response curve to the right in all subjects. The geometric mean shift of the dose-response curve being 3.8 fold both for the PC_{35}sGaw and $PC_{30}\dot{V}max_{30}$. There was considerable intra- and intersubject variation in the plasma levels of the drug achieved at the time of maximum bronchoconstriction but the plasma levels would have been sufficient to cause significant LTD_4 antagonism in the animal models studied. The only side effect of the drug was colicky abdominal pain and watery diarrhoea which occurred on 10 of the 22 occasions when active drug was ingested.

The effect of the same dose of L649,923 on the bronchoconstriction caused by antigen challenge in atopic asthmatic patients has been investigated by Britton et al (1987). Seven patients completed a double blind two part study in which they took 1g of L649,923 or matching placebo two hours before inhaling a dose of antigen which had previously been shown to cause a 20% fall in FEV_1. The drug had a small protective effect against the early response; the FEV_1 falling by 1.3 litres after active drug and 1.78 litres after placebo. There was no protection against the late phase response but plasma drug levels at the time of the late response were probably too low to test the drugs effectiveness at that time. The same side effects of abdominal pain and diarrhoea were noted in this study.

We have investigated REV5901 (R,S-2-[3'-(1"-hydroxyhexyl)-phenoxy methyl]quinoline) which in animal models is an orally active LT antagonist with some 5-lipoxygenase inhibitory actions. This drug is not structurally related to FPL 55712. REV5901 was investigated for its actions against histamine and LTD_4-induced bronchoconstriction in eight normal subjects (Evans et al, in press a). Overall, there was no protective action of the drug against either histamine or LTD_4-induced bronchoconstriction. The only side-effect noted was of nausea and noisy borborygmi on 4 of the 16 occasions when active drug was ingested. This study illustrates that LT-antagonism in animal models may not predict activity in man.

The other oral LT antagonist which has been studied in man and reported is LY171883 (Fleisch et al, 1986). This drug is also structurally related to FPL 55712. At a single dose of 400mg LY171883 has been shown to cause a shift to the right of the LTD_4 dose response curve in normal subjects (Phillips, Rafferty and Holgate, 1987). When FEV_1 was considered the mean shift in the dose response curve was 4.6 fold and when $\dot{V}max_{30}$ was assessed a 6.3 fold shift occurred. LY171883 is the first LT antagonist in which the effect of long term administration in asthmatic patients has been reported (Fleisch, Cloud and Marshall, in press). One hundred and thirty eight patients participated in a double blind, parallel group study, they took active drug or placebo for six weeks. A dose of LY171883 400mg twice a day was used, symptom scores, peak expiratory flow rate (PEFR) and concomitant bronchodilator usage was assessed daily by the patient and FEV_1 was measured at two weekly intervals in the laboratory. There was a statistically significant improvement in symptom scores and a decrease in concomitant use of β_2 agonists but only in those patients using greater amounts of inhaled bronchodilators. The most significant result was that the FEV_1 measured two weekly gradually rose in the actively treated group from 3.1 to 3.4 litres at the end of six weeks while remaining unchanged in the placebo group.

Of the new LT antagonists the results of human studies with only one inhaled drug have been reported. L648,051 is structurally related to FPL55712 and is very similar to L649,923 (Jones et al, 1986b), however, it is active by the inhaled rather than the oral route of administration. We have studied the effect of L648,051 on LTD_4-induced bronchoconstriction in nine normal subjects (Barnes et al, 1987). As L648,051 is inhaled plasma levels could not be used to obtain any clue about the likely duration of action of the drug. In view of this we did not feel that it would be possible initially to perform complete LTD_4 dose response curves with any certainty that the drug would still be active. The effect of 1.6mg L648,051 or matching placebo inhaled from a pressurised aerosol on the subsequent inhalation of a single bronchoconstricting concentration of LTD_4 was evaluated. L648,051 partially inhibited the bronchoconstriction caused by LTD_4. The maximum fall in $\dot{V}max_{30}$ was diminished (L648,051 - 23% vs placebo - 33%, $p = 0.03$), the duration of LTD_4-induced bronchoconstriction was shortened (L648,051 - 13.3 mins vs placebo - 19.4 mins, $p < 0.02$) and the fall in $\dot{V}max_{30}$ at 3.5 and 8.5 mins after LTD_4 inhalation was less. The drug was well tolerated with no side effects.

We have also investigated the acute effect of a single inhalation of L648,051 in wheezy asthmatics (Evans et al, in press b). Eight patients with asthma controlled on inhaled corticosteroids and bronchodilators refrained from taking inhaled B_2 agonists for six hours and oral theophyllines for 36 hours prior to study. On the two study days they has a baseline FEV_1 of between 50 and 70% of predicted normal. On the two study days they inhaled 1.6 mg L648,051 or matching placebo and FEV_1, sGaw and $\dot{V}max_{30}$ were monitored for four hours. There was no effect of drug on FEV_1, there was a trend to the sGaw and $\dot{V}max_{30}$ being higher after active drug but this failed to reach statistical significance.

LEUKOTRIENE SYNTHESIS INHIBITORS

Few LT synthesis inhibitors have been investigated in man. The effect of inhaled piriprost (1mg) on antigen and exercise induced bronchoconstriction in asthmatic subjects has been reported (Mann et al, 1986). Piriprost had no effect on either cause of bronchoconstriction, however there was no in vivo assay to prove the drug was effectively preventing the productin of LTs in man. Proof that any putative 5-lipoxygenase inhibitor is blocking LT production is an important stage in assessing any such drugs. The ability of enzyme inhibitors to prevent LT production in nasal discharge fluid following intra-nasal antigen challenge may provide such a model (Creticos et al, 1984).

DISCUSSION

What conclusions about the role of LTs in asthma, the potential therapeutic effects of drugs acting against LTs and the future development of such drugs can be reached from the present studies? The first and most basic observation is that antagonism of the cysteinyl-LTs in man can be achieved with both oral and inhaled LT antagonists. However, the results of animal studies have tended to overestimate the potency of LT antagonists in man. REV5901 was active as an LT antagonist in animals but not man and the potency of L649,923 and L648,051 was less in man than results from animal studies would have suggested. This emphasises the importance of the early evaluation of the activity of any LT antagonist in man. Shifts of the order of 50-fold in LTD_4 dose response curves in man would seem desirable to achieve effective receptor blockade. If increased potency in animal tissues translates into greater potency in man then SK&F104353 (Wasserman et al, 1987) and ICI 198,615 (Aharony et al, in press) which are about 100 times more active than the currently studied compounds may be of suitable potency in man. These drugs will also be of interest as they are not related to FPL55712. SK&F 104353 is a structured analogue of LTD_4 and ICI 198,615 is an indazoline.

The results of the study by Britton et al (1987) in atopic patients with asthma showed a slight protective effect of L649,923 on the early bronchoconstrictor response to antigen challenge. Two interpretations of this study are possible, (1) that the drug was not sufficiently active to antagonise the effects of the endogenously produced LTD_4 or (2) that LTs are relatively unimportant mediators in asthma and even more potent antagonists will only be of minor use.

Perhaps the most intriguing result has been with the LT antagonist L7171883. This drug caused only a five-fold shift in the LTD_4-dose-response curve. However, when given to asthmatic patients for six weeks it caused a gradual improvement in lung function with the mean FEV_1 improving from 3.1 to 3.4 litres. This is in some regards a slightly surprising result. A group of asthmatics who have only slightly impaired lung function have shown an improvement in FEV_1 with an LT antagonist of the same order as might be expected with inhaled corticosteroids. This would suggest that either the main role of the cysteinyl-LTs in asthma is not as endogenous bronchoconstrictors but that some other property such as formation of bronchial wall oedema or sensitisation to other mediators is important or that LY171883 has another therapeutic action apart from LT receptor antagonism. Studies with other structurally unrelated LT antagonists should help resolve these questions.

REFERENCES

Aharony P, Falcone RC, Yee YK, Hesp B, Giles RE, Krell RD. Ligand binding studies with 3H-ICI 198,615 a new peptide leukotriene receptor antagonist. Ann N Y Acad Sci: in press.

Ahmed T, Greenblatt DW, Birch S, Marchette B, Wanner A (1981). Abnormal mucociliary transport in allergic patients with antigen-induced bronchospasm: role of slow reacting substance of anaphylaxis. Am Rev Respir Dis 124: 110.

Augstein J, Farmer JB, Lee TB, Sheard P, Tattersall ML (1973). Selective inhibitor of slow reacting substance of anaphylaxis. Nature New Biol 245: 215-217.

Barnes NC, Evans JM, Zakrzewski JT, Piper PJ, Costello JF (1987). L648,051 a leukotriene D_4 antagonist is active by the inhaled route in man. Abstracts of the Tenth International Congress of Pharmacology (IUPHAR) 034.

Barnes NC, Piper PJ, Costello JF (1987). The effect of an oral leukotriene antagonist L649,923 on histamine and leukotriene D_3-induced bronchoconstriction in normal man. J Allergy Clin Immunol 79: 816.

Britton JR, Hanley SP, Tattersfield AE (1987). The effect of an oral leukotriene D_4 antagonist L649,923 on the response to inhaled antigen in asthma. J Allergy Clin Immunol 79: 811.

Creticos PS, Peters SP, Adkinson NF, Naclerio RM, Hayes EC, Norman PS, Lichtenstein LM (1984). Peptide leukotriene release after antigen challenge in patients sensitive to ragweed. New Engl J Med 310: 1626.

Evans JM, Barnes NC, Piper PJ, Costello JF. The effect of REV5901 on histamine and leukotriene D_4 induced bronchoconstriction in man. Br J Clin Pharmacol: Abstract in press a.

Evans JM, Barnes NC, Piper PJ, Costello JF. The effect of a single dose of an inhaled leukotriene antagonist L648,051 in mild asthma. Br J Clin Pharmacol: Abstract in press b.

Fleisch JH, Rinkema LE, Whitesitt CA, Marshall WS (1986). Pharmacologic antagonism of leukotriene mediated events. In Piper PJ (ed): "The leukotrienes - their biological significance" New York: Raven Press, p109.

Fleisch JM, Cloud ML, Marshall WS. Preclinical and clinical studies with LY171883 and other leukotriene (LT) receptor antagonists. Ann NY Acad Sci: in press.

Hammarström S, Murphy RC, Samuelsson B, Clark DA, Mioskowski C, Corey EJ (1979). Structure of leukotriene C: Identification of the amino acid part. Biochem Biophys Res Commun 91: 1266.

Holroyde MC, Altounyan REC, Cole M, Dixon M, Elliot EV (1981). Bronchoconstriction produced in man by leukotrienes C and D. Lancet 2: 17.

Jones TR, Young R, Champion E, Charette L, Denis D, Ford-Hutchison AW, Frenette R, Gauthier J-Y, Guindon Y, Kakushima M, Masson P, McFarlane C, Piechuta H, Rokach J, Zamboni R, De Haven RN, Maycock A, Pong SS (1986a). L-649,923, sodium (βS*, R*)-4-(3-(4-acetyl-3-hydroxy-2-propylphenoxy)-propylthio)-γ-hydroxy-B-methylbenzene butanoate, a selective, orally active-leukotriene receptor antagonist. Can J Physiol Pharmacol 64: 1068.

Jones TR, Guindon Y, Young R, Champion E, Charette L, Denis D, Ethier D, Hamel R, Ford-Hutchison AW, Fortin R, Letts G, Masson P, McFarlane C, Piechuta H, Rokach J, Yoakin C, De Haven RN, Maycock A, Pong SS (1986b). L648,051, sodium 4-[3-(4-acetyl-3hydroxy-2propylphenoxy)-propylsulphonyl]-γ-oxo-benzene butanoate: A leukotriene D_4 receptor antagonist. Can J Physiol Pharmacol 64: 1535.

Lewis RA, Austen KF, Drazen JM, Clark DA, Marfat A, Corey EJ (1980). Slow-reacting substance of anaphylaxis: Identification of leukotrienes C-1 and D from human and rat sources. Proc Nat Acad Sci 77: 3710.

Mann JS, Robinson C, Sheridan AQ, Clement P, Bach MK, Holgate ST (1986). Effect of inhaled piriprost (U-60257) a novel leukotriene inhibitor, on allergen and exercise induced bronchoconstriction in asthma. Thorax 41: 746.

Morris HR, Taylor GW, Piper PJ, Tippins JR (1980). Structure of slow-reacting substance from gunea-pig lung. Nature 285: 104.

Phillips GD, Rafferty P, Holgate ST (1987). LY171883 as an oral leukotriene D_4 antagonist in non-asthmatic subjects. Thorax 42: 723 (Abstract).

Wasserman MA, Torphy TJ, Hay DWP, Muccitelli RM, Tucker SS, Wilson KA, Osborn RR, Vickery-Clark L, hall RF, Erhard KF, Gleason JG (1987). Pharmalogic profile of

SK&F 104353, a novel, highly potent and selective peptidoleukotriene antagonist. In Samuelsson B, Paoletti R, Ramwell PW (eds) "Advances in prostaglandins, thromboxane and leukotriene research" vol 17a New York: Raven Press, p532.
Walker JL (1973). The regulatory function of prostaglandins in the release of histamine and SRS-A from passively sensitised human lung tissue. "Advances in the biosciences". Oxford: Pergamon, p235.

DISCUSSION

Paterson: It would seem that we are awaiting information on the effects of more potent PAF and leukotriene antagonists in man; discussion of these compounds should wait until this is available.

Barnes: Dr Seale, you didn't tell us that beta agonists are completely ineffective in blocking both the late response to allergen and the bronchial hyperresponsiveness. We know that beta agonists are effective in stablizing mast cells since they block the acute response to allergen. I believe this shows, firstly, that beta agonists have no effect on the chronic inflammation of asthma, which needs other treatment, and because they are bronchodilators they mask the inflammation which could be dangerous and may be responsible for increased asthma deaths. Secondly, it shows convincingly that the mast cell has absolutely nothing to do with the chronic inflammation associated with asthma. The only mast cell stabilizer effective in chronic asthma is disodium cromoglycate and this probably works by another mechanism. We've recently found that there are no beta receptors on the human eosinophil and Dr R. Fuller has shown there are none on the macrophage, and so this may be the reason why beta agonists are useless in asthma.

Paterson: Do you really consider that beta agonists are useless in asthma?

Barnes: They are useless for the chronic inflammation, but they are the best bronchodilators available. However, this is their danger, they mask the symptoms of asthma. The treatment of asthma requires bronchodilator therapy and an anti-inflammatory agent. When we find a suitable dose of anti-inflammatory drug we won't need a beta agonist because there will be no bronchodilation needed.

Seale: I agree with your comments. If you believe there is a close association between inflammation and bronchial hyperreactivity, then you should consider that beta agonists do not alter long term bronchial hyperreactivity. Unless you can demonstrate that these drugs have some activity on the cellular component of inflammation it may be that they are not going to do a lot to bronchial hyperreactivity. I think Dr Nijkamp could comment on this, since he has some data on the effects of beta agonists on macrophage function.

Nijkamp: In guinea-pig alveolar macrophages we have found that β_1 agonists suppress hydrogen peroxide release, but this effect is not inhibited by beta antagonists, so it seems that it is not mediated by the beta-adrenoceptor. I think there are many recent reports showing that some effects of beta agonists are not mediated by the beta-adrenoceptor.

Kerrebijn: We have completed a 6 months study in which we looked at the effects of beta agonists on bronchial hyperresponsiveness in children and found no effect. In addition, we have just completed a 5 months study looking at the effects of ipratropium bromide on bronchial hyperresponsiveness and found absolutely no effect. So Dr Barnes' comments regarding beta agonists and inflammation seem to be true for the anticholinergics as well. I am also in favour of combining a bronchodilator with an anti-inflammatory drug.

Daniel: I think it may be a bit premature to make these conclusions about beta agonists. We should take into account the pharmacokinetics of beta agonists versus the corticosteroids. Until we have a long-acting beta agonist we can't be so sure that they are ineffective.

Barnes: Disodium cromoglycate has an extremely short action and yet it can completely block the late response and the increased responsiveness, so I don't think that this is a good explanation for the difference between beta agonists and corticosteroids.

Zimmerman: I would like to comment on the ipratropium-induced bronchoconstriction in asthma; it may not be an isolated phenomenon. A paper presented at the British Thoracic Society Meeting in Edinburgh showed that 5 out of 30 asthmatic patients had falls in FEV_1 of 20% or more with the preservative-containing solution. This did not occur when they used the preservative-free solution. When the preservative-free solution becomes available we may need to re-evaluate this potential problem.

Mechanisms in Asthma: Pharmacology,
Physiology, and Management, pages 405–419

ACUTE EFFECTS OF FENOTEROL (BEROTEC) AND IPRATROPIUM BROMIDE (ATROVENT) ALONE AND IN COMBINATION ON BRONCHIAL HYPERRESPONSIVENESS IN ASTHMATIC SUBJECTS

Cheryl M. Salome, Wendy Wright,
Cheryl J. Sedgwick and Ann J. Woolcock

Department of Medicine,
University of Sydney, NSW 2006
Australia

INTRODUCTION

The underlying abnormalities in the airways of subjects with asthma are manifested clinically as bronchial hyperresponsiveness (BHR) and the severity of BHR correlates with the severity of asthma (Yan et al., 1983; Cockcroft et al., 1977a). Subjects with severe BHR are more susceptible to attacks of asthma provoked by allergens (Cockcroft et al., 1979) and exercise (Chatham et al., 1982) than subjects with mild BHR. The requirements for effective treatment of asthma are to decrease the level of BHR, to prevent attacks from occurring and to reverse attacks when they occur. It seems likely that the prevention of attacks is an important component in decreasing BHR (Woolcock et al., In press).

Both fenoterol and ipratropium bromide dilate the airways of asthmatic subjects, although fenoterol has a greater effect than ipratropium (Serra et al., 1986). When given in combination they achieve a greater degree and duration of bronchodilatation than either drug alone (Marlin et al., 1979). The two drugs work via different mechanisms, fenoterol via the B_2-adrenergic receptors and ipratropium via the cholinergic receptors and have an additive bronchodilating effect. It is not known if these two drugs given in combination have an additive protective effect against histamine induced bronchoconstriction. Studies have shown that B_2-adrenergic drugs are more effective than anticholinergic drugs in reducing bronchial responsiveness (Anderson et al., 1979; Cockcroft et al., 1977b). We have shown previously that fenoterol aerosol reduces responsiveness to histamine for up to five hours (Salome et al., 1983) and its effectiveness as an inhibitor of responsiveness is dose dependent. On the other hand, ipratropium appears to be a poor inhibitor of induced attacks but, because of its slow onset of action, may have an effect up to five hours after treatment (Crimi et al., 1986).

This study was designed to determine if the combination of fenoterol and ipratropium bromide provides a greater degree or duration of protection against histamine challenge than either drug alone. In addition, the effect of salbutamol on the acute response to histamine was studied in order to determine if there are differences between different B_2-adrenergic drugs.

METHODS

Subjects

Nine subjects with stable asthma, attending outpatient clinics at Royal Prince Alfred Hospital, were studied. All subjects were atopic, with one or more positive skin test from a standard battery of thirteen, and all were lifelong nonsmokers. None were taking ipratropium bromide and none had ever taken oral steroids. All had baseline values for one second forced expiratory volume (FEV_1) greater than 60% of predicted (Morris et al., 1971) and had demonstrated increases in FEV_1 >20% after 200 ug fenoterol aerosol. Prior to the study all subjects underwent a histamine challenge test and were shown to have severe or moderate BHR. The study was approved by the Ethics Review committee of the hospital and all subjects gave written informed consent to the study.

Study Design

The study was carried out on five separate days within one week and all subjects refrained from taking aerosol bronchodilators for six hours and oral bronchodilators for twelve hours prior to attending. Subjects came to the laboratory at 9.00am each day and, after resting for thirty minutes, had their baseline spirometric function and heart rate measured. They were then given one of five treatments described below. Treatments were given in random order over the five days and were given double blind. Five minutes after the treatment subjects again had spirometric function and heart rate measured and they were then given a histamine challenge test to measure BHR. Measurements of spirometric function, heart rate and BHR were repeated at hourly intervals for six hours.

Trial Treatments

The five treatments were:

A: fenoterol (1x200ug) + ipratropium bromide (4x20ug) + placebo salbutamol (2 puffs).

B: placebo fenoterol (1 puff) + ipratropium bromide (4x20ug) + placebo salbutamol (2 puffs).

C: fenoterol (1x200ug) + placebo ipratropium bromide (4 puffs) + placebo salbutamol (2 puffs).

D: placebo fenoterol (1 puff) + placebo ipratropium bromide (4 puffs) + placebo salbutamol (2 puffs).

E: placebo fenoterol (1 puff) + placebo ipratropium bromide (4 puffs) + salbutamol (2x100ug).

Lung function

Spirometric function was measured on a Vitalograph dry spirometer (Vitalograph Ltd, Buckingham, England) while the subject was standing. Forced expiratory manoeuvres were repeated until two values for the one second forced expiratory volume (FEV_1) were obtained which were reproducible to within 100ml and the higher value recorded.

Histamine Challenge Test

The histamine challenge tests were performed according to our standard method (Yan et al., 1983). Briefly, DeVilbiss No 40 hand held nebulisers (DeVilbiss Co, Somerset PA, USA) were used to deliver increasing doses of histamine, in doubling increments, from four stock solutions. Doses ranged from 0.03 umol to 7.8 umol. The challenge was stopped when the FEV_1 fell by 20% from the baseline value recorded immediately prior to the challenge.

Data Expression and Analysis

Values for FEV_1 were expressed as percent of the predicted values (Salome et al., 1983). Improvement in FEV_1 after treatment was determined as the difference between values before and after treatment as a percentage of the value before treatment. Dose response curves were plotted for each histamine challenge test and the dose which caused a 20% fall in FEV_1 ($PD_{20}FEV_1$) was read from the curve by interpolation. Improvement in $PD_{20}FEV_1$ after treatment was determined by dividing values on the treatment days by the value measured at the same time of the day on the placebo day. Values for $PD_{20}FEV_1$ and improvement in $PD_{20}FEV_1$ were log transformed before undergoing further analysis. Analysis of variance and paired t-tests were used to determine significance of differences and these were considered significant when $p<0.05$.

RESULTS

Details of individual subjects, including current medications, are shown in Table 1.

TABLE 1
Details of subjects, with baseline values for FEV_1 and $PD_{20}FEV_1$ determined as the mean of all measurements made on the placebo study day. Figures in parentheses are standard deviation for FEV_1 and lower and upper limits of the standard deviation about the geometric means for $PD_{20}FEV_1$.

Subject No	Age	Sex	FEV_1 (% pred)	$PD_{20}FEV_1$ (umol)	Current medication⁺
1	32	M	62.4 (8.2)	0.11 (0.07-0.18)	S*, B*
2	29	M	71.0 (4.1)	0.09 (0.06-0.12)	S*
3	29	F	88.6 (1.5)	0.13 (0.07-0.22)	S, B
4	55	M	79.3 (2.5)	0.12 (0.08-0.17)	S, T
5	34	M	81.8 (2.9)	0.11 (0.09-0.14)	S
6	22	M	78.0 (3.3)	0.23 (0.19-0.27)	O, B, T*
7	18	M	65.9 (8.9)	0.14 (0.10-0.21)	S
8	21	F	100.1 (5.2)	0.31 (0.15-0.63)	S, C
9	24	M	97.4 (2.0)	0.44 (0.28-0.69)	S, C
Mean SD			80.5 (13.1)	0.16 (0.09-0.27)	

⁺ S = salbutamol, B = beclomethasone, T = theophylline, C = sodium cromoglycate, O = orciprenaline.

* = therapy taken as needed.

Baseline values for $PD_{20}FEV_1$ and FEV_1 were determined by taking the mean of all values measured during the placebo day. The subjects had mean $PD_{20}FEV_1$ values on the placebo day ranging from 0.09 to 0.44 umol, and a mean value for the group of 0.16 umol. Values for $PD_{20}FEV_1$ measured hourly for six hours were extremely reproducible, with only two subjects having values more than plus or minus one doubling dose from their mean. Mean values for FEV_1 on the placebo day ranged from 62.4 to 100.1% of predicted, with a mean value for the group of 80.5 ± 13.1 %. Values for FEV_1 were also very reproducible with a coefficient of variation for the group of 5.6%. None of the treatments caused a significant change in heart rate at any time.

Table 2 shows the mean $PD_{20}FEV_1$ values on the four treatment days and on the placebo day during the six hours following the administration of treatment.

Table 2
Geometric mean $PD_{20}FEV_1$ values after treatment with fenoterol plus ipratropium, fenoterol, salbutamol, ipratropium and placebo. Figures in parentheses are upper and lower limits of the standard deviations.

	Time after treatment (hours)						
	0.1	1	2	3	4	5	6
Fenoterol plus Ipratropium	5.27 (10.0- 2.75)	3.69 (9.55- 1.45)	2.08 (8.5- 0.51)	1.22 (2.99- 0.5)	0.55 (1.58- 0.19)	0.32 (1.2- 0.09)	0.21 (0.66- 0.07)
Fenoterol	3.23 (11.75- 0.89)	2.02 (6.1- 0.68)	1.03 (3.04- 0.35)	0.47 (1.74- 0.13)	0.35 (1.31- 0.10)	0.24 (1.05- 0.05)	0.24 (0.87- 0.07)
Salbutamol	3.68 (12.88- 1.1)	1.79 (5.6- 0.56)	1.08 (3.92- 0.30)	0.65 (1.62- 0.26)	0.37 (0.87- 0.16)	0.22 (0.56- 0.09)	0.18 (0.51- 0.09)
Ipratropium	0.54 (1.62- 0.18)	0.42 (1.58- 0.11)	0.34 (1.55- 0.07)	0.43 (1.58- 0.11)	0.27 (0.93- 0.08)	0.17 (0.48- 0.06)	0.13 (0.45- 0.04)
Placebo	0.27 (0.60- 0.12)	0.25 (0.48- 0.13)	0.19 (0.39- 0.09)	0.17 (0.41- 0.07)	0.13 (0.27- 0.07)	0.14 (0.30- 0.07)	0.13 (0.22- 0.07)

Values for $PD_{20}FEV_1$ five minutes after treatment were, on all four treatment days, significantly greater than those five minutes after placebo ($p<0.001$ for fenoterol plus ipratropium, fenoterol, salbutamol; $p<0.05$ for ipratropium). After fenoterol plus ipratropium the $PD_{20}FEV_1$ values remained significantly greater than on the placebo day for five hours. After fenoterol and after salbutamol the $PD_{20}FEV_1$ values were increased for four hours. One hour after ipratropium there was no significant increase in $PD_{20}FEV_1$ over placebo values. However, ipratropium had variable effects on individual subjects. Five subjects (#1,4,5,7,8) had an increase in mean $PD_{20}FEV_1$ to 1.1 umol five minutes after treatment compared with 0.23 umol five minutes after placebo. The other four subjects had a mean $PD_{20}FEV_1$ value of 0.23 umol five minutes after ipratropium compared 0.22 umol after placebo. There were no significant differences in response to the combination of fenoterol and ipratropium between those who responded to ipratropium and those who did not.

The improvement in $PD_{20}FEV_1$ was expressed as the dose ratio, calculated by dividing the value on the treatment day by the value at the same time on the placebo day. Improvement in $PD_{20}FEV_1$ on four treatment days is shown in Figure 1.

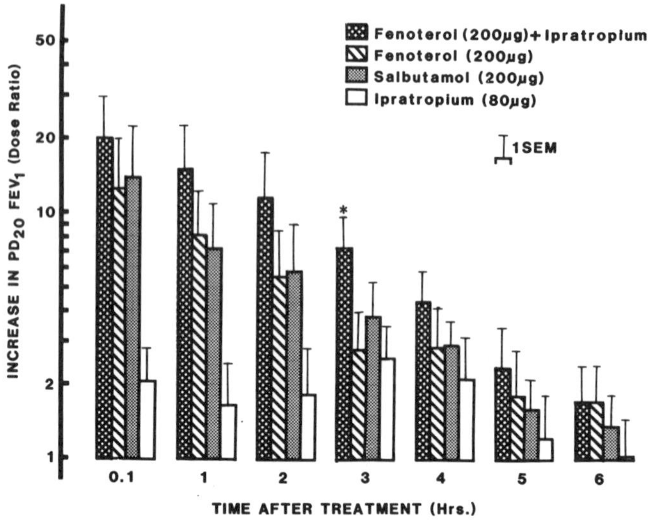

Figure 1
Mean increase in $PD_{20}FEV_1$, as the dose ratio of $PD_{20}FEV_1$ on active treatment to $PD_{20}FEV_1$ on placebo, for six hours after treatment.
* $p < 0.05$ for difference between fenoterol plus ipratropium and all other treatments.

Five minutes after treatment with fenoterol plus ipratropium the mean increase in $PD_{20}FEV_1$ was 19.8 fold, which was not significantly different from the mean improvement after fenoterol (12.1 fold) or the mean improvement after salbutamol (13.8 fold). Three hours after treatment, however, fenoterol plus ipratropium maintained a mean 7.1 fold improvement, which was significantly greater than the mean 2.8 fold improvement ($p<0.05$) elicited by fenoterol and the mean 3.8 fold improvement ($p<0.05$) elicited by salbutamol. After six hours, mean $PD_{20}FEV_1$ values on all treatment days were within the two fold range which represents the limit of sensitivity of the histamine challenge test.

Figure 2 shows the increase in FEV_1 (percent increase over the baseline value) on the four treatment days.

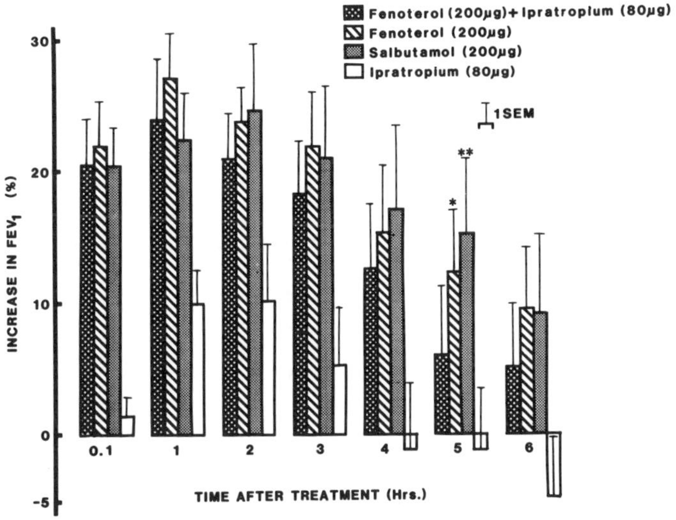

Figure 2
Mean percentage increase in FEV_1 over pretreatment values for six hours after treatment. Significance of differences between fenoterol plus ipratropium, fenoterol and salbutamol are * $p < 0.05$, ** $p < 0.01$.

Maximal increase was not reached until 1 to 2 hours after treatment and, after 2 hours both fenoterol alone and salbutamol alone caused larger increases in FEV_1 than did fenoterol plus ipratropium. Five hours after treatment the mean percentage increase in FEV_1 with fenoterol plus ipratropium (5.9%) was less than that with fenoterol (12.2%) ($p<0.05$) or with salbutamol (15.1%) ($p<0.01$). Ipratropium alone caused a small but significant increase at one (9.8%) and two (10.1%) hours ($p<0.05$).

Differences in the time course for bronchodilatation and protection against histamine challenge are shown in Figure 3.

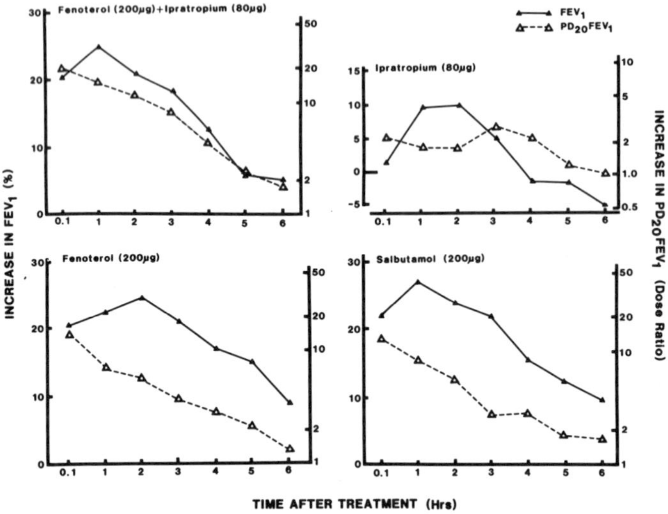

Figure 3
Comparison of the time course of bronchodilating effects and protective effects of the four active treatments.

For fenoterol and salbutamol their protective effect, as measured by the fold change in $PD_{20}FEV_1$, decreased during the first one to two hours while FEV_1 was still improving. Five hours after treatment bronchodilation was still significant whereas protection was not. Ipratropium had little effect on either $PD_{20}FEV_1$ or FEV_1 and after four hours most subjects had worse lung function than on the placebo day. After fenoterol plus ipratropium the fall off in protection was similar to the fall off in bronchodilating effect.

There was a significant correlation between improvement in $PD_{20}FEV_1$ and improvement in FEV_1 (as percent predicted) after fenoterol plus ipratropium, fenoterol alone and salbutamol alone ($p<0.001$ in all cases), but not after ipratropium alone. There was no relation between the degree of improvement in $PD_{20}FEV_1$ on any treatment and baseline severity of BHR, measured as $PD_{20}FEV_1$ on the placebo day.

DISCUSSION

The study has shown that a combination of fenoterol and ipratropium bromide sustains protection against histamine challenge for longer than either drug alone or salbutamol alone, but does not increase the degree of protection. The time course of the protection differs from the time course of bronchodilatation. Fenoterol and salbutamol do not differ in the degree or duration of protection afforded.

The stability of baseline $PD_{20}FEV_1$ and FEV_1 was determined on the placebo study day. Despite the fact that the subjects had either moderately severe or severe asthma their values for both $PD_{20}FEV_1$ and FEV_1 were very reproducible. Thus, it is unlikely that the differences seen in the study were due to spontaneous fluctuations in the severity of BHR or in baseline lung function.

There were no differences in the maximum level of improvement in $PD_{20}FEV_1$, measured five minutes after the administration of treatment, between the combination treatment and treatment with either fenoterol or salbutamol. This suggests that there was no additive effect of the slight protection afforded by ipratropium five minutes after administration. This suggestion is supported by examination of data from individual subjects which shows no significant differences in the improvement in $PD_{20}FEV_1$ after the combination treatment between those subjects who were protected by ipratropium (#1,4,5,7,8) and those who were not.

The combination treatment of fenoterol and ipratropium sustained a significant level of protection for five hours after treatment. Only after the combination treatment were the $PD_{20}FEV_1$ values still significantly above those on the placebo day five hours after treatment. Of greater importance, however, is the fact that three hours after the combination treatment this group of severe asthmatics had a mean $PD_{20}FEV_1$ value which was greater than 1.0 umol. Values in this range are not usually associated with current symptoms of asthma (Yan et al., 1983; Woolcock et al., 1985), suggesting that the average 7 fold improvement over baseline values is clinically important. Subjects were significantly better protected at this time than they were by either fenoterol or salbutamol. These findings are in concurrence with the findings of Fontana et al., 1986 who showed a difference between $PD_{20}FEV_1$ to histamine 4 hours after a combination of fenoterol and ipratropium and after salbutamol.

The combination treatment was less effective in sustaining increases in FEV_1 than either fenoterol or salbutamol. This finding is in marked contrast to the findings of other studies. Marlin et al., 1979, have shown an additive effect of ipratropium and beta agonists which not only increases the extent of bronchodilation but also increases its duration. Some asthmatic subjects have been reported to react adversely to ipratropium bromide (Mann et al., 1984), but in the present study no subject had a fall in FEV_1 when given ipratropium alone. It is not clear why, in this study, the bronchodilatation induced by the combination of fenoterol and ipratropium was not sustained as long as that induced by either fenoterol or salbutamol alone.

In the present study, while there was a good relationship between improvement in $PD_{20}FEV_1$ and improvement in FEV_1 it is clear that they are not directly related. Firstly, the time course of the changes in $PD_{20}FEV_1$ and FEV_1 are different. Improvement in $PD_{20}FEV_1$ was maximal five minutes after treatment, whereas maximal improvement in FEV_1 did not occur until 1-2 hours after treatment. Secondly, treatment with ipratropium produced a small, but significant, improvement $PD_{20}FEV_1$ at five minutes when there was no significant change in FEV_1. Thirdly, both fenoterol and salbutamol continued to maintain significant improvement in FEV_1 above baseline five hours after treatment, but at this time they provided no significant protection against histamine.

The mechanisms by which the combination of fenoterol and ipratropium cause increased duration of protection against histamine challenge are unclear. It appears not to be due to an additive protective effect of the two drugs and is probably not related to changes in baseline lung function.

Since sensitivity to such provoking stimuli as allergens (Cockcroft et al., 1979) and exercise (Chatham et al., 1982) is related to the severity of BHR, improvement in $PD_{20}FEV_1$ to histamine should be associated with reduced sensitivity to these stimuli. It is possible that the improved protection against histamine challenge provided by the combination of fenoterol and ipratropium allows improved control of asthmatic symptoms. It is yet to be determined if long term treatment with a combination of fenoterol and ipratropium can lead to lasting improvement in BHR.

REFERENCES

Anderson SD, Seale JP, Ferris L, Schoeffel R, Lindsay DA (1979). An evaluation of pharmacotherapy for exercise-induced asthma. J Allergy Clin Immunol 64:612-624.

Chatham M, Bleecker ER, Smith PL, Rosenthal RR, Mason P, Norman PS (1982). A comparison of histamine, methacholine, and exercise airway reactivity in normal and asthmatic subjects. Am Rev Respir Dis 126:235-240.
Cockcroft DW, Killian DM, Mellon JJA, Hargreave FE (1977a). Bronchial reactivity to inhaled histamine: a method and clinical survey. Clin Allergy 7:235-243.
Cockcroft DW, Killian DN, Mellon JJA, Hargreave FE (1977b). Protective effects of drugs on histamine-induced asthma. Thorax 32:429-437.
Cockcroft DW, Ruffin RE, Frith PA, Cartier A, Juniper EF, Dolovich J, Hargreave FE (1979). Determinants of allergen-induced asthma: Dose of allergen, circulating IgE antibody concentration, and bronchial responsiveness to inhaled histamine. Am Rev Respir Dis 120:1053-1058.
Crimi N, Palermo F, Ciccarello C, Distefano SM, Vancheri C, Cacopardo B, Mistretta A (1986). Effect of Duovent (ipratropium bromide and fenoterol) on non-specific bronchial hyperreactivity. Respiration 50 (Suppl 2) :206-208.
Fontana G, Mugnai M, Cresci F, Panuccio P (1986). Histamine-induced bronchial response after administration of placebo, salbutamol and a combination of a beta-2-adrenergic drug (Fenoterol) with an anticholinergic agent (Ipratropium bromide) in asymptomatic asthma patients. Respiration 50 (Suppl 2):201-205.
Mann JS, Howarth PH, Holgate ST (1984). Bronchoconstriction induced by ipratropium bromide in asthma: relation to hypotonicity. Br Med J 289:469.
Marlin GE, Berend N, Harrison AC (1979). Combined cholinergic antagonist and B_2-adrenoceptor agonist bronchodilator therapy by inhalation. Aust NZ J Med 9:511-514.
Morris JF, Koski A, Johnson LC (1971). Spirometric standards for healthy nonsmoking adults. Am Rev Respir Dis 103:57-67.

Salome CM, Schoeffel RE, Yan K, Woolcock AJ (1983). Effect of aerosol fenoterol on the severity of bronchial hyperreactivity in patients with asthma. Thorax 38:854-858.

Serra C, Giacopelli A, Luciani G (1986). Acute controlled study of the dose response relationships of fenoterol, ipratropium bromide and their combination. Respiration 50 (suppl 2):144-147.

Woolcock AJ, Yan K, Salome CM (In press). The effect of therapy on bronchial hyperresponsiveness in the long term management of asthma. Clin Allergy.

Woolcock AJ, Yan K, Salome CM, Sedgwick CJ, Peat J (1985). What determines the severity of asthma? Chest 87:209s-213s.

Yan K, Salome CM, Woolcock AJ (1983). Rapid method for measurement of bronchial responsiveness. Thorax 38:760-765.

ACKNOWLEDGEMENTS

We wish to thank our subjects, who gave up a week of their holidays to participate in the study, Boehringer Ingelheim Pty Ltd who funded the study, Glaxo Australia Pty Ltd, who supplied the active and placebo salbutamol and Ms Victoria Keena of the Institute of Respiratory Medicine, who prepared the manuscript.

Mechanisms in Asthma: Pharmacology, Physiology, and Management, pages 421–425

FIXED DOSE COMBINATION THERAPY IN THE TREATMENT OF ASTHMA - THE CASE AGAINST IT.

DAVID A. LINDSAY

DIRECTOR OF MEDICINE,

GOLD COAST HOSPITAL, NERANG ST., SOUTHPORT. QLD.

The airflow limitation which characterises asthma results from contraction of bronchial smooth muscle in all patients; in some, those with the most severe asthma clinically, excessive endobronchial secretions, and inflammatory exudate in the bronchial lumina and mucosa contribute significantly. In these latter patients, the airflow limitation is then understandably unresponsive or incompletely responsive to medications which effect relaxation of smooth muscle.

Since there is no currently available medication with both bronchial smooth muscle relaxing and anti-inflammatory properties, combinations of two or more agents are necessary for optimal treatment of many asthmatic patients.

Only two of the last 100 patients with asthma treated by the author were prescribed one drug - a beta-agonist aerosol. Various combinations of beta-agonist, steroid, sodium cromoglycate, or ipratropium bromide as metered dose aerosols, dry powder or nebulising solutions with or without theophylline (as sustained release oral preparations or as Aminophylline intravenously) and systemic steroids (orally or intravenously) were prescribed for the other 98!

Since therapy for these asthmatic patients was complicated by the need to use two or more drugs in most, delivery of these from a single container, tablet or capsule to uncomplicate treatment, is intuitively attractive.

In considering the possible role of combinations of drugs for asthma treatment, and, in particular, fixed combinations, it is helpful to consider two types of combination. Firstly the combination of two "muscle" drugs e.g. beta-agonist plus anticholinergic, or beta-agonist plus theophylline; secondly that of a "mucosal" drug with "muscle" one e.g. beclomethasone diproprionate (BDP) and a beta-agonist or sodium cromoglycate and a beta-agonist.

For discussion purposes, fenoterol plus ipratropium bromide ('Duovent') and salbutamol plus BDP ('Ventide') will be used as examples, the major emphasis being on the place in asthma therapy of fixed dose combinations of these, as metered aerosols.

In vitro studies suggest that there is synergism between beta-agonists and anti-cholinergics. Synergism also has been shown in vitro between theophylline and beta-agonists and clinical experience supports their concomitant use; theophylline is not effective via the aerosol route and therefore its use in combination is not further discussed in this paper.

A number of clinical studies have shown the benefit of adding anticholinergics such as ipratropium bromide to a beta-agonist, as wet nebulising solutions. Studies using metered doses of these anti-asthma agents from separate cannisters have also indicated beneficial interaction.

Flint, Johnson and Hockley (1983) concluded that the bronchodilator efficacy of 2 puffs of a combination inhaler of ipratropium bromide and fenoterol was greater than that which was achieved by 2 puffs of salbutamol, in 12 asthmatic patients. An experienced clinician might ask : Would a larger dose of the combination therapy have effected even more improvement in lung function or, would perhaps, a larger dose of salbutamol alone have effected a better response, equal to or better than the combination? And would this experience in 12 patients aged 24-75 years be reproducible in more and younger asthmatic patients?

Finally, would the minor difference in after treatment FEV 1.0 (mean 1.88 litres for salbutamol and 1.98 litres for the combination) be of enough clinical significance to justify any additional cost of the combination therapy?

Tang and Flatley (1984) used combination therapy (ipratropium bromide and fenoterol) in 24 patients - 20 described as having "chronic bronchitis" and 4 with "chronic stable asthma". They compared changes in peak expiratory flowrate in patients treated with the combination with changes following fenoterol or salbutamol. The same or similar questions might be asked of their study, plus : "Would the additional 1 hour (from six to seven) of "significant effect" be sufficient to justify the use of the combination therapy? In the same journal, Fishbacher, Giannini, Milroy and Monie reported the results of a study comparing the bronchodilator efficacy of 'Duovent' and salbutamol aerosols in 16 asthmatic patients. They concluded that "improvement in $FEV_{1.0}$ was better (their value judgement) and longer lasting with 'Duovent'. They tempered this enthusiasm by stating in their discussion : "Although the improvement in $FEV_{1.0}$ with 'Duovent' was significantly better than that with salbutamol, in absolute terms the mean difference between the two inhalers was only 118 mls averaged over the study period", and concluded : "that in the doses used in this study the difference between the two drugs is small".

In his review of combination therapy with beta-adrenergic and anticholinergic agents Boushey (1987) concluded that the combination was "justified for elderly bronchitic or emphysematous patients and for young asthmatic patients intolerant of adrenergic therapy". It should be noted that none of the studies to which he referred used fixed dose combination metered dose ('Duovent') therapy.

Whilst the evidence for the efficacy of combination therapy with anticholinergic and beta-adrenergic therapy in asthmatic patients is good, most does not relate to fixed dose combinations. It is appropriate to similarly criticise the data relating to combination therapy with salbutamol and BDP ('Ventide') aerosols.

It is sufficient to refer to a recent study by Plit and Pover (1984) without discussing the considerable body of data supporting the use of beclomethasone dipropionate plus a beta-agonist using separate containers in asthma treatment, to demonstrate the efficacy of the combination inhaler ('Ventide') in asthma treatment. In 15 patients with chronic asthma, the combination therapy was shown to "provide an alternative in the management of asthma which is at least as effective as treatment with salbutamol and beclomethasone diproprionate from two separate inhalers". The authors and other protagonists of combination therapy for asthma imply that there may be advantages in ensuring treatment with the steroid by simplification of the treatment regimen.

Whilst the efficacy of the combination is certain, its safety is not. The most pressing potential problem of fixed dose combination therapy with 'Ventide' is overdosage with BDP with consequent unwanted systemic steroid side effects, the most life threatening of these being the one most sensitive to overdosage - suppression of the hypothalamic pituitary adrenal axis (HPA). Many patients prescribed standard (2 puffs four times daily) regimens of beta-agonist bronchodilator aerosols take many more puffs than prescribed. With 50 micrograms of BDP "tied" immutably to each 100 micrograms of salbutamol the potential for exceeding safe doses of the steroid is considerable.

Mikhail and Daly (1986) demonstrated in an 8 week study of 20 stable asthmatic patients, that a twice daily dose schedule from a combination inhaler ('Ventide') was as effective as a 4 times daily regimen. The advantage to the patient is the need to use only one metered dose container instead of two. However, if additional beta-agonist bronchodilator is required for symptoms occurring after the scheduled two doses or for prophylaxis of exercise induced asthma, either "unnecessary" BDP will be inhaled or a separate "salbutamol only" inhaler must be carried for such exigencies, thus negating the convenience of one container therapy!

Amongst the 100 asthmatic patients mentioned previously, one was taking only 200 micrograms of beclomethasone dipropionate daily (with 800 micrograms of salbutamol) and several were prescribed more than 1200 micrograms of BDP with 800 micrograms of salbutamol (2 puffs every 6 hours). None of these patients could have been treated with their optimal regimen of salbutamol and BDP using only a 'Ventide' inhaler.

Combination chemotherapy with inhalers such as 'Duovent' and 'Ventide' is intuitively attractive for asthmatic patients. However, for a classically variable disorder characterised by airflow limitation due to widely different pathology, maximum flexibility of drug type ("muscle" or "mucosal") and dosage by the use of separate containers is the only rational alternative.

Combinations of drugs with different mechanisms of action are necessary for optimal therapy for most asthmatic patients. Fixed dose combinations offer insufficient advantage to outweigh their considerable disadvantages in the ordinary clinical context.

In an excellent review paper, Gillian Shenfield (1982) stated : "There is no longer any place for fixed combination bronchodilators...." ; I agree with her, and believe that a similar statement is appropriate for fixed combinations of BDP and beta-agonists.

REFERENCES

Boushey HA, Combination therapy with anticholinergic agents for airflow obstruction. Postgraduate Medical Journal (1987) 63 (suppl 1) 69-74.

Fishbacher CM, Giannini D, Milroy R, Monie RDH. Comparison of Duovent and salbutamol inhalers in chronic stable asthma. Postgraduate Medical Journal (1984). 60 (suppl 1) 28-34.

Flint KC, Johnson NMcI, Hockley B. A comparison between a combination of ipratropium bromide plus fenoterol in a single metered dose inhaler (Duovent) and salbutamol in asthma. Postgraduate Medical Journal. (November 1983) 59 724-25.

Mikhail JR, Daly S. Is twice daily prophylaxis with salbutamol and beclomethasone dipropionate effective in the management of asthma. Pharmatyerapeutica 1986 4 (10) 648-654.

Plit M, Pover GM. Assessment of a new combination inhaler containing salbutamol and beclomethasone diproprionate in the management of asthmatic patients. S.A. Mediese Tydskrif Deel 65 12 Mei 1985.

Shenfield Gillian M. Combination Bronchodilator Therapy Drugs 24 (1982) 414-439.

Tang OT, Flatley M. A comparison of effects of inhaling a combined preparation of fenoterol with ipratropium bromide (Duovent) with those of fenoterol and salbutamol. Postgraduate Medical Journal 1984 60 (suppl 1) 24-27.

Mechanisms in Asthma: Pharmacology,
Physiology, and Management, pages 427–435

FIXED DOSE COMBINATION THERAPY IN ASTHMA. THE POSITIVE CASE FOR FUTURE THERAPY

Richard E Ruffin

Department of Respiratory Medicine
Flinders Medical Centre
Bedford Park
South Australia, Australia 5042

General reviews of fixed dose drug combinations (Shenfield 1986) and of fixed combination treatment for asthma (Shenfield 1982) have suggested that there is no place for this form of treatment for asthma. However new knowledge about the implications of airway hyperresponsiveness for patients and a possible change in attitude to asthma therapy provides the stimulus to re-examine the case for fixed dose combination treatment in asthma.

Asthma treatment aims

It is my impression that Australian aims of asthma treatment have changed in the last decade. The earlier aims were to try to achieve a normal lifestyle for patients with the minimum dose of medications (Paterson, Woolcock, Shenfield, 1979). My treatment aims are now to achieve (i) symptom control, (ii) normal airway function measurements, and (iii) a reduction in airway hyperresponsiveness in asthmatics. Aims (i) and (ii) mean achieving a normal lifestyle for patients. The reasons for introducing aim (iii) need to be reviewed briefly because fixed dose combination therapy holds the key to achieving this aim.

Airway hyperresponsiveness

Increased airway hyperresponsiveness is associated with a greater potential for bronchoconstriction occurring with exercise (Anderton et al 1979), allergen inhalation (Cockcroft et al 1979) and cold air inhalation (O'Byrne et al 1982). Therefore reducing airway hyperresponsiveness will reduce the likelihood of acute episodes enabling continuation of a normal lifestyle and lower morbidity from asthma. Local experience has shown that patients experiencing a near miss death episode from acute asthma have often had two trigger factors such as a viral respiratory infection and exercise or a viral respiratory infection and ingestion of aspirin. Reducing airway hyperresponsiveness is likely to reduce the occurrence of life threatening episodes of asthma and potentially reduce asthma mortality.

There is accumulating evidence that asthmatics have a more rapid decline in lung function than normals (Buist and Vollmer 1987, Peat et al 1987). A recent cross sectional study showed that airway responsiveness was related to a faster decline in lung function (Sparrow et al 1987). Reducing airway hyperresponsiveness is therefore likely to slow the rate of decay of lung function in asthmatics.

Reducing airway hyperresponsiveness offers significant benefits to asthmatics, but how should airway hyperresponsiveness be reduced? There is evidence that the regular use of inhaled steroids can reduce non-specific airway responsiveness. Kraan et al 1985 showed that 400 mcg of inhaled budesonide daily for 4 weeks in 17 asthmatics increased the mean provocative concentration of histamine to cause a 20% fall in FEV_1 (PC_{20}), from 4.0 mg/ml to 9.5 mg/ml.

Jenkins and Woolcock (1987) have shown that 1200 mcg of inhaled beclomethasone diproprionate daily increased the geometric mean PD_{20} from 0.38 to 1.01 mmol after 3 weeks of treatment in 18 asthmatic patients.

Regular inhaled corticosteroids offer a means of reducing non-specific responsiveness, and the effect occurs within 2 weeks and may be a progressive reduction over at least 4 weeks.

Combination treatment

How best to administer these corticosteroid aerosols? In order to achieve good compliance and avoid the potential of aerosol particles triggering bronchoconstriction, a fixed dose combination of inhaled beta 2 adrenergic agonist + corticosteroid combination in a single metered dose inhaler will provide the best treatment. This combination fulfils both criteria of the FDA guidelines for combination drugs i.e. each agent makes a contribution and that each component dosage is safe and effective for a significant patient population (Crout 1974). Undertreatment of asthma has been blamed for mortality (Read 1968) and morbidity (Speight et al 1983). Therefore the time has come to reject borderline or inadequate asthma treatment and relatively overtreat on a patient symptom basis to enable reduction of airway hyperresponsiveness. Since the prevalence, morbidity and mortality of asthma appears to be increasing, there is a large number of patients who should be treated in this fashion and who will benefit (Evans et al 1987). The benefit of fixed dose beta 2 agonist + corticosteroid aerosol has implications nationally and internationally as well as for individual asthmatics.

For the individual asthmatic the benefits of a combined aerosol include:

(i) better compliance with one metered dose inhaler rather than following current manufacturers instruction of waiting 10 min between the use of Ventolin (R) and Becotide metered dose inhalers. Since poor compliance has been raised as an issue with asthma mortality (Beaupré 1987), the combined aerosol could be lifesaving for some patients.

(ii) reduced patient exposure to fluorocarbon propellant by using one inhaler preferably with a low volume valve. These substances do have toxic potential (Dollery 1974).

(iii) reduced patient exposure to the dispersal agents in aerosols. Toogood et al (1985) report that some aerosols use oleic acid as the dispersal agent. Since oleic acid causes lung injury in some animal models (Albert et al 1987) it is appropriate to minimise exposure of patients to this substance. A single inhaler will enable such a reduction.

(iv) the advantages of reduced airway responsiveness i.e. a reduction in morbidity, mortality and decay of lung function.

This latter point is important at a national level because the reduced disability and mortality will be an economical saving. Further, it is likely that the combined inhaler will be cheaper than two separate inhalers.

At an international level it is important to minimise the release of fluorocarbons into the atmosphere because of the risk of further depleting the ozone layer (Anderson 1987). The impact of destruction of the ozone layer could have far reaching economic consequences from increased melanoma incidence in man to a destruction of animal and plant life. In 1985-1986 there were prescriptions for > 3 x 10^6 metered dose aerosol canisters written in Australia (Murtagh 1987). This is a conservative estimate and halving this number of canisters releasing their fluorocarbon contents into the atmosphere would be wise and a useful means of trying to maintain our environment.

The fixed dose combination of beta 2 agonist and corticosteroid can be applied to most asthmatics.

Combination bronchodilator treatment

The fixed dose combination of a beta 2 adrenergic agonist and anticholinergic has the potential of limited use in selected asthmatics in contrast to the almost universal application of the beta 2 adrenergic agonist + corticosteroid aerosol. Although an attractive concept because of the two different actions and the potential of reduced side effects, the combination bronchodilator has shown small benefits in some asthmatics (Ruffin et al 1982) or no advantage over a beta 2 adrenergic agonist in other asthmatics (Ullah, Newman, Saunders 1981). There is a need to identify patients who will do better on the combination by doing a controlled clinical observation of n = 1 (Guyatt et al 1986). The older asthmatic may benefit more (Ullah, Newman, Saunders 1981) as well as those with sensitivity to beta 2 adrenergic agonist unwanted effects. In those patients who have a demonstrated benefit from the combination, the combination of drugs in one inhaler avoids potential toxic effects of fluorocarbons and dispersal agents.

CONCLUSION

If we are to reduce morbidity and mortality of asthma we must educate patients and doctors and aim to reduce airway hyperresponsiveness. A combined beta 2 adrenergic agonist and corticosteroid aerosol will be appropriate for most asthmatics and we must think in terms of overtreating symptoms to enable a reduction in airway responsiveness. Combination bronchodilator is indicated in those patients in which it is better than either drug alone or results in a significant prolongation of effect. The patients need to be identified or selected by a clinical trial.

REFERENCES

Albert RK, Leasa D, Sanderson M, Robertson HT, Hlastala MP (1987). The prone position improves arterial oxygenation and reduces shunt in oleic-acid-induced acute lung injury. Am Rev Respir Dis 135:628-633.

Anderson A (1987). Expedition faces Antarctic ozone hole mysteries. Nature 328:463.

Anderton RC, Cuff MT, Frith PA, Cockcroft DW, Morse JLC, Jones NL, Hargreave FE (1979). Bronchial responsiveness to inhaled histamine and exercise. J Allergy Clin Immunol 63:315-320.

Beaupré A (1987). Death in asthma. Eur J Respir Dis 70:259-260.

Buist AS, Vollmer WM (1987). Prospective investigations in asthma. What have we learned from longitudinal studies about lung growth and senescence in asthma? Chest 91 (Suppl):119S-126S.

Cockcroft DW, Ruffin RE, Frith PA, Cartier A, Juniper EF, Dolovich J, Hargreave FE (1979). Determinants of allergen-induced asthma: dose of allergen, circulating IgE antibody concentration and bronchial responsiveness to inahled histamine. Am Rev Respir Dis 120:1053-1058.

Crout JR (1974). Fixed combination prescription drugs: FDA policy. J Clin Pharm 14:249-254.

Dollery CT (1974). The toxicity of propellant gases. In: An evaluation of bronchodilator drugs, an Asthma Research Council Symposium, London. Trust for Education and Research and Therapeutics p 183-189.

Evans R, Mullally DI, Wilson RW, Gergen PJ, Rosenberg HM, Grauman JS, Chevarley FM, Feinleib M (1987). National trends in the morbidity and mortality of asthma in the US. Prevalence, hospitalization and death from asthma over two decades: 1965-1984. Chest 91 (Suppl):65S-74S.

Guyatt G, Sackett D, Taylor W, Chong J, Roberts R, Pugsley S (1986). Determining optimal therapy - randomized trials in individual patients. N Engl J Med 314:889-892.

Jenkins CR, Woolcock AJ (1987). A comparative study of the effect of prednisolone and beclomethasone on airway responsiveness in asthma. Aust NZ J Med: in press.

Kraan J, Koeter GH, Mark TW, Sluiter HJ, deVries K (1985). Changes in bronchial hyperreactivity induced by 4 weeks of treatment with antiasthmatic drugs in patients with allergic asthma: A comparison between budesonide and terbutaline. J Allergy Clin Immunol 76: 628-636.

Murtagh J (1987). Prescribing patterns in Australia. Aust Family Phys 16:902-906.
O'Byrne PM, Ryan G, Morris M, McCormack D, Jones NL, Morse JLC, Hargreave FE (1982). Asthma induced by cold air and its relation to nonspecific bronchial responsiveness to methacholine. Am Rev Respir Dis 125: 281-285.
Paterson JW, Woolcock AJ, Shenfield GM (1979). Bronchodilator drugs. Am Rev Respir Dis 120:1149-1188.
Peat JK, Woolcock AJ, Cullen K (1987). Rate of decline of lung function in subjects with asthma. Eur J Respir Dis 70:171-179.
Read J (1968). The reported increase in mortality from asthma: a clinico-functional analysis. Med J Aust 1:879-891.
Ruffin RE, McIntyre E, Crockett AJ, Zielonka K, Alpers JH (1982). Combination bronchodilator therapy in asthma. J Allergy Clin Immunol 69:60-65.
Shenfield GM (1982). Combination bronchodilator therapy. Drugs 24:414-439.
Shenfield GM (1986). Fixed drug combinations. Which ones can be recommended? Current Therapeutics 27:15-29.
Sparrow D, O'Connor G, Colton T, Barry CL, Weiss ST (1987). The relationship of nonspecific bronchial responsiveness to the occurrence of respiratory symptoms and decreased levels of pulmonary function. The normative aging study. Am Rev Respir Dis 135:1255-1260.
Speight ANP, Lee DA, Hey EN (1983). Underdiagnosis and undertreatment of asthma in childhood. Br Med J 286:1253-1256.
Toogood JH, Jennings B, Baskerville JC (1985). Aerosol corticosteroids. In Weiss EB, Segal MS, Stein M (eds) : "Bronchial Asthma: Mechanisms and Therapeutics" 2nd Ed. Boston. Little Brown and Co. p 698-713.
Ullah MI, Newman GB, Saunders KB (1981). Influence of age on response to ipratropium and salbutamol in asthma. Thorax 36:523-529.

DISCUSSION

Paterson: When intal co was introduced i.e. intal combined with isoprenaline, it caused total confusion amongst patients who used it as bronchodilator even though it had all been explained to them. Compliance in terms of intal therapy was apalling.

Ruffin: I think this is a problem with patient education. Many patients toss away their becotide because it hasn't had an effect in the first two days. We are not educating the patient properly.

Paterson: If you really think fluorocarbons are a problem, which I don't, then surely you should be recommending that all patients take dry powders. On another point, there are two drugs, atrovent and theophylline, with which we have populations of patients who do extremely well and others who don't. If you have made the measurement and you have a patient who does well with two bronchodilators then for the sake of compliance there is a point in combined therapy. I'd be unhappy if everyone were getting the combination in order to get to the unknown proportion that need the combination, so maybe there should be a select clinical trial and then there's a case for it.

Sutherland: We have to consider the situation in the 'real world', i.e. when we treat asthmatics in the community. One-shot studies in casualty and our controlled clinical trials where there's a certain amount of bias with patient selection don't reflect the 'real world' - these studies haven't been done. When we looked at mortality studies the message was always the same - delayed perception of severity, too little too late, overreliance on $beta_2$ agonists. David Henry and I have just completed a study in Newcastle where we used retail pharmacy computers to identify cohorts of asthmatics nonselected and we followed them. We found what every clinician knows - people like one drug, and because it's instant gratification that's a $beta_2$ agonist. You cannot distinguish those on one drug from those on multiple therapy by any of the standard parameters of disease severity - hospital admissions, emergency visits, noctural wakenings, limitation of day-to-day activities. These people take only one drug and that's the problem we must address.

Woolcock: I think it's a very good point - we have little

data about compliance.

Lindsay: I think this is a problem of patient education again. I tell my patients who take two drugs, i.e. a beta agonist and beclomethasone, that the more important drug is beclomethasone and explain to them why I believe this. We need to emphasise this and this takes time and often insufficient time is spent with the patient in the 'real world'.

Seale: Regarding compliance - if we try to solicit information from our patients on compliance it may be inacurate - they have an inordinate desire to please us. The only way to find out about compliance is to get an independent observer and that's what Nerida Smith did at the Children's Hospital in Sydney. She found that 70% of patients didn't take their medication according to directions. The optimistic view is that by embarking on an intense program of education and distribution of information, she was able to improve that. We don't know the duration of the improvement but there is some hope that if you try hard, you can improve the situation.

O'Byrne: Although there are few studies on compliance in asthma, there are a number for other medications especially anti-hypertensives. Brian Haynes from McMaster years ago studied large groups of patients and tried a large number of strategies to improve compliance including education, time with the patient, formal pill counts at each clinic visit - nothing really worked long-term. They got short transient improvements but nothing was maintained. So I think a rather simplistic attitude of spending more time with patients is not going to work.

Nogrady: Perhaps the ideal form of combination fixed dose therapy should be medication plus their doctor. The question raised is - should we be removing drugs from over-the-counter sale?

Fuller: The management of hospitals in the U.K. won't allow the use of the present fixed dose combination therapy because it's more expensive than the generic salbutamol which we prescribe. I think it's unlikely that fixed dose combinations will be cheaper because they're patent - protected and therefore by definition will be more expensive.

Barnes: There is actually some data on compliance in asthma

from Mac Cochrane at Guy's Hospital in London. He has shown that asthmatics take more inhaled steroids than they should be taking. It's a sensible idea to get steroids into patients. At the present time they are the only drugs that reduce bronchial hyperresponsiveness in all patients effectively. If you have to make compromises, you should think about giving combinations of inhaled steroids and beta agonists. The patients will take the drug because they get immediate symptom relief, but the important thing is you actually get the useful drug into the patients.

Lindsay: The problem is that when they don't have symptoms they won't take anything and then they'll go from crisis to crisis.

Berend: With the introduction of the higher dose inhaled steroid aerosols, we have for the first time the opportunity to realistically alter the dose of inhaled steroids for the individual patients - I'd hate to give that up with fixed dose therapy. The only alternative would be to have multiple fixed combinations and that might be worse than the present situation.

Mapp: We must teach our patients to try to correlate the drugs and perception of disease with measurement of lung function using peak flow meters. When patients see satisfactory peak flow meter readings after medication they are much more compliant. So it's not just a question of use of drugs.

Landau: Professor Woolcock, everyone knows of your work on the effect of steroids on bronchial hyperresponsiveness and it has been confirmed by lots of others. We are now saying that this reduction in bronchial hyperresponsiveness will reduce morbidity. If you look at the deaths from asthma, some of them occur in patients who should have been treated more intensively, but another large group are those on chronic high dose steroids and another group are those who have very labile asthma, who can have normal lung function and then rapidly deteriorate. In my experience and that of others, this group does not respond very well to steroids. I think we have to await the results of studies that you and others are doing of the clinical significance of attempting to control reactivity by steroid treatment. Therefore using this as an argument for fixed dose therapy has some limitations.

Index